Clinical Fluid Therapy in the Perioperative Setting

Second Edition

Clinical Fluid Therapy in the Perioperative Setting

Second Edition

Edited by

Robert G. Hahn

Research Director, Södertälje Hospital, Södertälje, Sweden

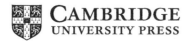

CAMBRIDGE
UNIVERSITY PRESS

CAMBRIDGE
UNIVERSITY PRESS

University Printing House, Cambridge CB2 8BS, United Kingdom

One Liberty Plaza, 20th Floor, New York, NY 10006, USA

477 Williamstown Road, Port Melbourne, VIC 3207, Australia

314-321, 3rd Floor, Plot 3, Splendor Forum, Jasola District Centre, New Delhi - 110025, India

103 Penang Road, #05-06/07, Visioncrest Commercial, Singapore 238467

Cambridge University Press is part of the University of Cambridge.

It furthers the University's mission by disseminating knowledge in the pursuit of
education, learning and research at the highest international levels of excellence.

www.cambridge.org
Information on this title: www.cambridge.org/9781107119550

© Cambridge University Press 2016

First published 2011
Second edition 2016

A catalogue record for this publication is available from the British Library

Library of Congress Cataloging in Publication data
Names: Hahn, Robert G., editor.
Title: Clinical fluid therapy in the perioperative setting / edited by Robert G. Hahn.
Description: 2nd edition. | Cambridge ; New York : Cambridge University Press,
2016. | Includes bibliographical references and index.
Identifiers: LCCN 2015046421 | ISBN 9781107119550 (hardback : alk. paper)
Subjects: | MESH: Fluid Therapy | Perioperative Care | Rehydration Solutions –
therapeutic use
Classification: LCC RD51 | NLM WD 220 | DDC 617.9/6 – dc23
LC record available at http://lccn.loc.gov/2015046421

ISBN 978-1-107-11955-0 Hardback

Contents

Contents

Contributors

Şakir Akin, MD
Department of Intensive Care, Erasmus MC
University Hospital Rotterdam, Rotterdam, The
Netherlands

Jonathan Aron, MBBS BSc (Hons) MRCP (UK) FRCA FFICM
Intensive Care, St George's Healthcare Trust &
Medical School, Tooting, London, United Kingdom

João Batista Borges, MD, PhD, Senior Researcher
Section of Anesthesia and Intensive Care,
Department of Surgical Sciences, Uppsala University,
Uppsala, Sweden

Anna Bertram, MD
Department of Nephrology and Hypertension,
Medizinische Hochschule Hannover, Hannover,
Germany

Eileen M. Bulger, MD, FACS, Professor
General Surgery Clinic at Harborview, University of
Washington, Seattle, Washington, USA

Birgitte Brandstrup, MD, PhD
Department of Surgery, Holbaek University Hospital,
Smedelundsgade 60, 4300 Holbaek, Denmark

Maxime Cannesson, MD, PhD, Professor
Department of Anesthesiology and Perioperative
Care, University of California, Irvine, School of
Medicine, Irvine, USA

Maurizio Cecconi, Professor
Intensive Care, St George's Healthcare Trust &
Medical School, Tooting, London, United Kingdom

Nils Dennhardt, Dr. med.
Klinik für Anästhesiologie und Intensivmedizin,
Medizinische Hochschule Hannover, Hannover,
Germany

Robert A. Dyer, BSc (Hons), MBChB, PhD, FCA (SA)
Department of Anaesthesia, University of Cape Town
and Groote Schuur Hospital, Western Cape, South
Africa

Paul W. G. Elbers, MD, PhD, EDIC
Department of Intensive Care Medicine,
VU University Medical Centre Amsterdam,
Amsterdam, the Netherlands

Claes Frostell, MD, PhD, Professor
Department of Anesthesia and Intensive Care,
Karolinska Institutet at Danderyd Hospital,
Danderyd, Sweden

Tong J. Gan, MD, MHS, FRCA, Professor and Chairman
Department of Anesthesiology, Stony Brook
Medicine, Stony Brook, NY, USA

Per-Olof Grände, MD, PhD, Professor
Department of Anaesthesia and Intensive Care, Lund
University Hospital, Lund, Sweden

Oliver Habler, Professor
Department of Anesthesiology, Surgical Intensive
Care Medicine and Pain Therapy, Krankenhaus
Nordwest GmbH, Frankfurt am Main, Germany

Robert G. Hahn, MD, PhD, Professor
Södertälje Hospital, Södertälje, Sweden

Hermann Haller, Professor
Department of Nephrology and Hypertension,
Medizinische Hochschule Hannover, Hannover,
Germany

Göran Hedenstierna, MD, PhD, Professor
Section of Clinical Physiology, Department of
Medical Sciences, Uppsala University, Uppsala,
Sweden

Jan Hegermann, PhD
Department of Anatomy, Medizinische Hochschule
Hannover, Hannover, Germany

John B. Holcomb, MD, Professor
Department of Surgery, The University of Texas,
Houston, Texas, USA

Kathrine Holte, MD, DMSc
Department of Surgical Gastroenterology, Hvidovre
University Hospital, Hvidovre, Denmark

Can Ince, Professor
Department of Intensive Care, Erasmus MC
University Hospital Rotterdam, Rotterdam, The
Netherlands

Jan Jakobsson, Professor
Institution for Physiology and Pharmacology,
Department of Anaesthesia and Intensive Care,
Karolinska Institutet, Stockholm, Sweden

Michael F. M. James, MBChB, PhD, FRCA, FCA (SA)
Department of Anaesthesia, University of Cape Town
and Groote Schuur Hospital, Western Cape, South
Africa

Atilla Kara, MD
Department of Intensive Care, Erasmus MC
University Hospital Rotterdam, Rotterdam, The
Netherlands, and Intensive Care Unit, Hacettepe
University Medicine Faculty, Ankara, Turkey

Sibylle A. Kozek-Langenecker, MD, Professor, MBA
Sigmund Freud Private University Vienna,
Department of Anesthesia and Intensive Care,
Evangelical Hospital Vienna, Vienna, Austria

Alena Lira, MD
Department of Critical Care Medicine, University of
Pittsburgh, PA, USA

Dileep N. Lobo, MS, DM, FRCS, FACS, FRCPE
Gastrointestinal Surgery, Nottingham Digestive
Diseases Centre, National Institute for Health
Research Biomedical Research Unit, Nottingham
University Hospitals NHS Trust, Queen's Medical
Centre, Nottingham, United Kingdom

Giovanni Mariscalco, MD, PhD
University of Leicester, Clinical Sciences Wing,
Glenfield General Hospital, Leicester, United
Kingdom

**Timothy E. Miller, MBChB, FRCA, Associate
Professor**
Division of General, Vascular and Transplant
Anesthesiology, Department of Anesthesiology, Duke
University Medical Center, Durham, NC, USA

Joshua D. Person, MD
Department of Surgery, The University of Texas,
Houston, Texas, USA

Johan Persson, MD, PhD
Department of Anaesthesia and Intensive Care, Lund
University Hospital, Lund, Sweden

Michael R. Pinsky, MD, Dr. h.c.
Department of Critical Care Medicine, University of
Pittsburgh, PA, USA

Hemanshu Prabhakar, Professor
Department of Neuroanesthesiology, All India
Institute of Medical Sciences, New Delhi, India

Saqib H. Qureshi, MD
University of Leicester, Clinical Sciences Wing,
Glenfield General Hospital, Leicester, United
Kingdom

Katie E. Rollins, BM BS, MRCS
Gastrointestinal Surgery, Nottingham Digestive
Diseases Centre, National Institute for Health
Research Biomedical Research Unit, Nottingham
University Hospitals NHS Trust, Queen's Medical
Centre, Nottingham, United Kingdom

Niels H. Secher, MD, PhD
Department of Anaesthesia, Rigshospitalet,
University of Copenhagen, Copenhagen,
Denmark

Folke Sjöberg, MD, Professor
Burn Center, Linköping University Hospital and
Linköping University, Linköping, Sweden

Klaus Stahl, Dr. med.
Department of Nephrology and Hypertension,
Medizinische Hochschule Hannover, Hannover,
Germany

Robert Sümpelmann, Dr. med., Professor
Klinik für Anästhesiologie und Intensivmedizin,
Medizinische Hochschule Hannover, Hannover,
Germany

Palle Toft, MD, Professor
Department of Anaesthesiology and Intensive Care, Odense Universitetshospital, Odense, Denmark

Else Tønnesen, Professor
Department of Anaesthesiology and Intensive Care, Aarhus University Hospital, Kommunehospitalet, Århus, Denmark

Philippe van der Linden, MD, PhD
Department of Anesthesiology, CHU Brugmann-HUDERF, Université Libre de Bruxelles, Brussels, Belgium

Johannes J. van Lieshout, MD, PhD, Consultant
Department of Internal Medicine and the Laboratory for Clinical Cardiovascular Physiology, AMC Centre for Heart Failure Research, University of Amsterdam, Amsterdam, The Netherlands

Niels Van Regenmortel, MD
Intensive Care Unit and High Care Burn Unit, Ziekenhuis Netwerk Antwerpen, Campus Stuivenberg, Department of Intensive Care Medicine, Antwerp University Hospital, Antwerp, Belgium

Laurence Weinberg, MD, BSc, MBBCh, MRCP, FANZCA
Department of Anesthesia, Austin Hospital, Department of Surgery and Anesthesia, Perioperative Pain Medicine Unit, University of Melbourne, Australia

Preface

Intravenous fluid is a cornerstone in the treatment of the surgical patient. Perioperative management with intravenous fluids is a responsibility of the anesthetist, but many others, including the surgeon, must be oriented in the principles that guide the therapy.

The clinical use of infusion fluids has long been overlooked as a science. One of the main reasons for the neglect is that fluids have not been considered to be drugs. Many of the usual requirements for registration, such as the specification of a therapeutic window and detailed pharmacokinetics, have been overlooked. On the other hand, the experience of the anesthetist is indeed that infusion fluids are drugs. Their appropriate use can be life-saving, while inappropriate use might jeopardize the clinical outcome and even be a threat to the patient's life.

The scattered scientific basis for perioperative fluid therapy has necessitated the development of experience-based "rules-of-thumb" which still play an enormously important role in daily practice. They are usually based on a summation of perceived and measured losses and also include compensation for various factors, such as anesthesia-induced vasodilatation and protein losses due to inflammation.

Alongside the trial-and-error approach and theoretical calculations, scientific methods have been used to find evidence-based guidelines. This has resulted in a marked change over the past decade. The amount of fluid infused has been shown to affect the course of the postoperative follow-up greatly, at least after some types of operation. Another important insight is that guiding fluid therapy by dynamic hemodynamic measures reduces the risk of postoperative complications. A changeover from relying on the pulmonary artery catheter to less invasive and even non-invasive tools for the monitoring of fluid administration is in full swing.

I am extremely proud to welcome contributions from colleagues around the world who are among the highest-ranked researchers in the field of perioperative fluid therapy. I have taken great care to ask researchers and clinicians whom I respect and admire for outstanding contributions to our knowledge about how fluid therapy should be managed. They have written authoritative chapters about subjects in which every anesthetist should be updated when working with patients subjected to common types of surgery.

Each chapter should be read as an independent essay, which means that a topic discussed briefly by one author is often explored in more detail by another. As you will see, the experts take you by the hand and tell you not only what to do, but also why.

Overview of chapter summaries

Section 1: The fluids

Chapter 2. Crystalloid fluids

Robert G. Hahn

Crystalloid electrolyte solutions include isotonic saline, Ringer's lactate, Ringer's acetate, and Plasma-Lyte. In the perioperative period these fluids are used to compensate for anesthesia-induced vasodilatation, small to moderate blood losses, and urinary excretion. Although evaporation consists of electrolyte-free water, such fluid losses are relatively small during short-term surgery and may also be compensated by a crystalloid electrolyte solution.

These fluids expand the plasma volume to a lesser degree than colloid fluids as they hydrate both the plasma and the interstitial fluid space. However, the distribution to the interstitial fluid space takes 25–30 min to be completed, which is probably due to the restriction of fluid movement by the finer filaments in the interstitial gel. The slow distribution gives crystalloid electrolyte solutions a fairly good plasma volume-expanding effect as long as the infusion continues and shortly thereafter.

Isotonic saline is widely used, but has an electrolyte composition that deviates from that of the extracellular fluid ("unbalanced"). This fluid is best reserved for special indications, such as hyponatremia, hypochloremic metabolic alkalosis, and disease states associated with vomiting. Isotonic saline may also be considered in trauma and in children undergoing surgery. Hypertonic saline might be considered in neurosurgery and, possibly, in preoperative emergency care.

Ringer's lactate, Ringer's acetate, and Plasma-Lyte have been formulated to be more similar to the composition of the ECF ("balanced fluids"). They are the mainstay of fluid administration in the perioperative period and should be used in all situations where isotonic saline is not indicated.

Chapter 3. Colloid fluids

Robert G. Hahn

Colloid fluids are crystalloid electrolyte solutions with a macromolecule added that binds water by its colloid osmotic pressure. As macromolecules escape the plasma only with difficulty, the resulting plasma volume expansion is strong and has a duration of many hours. Clinically used colloid fluids include albumin, hydroxyethyl starch, gelatin, and dextran.

The plasma volume expansion shows one-compartment kinetics, which means that colloids, in contrast to crystalloids, have no detectable distribution phase. Marketed fluids are usually composed so that the infused volume expands the plasma volume by the infused amount. Exceptions include rarely used hyperoncotic variants and mixtures with hypertonic saline.

The main indication for colloid fluids is as secondline treatment of hemorrhage. Because of inherent allergenic properties, crystalloid electrolyte fluids should be used when the hemorrhage is small. A changeover to a colloid should be performed only when the crystalloid volume is so large that adverse effects may ensue (mild effects at 3 liters, severe at 6 liters). The only other clinical indication is that dextran can be prescribed to improve microcirculatory flow.

There has been lively debate about clinical use of colloid fluids after studies in septic patients have shown that hydroxyethyl starch increases the need for renal replacement therapy. This problem has not been found in the perioperative setting but the use of starch has still been restricted.

The colloids have defined maximum amounts that can be infused before adverse effects, usually arising from the coagulation system, become a problem.

Chapter 4. Glucose solutions

Robert G. Hahn

Glucose 5% is given after surgery to prevent starvation and to provide free water for hydration of the intracellular fluid space. Glucose is sometimes infused before surgery as well, in particular when surgery is started late during the day, and, in some hospitals, also as a 2.5% solution during the surgical procedure. Glucose infusion has also been used together with insulin to improve outcome in cardiac surgery and in intensive care.

Because of the risk of hyperglycemia, intravenous glucose infusions need to be managed with knowledge, attention, and responsibility. Hyperglycemia promotes wound infection and osmotic diuresis, by which the kidneys lose control of the urine composition. The anesthetist has to consider a four-fold modification in infusion rate of glucose to account for the perioperative change in glucose tolerance. The suitable rate of infusion when a glucose infusion is initiated can be predicted by pharmacokinetic simulation. A control plasma sample taken one hour later shows whether the prediction was correct, and also that plasma glucose will only rise by another 25% if no adjustment of the infusion rate is made.

Glucose solution is contraindicated in acute stroke and not recommended in operations associated with a high risk of perioperative cerebral ischemia, such as carotid artery and cardiopulmonary bypass surgery. Subacute hyponatremia is a postoperative complication that is promoted by infusing >1 liter of plain 5% glucose in the perioperative setting.

Chapter 5. Hypertonic fluids[1]

Eileen M. Bulger

Hypertonic fluids have an osmotic content that is higher than in the body fluids. When this content remains in the extracellular fluid space, such as with saline, the volume effect becomes very powerful owing to osmotic allocation of fluid from the intracellular to the extracellular fluid space. These fluids have also been found to favorably modulate the inflammatory response. The most studied preparations are saline 7.5% with and without a colloid (dextran or hydroxyethyl starch) added.

This chapter reviews the current clinical evidence regarding the use of hypertonic fluids for the early resuscitation of injured patients and for perioperative indications for a variety of procedures. While there is a wealth of preclinical data suggesting potential benefit from this resuscitation strategy, the clinical trial data have failed to show any clear benefit to the prehospital administration of these fluids in trauma patients, and the data for perioperative use is limited. More study is needed to define the best use of these fluids in a variety of patient populations and surgical procedures.

---

[1] For chapters 5, 12, 13, 15, 16, 20, 21, 25, 28, and 31, summary was compiled by the Editor.

Chapter 6. Fluids or blood products?

Oliver Habler

Thanks to the impressive anemia tolerance of the human body, red blood cell (RBC) transfusion may often be avoided despite even important blood losses – provided that normovolemia is maintained. While a hemoglobin (Hb) concentration of 60–70 g/l can be considered safe in young, healthy patients, older patients with preexisting cardiopulmonary morbidity should be transfused at Hb 80–100 g/l. Physiological transfusion triggers (e.g. decrease of VO_2, ST-segment depression in the ECG, arrhythmia, continuous increase in catecholamine needs, echocardiographic wall motion disturbancies, lactacidosis) appearing prior to the aforementioned Hb concentrations necessitate immediate RBC transfusion. In the case of unexpected massive blood losses and/or logistic difficulties impeding an immediate start of transfusion, the anemia tolerance of the patient can be effectively increased by several measures (e.g. hyperoxic ventilation, muscular relaxation, or adequate depth of anesthesia).

In cases of dilutional coagulopathy – often reflected by an intraoperatively diffuse bleeding tendency – a differentiated coagulation therapy can either be directed on the basis of viscoelastic coagulation tests (e.g. thromboelastometry/-graphy) or directed empirically by replacing the different components in the order of their developing deficiency (i.e. starting with fibrinogen, followed by factors of the prothrombin complex and platelets). The "global" stabilization of coagulation with fresh frozen plasma requires the application of high volumes and bears the risk of cardiac overload (TACO) and immunological alterations (TRIM).

Section 2: Basic science

Chapter 7. Body volumes and fluid kinetics

Robert G. Hahn

Body fluid volumes can be measured and estimated by using different methods. A key approach is to use a tracer by which the volume of distribution of an injected substance is measured. Useful tracers occupy a specific body fluid space only. Examples are radioactive albumin (plasma volume), iohexol (extracellular fluid space), and deuterium (total body water). The transit time from the site of injection to the site of elimination must be considered when using tracers with a rapid elimination, such as the indocyanine green dye. The volume effect of an infusion fluid can be calculated by applying a tracer method before and after the administration.

Guiding estimates of the sizes of the body volumes can be obtained by bioimpedance measurements and anthropometric equations.

The blood hemoglobin (Hb) concentration is a frequently used endogenous tracer of changes in blood volume. Hb is the inverse of the blood water concentration, and changes in Hb indicate the volume of distribution of the infused fluid volume. Certain assumptions have to be made to convert the Hb dilution to a change in blood volume. Volume kinetics is based on mathematical modeling of Hb changes over time which, together with measurements of the urinary excretion, can be used to analyze and simulate the distribution and elimination of infusion fluids.

Chapter 8. Acid–base issues in fluid therapy

Niels Van Regenmortel and Paul W. G. Elbers

Solutions such as NaCl 0.9% are an established cause of metabolic acidosis. The underlying mechanism, a reduction in plasma strong ion difference, [SID], is comprehensibly explained by the principles of the Stewart approach. Fluid-induced metabolic acidosis can be avoided by the use of so-called balanced solutions that do not cause alterations in plasma [SID]. Many balanced solutions are commercially available, their only drawback being their higher cost. Since NaCl 0.9% remains the first choice of resuscitation fluid in large parts of the world, there remains an important question over whether a large-scale upgrade to balanced solutions should be at hand. There is a lack of high-quality data at the time of writing, but there is increasing evidence that hyperchloremia has a detrimental effect on renal function and has an economic impact of its own. Therefore, until we have more definitive data, the use of balanced solutions in patients who need a relevant amount of fluid therapy seems to be a pragmatic choice.

Chapter 9. Fluids and coagulation

Sibylle A. Kozek-Langenecker

Infusion therapy is essential in intravascular hypovolemia and extravascular fluid deficits. Crystalloid fluids and colloidal volume replacement affect blood coagulation when infused intravenously. Questions remain over whether unspecific dilution and specific side effects of infusion therapy are clinically relevant in patients with and without bleeding manifestations, and whether fluid-induced coagulopathy is a risk factor for anemia, blood transfusion, mortality, and a driver for resource use and costs. In this chapter, pathomechanisms of dilutional coagulopathy and evidence for its clinical relevance in perioperative and critically ill patients are reviewed. Furthermore, medicolegal aspects are discussed. The dose-dependent risk of dilutional coagulopathy differs between colloids (dextran > hetastarch > pentastarch > tetrastarch > gelatins > albumin). Risk awareness includes monitoring for early signs of side effects. With rotational thromboelastometry/thromboelastography not only the deterioration in clot strength can be assessed but also in clot formation and platelet interaction. Fibrinogen concentrate administration may be considered in severe bleeding as well as relevant dilutional coagulopathy. Targeted doses of gelatins and tetrastarches seem to have no proven adverse effect on anemia and allogeneic blood transfusions. Further studies implementing goal-directed volume management and careful definition of triggers for transfusions and alternative therapies are needed.

Chapter 10. Microvascular fluid exchange

Per-Olof Grände and Johan Persson

There is always a continuous leakage of plasma fluid and proteins to the interstitium, called the transcapillary escape rate (TER). The transcapillary escape rate of albumin (TERalb) corresponds to 5–6% of total plasma albumin per hour. Plasma volume is preserved mainly because of recirculation via the lymphatic system and transcapillary absorption. During inflammation and after trauma, TER may increase up to 2–3 times and exceed the recirculation capacity, resulting in hypovolemia, low plasma concentration of proteins, and tissue edema. The present chapter discusses mechanisms controlling microvascular fluid exchange under physiological and pathophysiological conditions, including possible passive and active mechanisms controlling transcapillary fluid exchange. Options to reduce the need for plasma volume expanders while still maintaining an adequate plasma volume are presented. Consequently, this may simultaneously reduce accumulation of fluid and proteins in the interstitium. The effectiveness of available plasma volume expanders is also discussed.

Chapter 11. The glycocalyx layer

Anna Bertram, Klaus Stahl, Jan Hegermann, and Hermann Haller

Endothelial cells cover the inner surface of the vasculature and are essential for vascular homeostasis with regulation of vasodilation and vasoconstriction, permeability, inflammation, and coagulation. The endothelium is not a barren surface but is covered by a thick layer of so-called glycocalyx. The glycocalyx is built of heavily glycosylated proteins such as syndecans which are anchored in the cell membrane, freely associating proteoglycans such as hyaluronidase, and also a multitude of plasma molecules that bind and interact with the proteoglycans.

The glycoproteins collectively organize into the glycocalyx, which plays a vital role in several important vascular functions. It serves as a mechanotransductor mediating information on blood flow and cellular movement to the endothelium, it regulates permeability via its physical properties, it regulates binding of vascular factors to the endothelium, and it is the "habitat" of the resident components of the complement system and the coagulation cascade. In addition, the glycocalyx serves as a sink for small molecules and electrolytes in the plasma and generates chemokine gradients to guide leukocytes to sites of inflammation. The delicate structures of the glycocalyx can be easily disturbed and damaged by acute disease such as sepsis or ischemia, as well as chronic disease such as diabetes or hypertension. The proteoglycans and/or its sugar moieties can be shed by specific enzymes. Novel tools have been developed to better visualize the glycocalyx both *in vitro* and *in vivo*. An understanding and, possibly, a molecular manipulation of the glycocalyx will be important to improve our therapeutic strategies in patients.

Chapter 12. Monitoring of the microcirculation

Atilla Kara, Şakir Akin, and Can Ince

Perioperative fluid management requires comprehensive training and an understanding of the physiology of oxygen transport to tissue. Administration of fluids has a limited window of efficacy. Too little fluid reduces organ perfusion and too much fluid causes organ dysfunction from edema. In addition, isotonic saline carries the danger of hyperchloremia, whereas balanced crystalloid solutions are pragmatic choices of fluid in the majority of perioperative resuscitation settings.

The prime aim of fluid therapy is to improve tissue perfusion so as to provide adequate oxygen to the tissues. Macrohemodynamical parameters and/or surrogates of tissue perfusion do not always correspond to microcirculatory functional states, and especially not in states of inflammation. Even when targets for macrohemodynamics are reached, the microcirculation may still remain damaged and dysfunctional.

Observation of the microcirculation in the perioperative setting provides a more physiologically based approach for fluid therapy by possibly avoiding the unnecessary and inappropriate administration of large volumes of fluids.

Hand-held videomicroscopy is able to visualize microcirculatory perfusion sublingually. It can be used to monitor the functional state of the microcirculation by assessment and quantification of sublingual microvascular capillary density, and thus to guide fluid therapy. The Cytocam-IDF device might provide the needed clinical platform because of its improved imaging capacity in terms of density and perfusion parameters as well as providing on-line quantification of the microcirculation.

Chapter 13. Pulmonary edema

Göran Hedenstierna, Claes Frostell, and João Batista Borges

Pulmonary edema can be either hydrostatic (cardiac) or high-permeability (non-cardiac). In the first type, therapy should focus on a reduction of hydrostatic pressure. Pain relief and anxiety relief reduces vascular pressures by bringing down sympathetic nervous system drive. Treatment also consists in oxygen supplementation, furosemide, continuous positive airway pressure (CPAP) on a tight-fitting face-mask, and possibly venesection.

High-permeability pulmonary edema implies that the barrier function of the vasculature to larger molecules and cells is no longer intact. The permeability increase leads to a rapid and profound fluid leakage, followed by inflammation and destruction of lung parenchymal structure. Treatment consists of fluid restriction while maintaining adequate organ perfusion. Extracorporeal membrane oxygenation (ECMO) may be used in patients with severe non-cardiac pulmonary edema. Adequate treatment of the primary etiology of the condition is essential.

Resolution of pulmonary edema might include local reabsorption, clearance through the lymphatic system, clearance via the pleural space, or clearance through the airway. Maintaining spontaneous breathing, whenever possible, cannot be over-emphasized. Spontaneous breathing with CPAP both counteracts atelectasis formation in the lung and facilitates the ability to clear secretions with the re-emergence of cough.

Section 3: Techniques

Chapter 14. Invasive hemodynamic monitoring

Jonathan Aron and Maurizio Cecconi

The aim of hemodynamic monitoring is to enable the optimization of cardiac output and therefore improve oxygen delivery to the tissues, avoiding the accumulation of oxygen debt, in the perioperative period. Instigating goal-directed therapy based on validated optimization algorithms has been shown to reduce mortality in highrisk patients and complications in moderate-to high-risk patients.

A number of devices are available to facilitate this goal. The pulmonary artery catheter was the first hemodynamic monitor, but its invasive nature precludes its routine use in today's clinical practice. More recently, devices that continuously analyze the arterial pressure waveform to calculate various flow parameters have been developed and validated. These devices have facilitated the introduction of hemodynamic monitoring to the wider surgical population, providing useful clinical information that enables the judicious use of fluid therapy whilst avoiding hypervolemia.

This chapter explores the role that hemodynamic optimization plays in perioperative care, describes some of the commonly used invasive hemodynamic monitors, and explains how to use the information produced effectively. Used correctly, any monitor can be useful to improve outcome if applied to the right population, at the right time, and with the right strategy.

Chapter 15. Goal-directed fluid therapy

Timothy E. Miller and Tong J. Gan

Perioperative morbidity has been linked to the amount of fluid administered, with both insufficient and excess fluid leading to increased morbidity, resulting in a characteristic U-shaped curve. The challenge for us as clinicians is to keep our patients in the optimal range at all times during the perioperative period. Goal-directed therapy (GDT) is a term that has been used for nearly 30 years to describe methods of optimizing fluid and hemodynamic status. The arrival of a number of minimally invasive cardiac output monitors enables clinicians to guide perioperative volume therapy and cardiocirculatory support.

The most widely used monitor is the esophageal Doppler. There are several others that are able to analyze the arterial waveform to calculate stroke volume and cardiac output, and therefore use the "10% algorithm" in response to a fluid challenge. There are a number of studies that show improved outcomes with GDT-guided fluid optimization, as demonstrated by a faster return in gastrointestinal function, a reduction in postoperative complications, and reduced length of stay. The underlying mechanisms for the success of GDT are thought to relate to avoidance of episodes of hypovolemia, hypoxia, or decreased blood flow that may cause mitochondrial damage and subsequent organ dysfunction.

Chapter 16. Non-invasive guidance of fluid therapy

Maxime Cannesson

Optimization of oxygen delivery to the tissues during surgery cannot be conducted by monitoring arterial pressure alone. Therefore, apart from cardiac output monitoring, functional hemodynamic parameters have been developed. These parameters indicate "preload dependence," which is defined as the ability of the heart to increase stroke volume in response to an increase in preload. The Frank–Starling relationship links preload to stroke volume and presents two distinct parts: a steep portion and a plateau. If the patient is on the steep portion of the Frank–Starling relationship, then an increase in preload (induced by volume expansion) is going to induce an important increase in stroke volume. If the patient is on the plateau of this relationship, then increasing preload will have no effect on stroke volume. The functional hemodynamic parameters rely on cardiopulmonary interactions in patients under general anesthesia and mechanical ventilation and can be obtained invasively from the arterial pressure waveform or non-invasively from the plethysmographic waveform. Here, the effects of positive-pressure ventilation on preload and stroke volume are used to detect fluid responsiveness. If mechanical ventilation induces important respiratory variations in stroke volume (SVV) or in pulse pressure (PPV) it is more likely that the patient is preload-dependent. These dynamic parameters, including passive leg raising, have consistently been shown to be superior to static parameters, such as central venous pressure, for the prediction of fluid responsiveness.

Chapter 17. Hemodilution

Philippe van der Linden

Acute normovolemic hemodilution entails the removal of blood either immediately before or shortly after the induction of anesthesia and its simultaneous replacement by an appropriate volume of crystalloids and/or colloids to maintain "isovolemic" conditions. As a result, blood subsequently lost during surgery will contain proportionally fewer red blood cells, thus reducing the loss of autologous erythrocytes. Although still frequently used in some surgical procedures, the real efficacy of acute normovolemic hemodilution in reducing allogeneic blood transfusion remains discussed. The aim of this article is to describe the physiology, limits, and efficacy of acute normovolemic hemodilution.

Chapter 18. The ERAS concept

Katie E. Rollins and Dileep N. Lobo

Optimum perioperative fluid administration as part of an Enhanced Recovery After Surgery (ERAS) program is dependent on a range of factors which are becoming increasingly well documented. Following previous ambiguous terms and definitions for fluid management strategies, appreciation of the importance of "zero balance" (where amount infused equals the amount lost from the body) of both water and salt is increasing, with both over- and underhydration resulting in significantly worse clinical outcomes (in a U-shaped distribution). Excessive fluid loads have a significant negative impact upon outcome. Electrolyte balance, from pre- to postoperative stages, is also now understood to play a key role.

Section 4: The clinical setting

Chapter 19. Spinal anesthesia

Michael F. M. James and Robert A. Dyer

Fluid therapy is widely used in conjunction with spinal anesthesia to minimize hypotensive events. The use of crystalloids for this purpose seems to be only minimally effective, particularly when given prior to the administration of the spinal anesthetic. To be effective, substantial fluid boluses must be administered – of the order of 20 ml/kg – and then preferably as a rapid coload simultaneously with the induction of spinal anesthesia. Several studies and meta-analyses suggest that colloids, either as preload or coload, are more effective than crystalloids and may result in a smaller volume of fluid loading being required. However, fluids alone, whether crystalloid or colloid, are generally inadequate to prevent or treat significant hypotension associated with spinal anesthesia, and the concomitant use of a vasopressor will frequently be necessary, particularly in obstetrics. The best that can be achieved with optimal fluid therapy is an overall reduction in the total dose of vasopressor required. The best available management of spinal hypotension would appear to be optimal fluid therapy combined with carefully graded administration of the appropriate vasopressor. It is possible that goal-directed fluid therapy, using an appropriate analysis of cardiac performance to assess the response dynamic indices to a fluid challenge, may improve fluid therapy in the future, but, at present, the evidence for this is insufficient to make a firm recommendation.

Chapter 20. Day surgery

Jan Jakobsson

Rapid recovery and a minimum of residual effects are factors of utmost importance when handling the daycase patient. Prolonged preoperative fasting should be avoided. Many countries have adopted revised fasting guidelines that allow patients without risk factors to eat a light meal up to 6 hours and to ingest clear fluids up to 2 hours prior to the induction of anesthesia. Postoperative fatigue can be reduced by fluid intake up to 2–3 hours prior to surgery.

Perioperative intravenous fluid therapy should be instituted on the basis of the case profile. In general, fluid infused during minor surgery may not exert a major effect, but during intermediate surgery, such as laparoscopic cholecystectomy, a liberal fluid program has been shown to improve recovery and reduce postoperative fatigue. Administration of about 1 liter isotonic electrolyte solution to compensate for the fasting, and a further 1 liter during surgery, improves the postoperative course. Liberal fluid administration also reduces the risk for postoperative nausea and the risk vs. benefit seems to be in favor for its routine use in ASA 1–2 patients. The potential benefit in adding dextrose to the intravenous fluid during the early postoperative phase has been assessed, but the benefit seems to be very minor.

Resumption of oral intake, drinking, and eating are traditional variables for the assessment of eligibility for discharge and thus an essential part of day surgery. However, there is no need for patients to drink before discharge; intake of fluid and food should be recommended but not pushed.

Chapter 21. Abdominal surgery

Birgitte Brandstrup

Normal as well as pathological fluid losses should be replaced with a fluid resembling the loss in quantity and quality (electrolyte composition). Elective surgical patients can be allowed to eat until 6 hours and drink up to 2 hours before surgery without increasing the risk of fluid aspiration. Preoperative administration of sugarcontaining fluids, intravenous or by mouth, improves postoperative well-being and muscle strength, and lessens the postoperative insulin resistance. It does not, however, reduce the number of patients with wound- or other complications, length of stay, or mortality. Surgery does not increase the normal fluid and electrolyte losses, but causes perspiration from the abdominal wound that approximately equals the decreased water loss from the lungs because of ventilation with moist air. It is not possible to treat a decrease in blood pressure caused by the use of epidural analgesia with fluid.

The goal of zero fluid balance (formerly called "restrictive") reduces postoperative complications and the risk of death in major abdominal surgery. The goal of zero balance in combination with a goal of nearmaximum stroke volume provides equally good outcome. During outpatient surgical procedures the wellbeing of the patient is improved by giving approximately 1 liter of fluid. The role of glucose-containing fluid in this setting may be beneficial, but the evidence is sparse. "Postoperative restricted fluid therapy," allowing the patients to drink no more than 1,500 ml/day, is not recommended. To measure the body weight is the best way to monitor the postoperative fluid balance. Fluid charts are insufficient.

Chapter 22. Cardiac surgery

Saqib H. Qureshi and Giovanni Mariscalco

Cardiac surgical patients have altered vascular and immunological factors that dictate short- and long-term clinical outcomes. So far, the evidence does not favor any single choice of fluid therapy. In fact, volume replacement is a determinant of "filling pressures" in isolation but requires a critical balance with other determinants of tissue-oxygen debt such as vasomotor tone, fluid responsiveness, and cardiac contractility. Lastly, none of the available fluid therapies have been assessed for their comparative endothelial homeostatic potential. This leaves a significant knowledge gap and an incentive for researchers, clinicians, and industry to design and test safer and more efficacious choices for clinical use.

Chapter 23. Pediatrics

Robert Sümpelmann and Nils Dennhardt

The main aim of perioperative fluid therapy is to stabilize or normalize the child's homeostasis. Young infants have higher fluid volumes, metabolic rates, and fluid needs than adults. Therefore, short perioperative fasting periods are important to avoid iatrogenic dehydration, ketoacidosis, and misbehavior. Balanced electrolyte solutions with 1–2.5% glucose are favored for intraoperative maintenance infusion. Glucose-free balanced electrolyte solutions should then be added as needed to replace intraoperative fluid deficits or minor blood loss. Hydroxyethyl starch or gelatin solutions are useful in hemodynamically instable patients or those with major blood loss, especially when crystalloids alone are not effective or the patient is at risk of interstitial fluid overload. The monitoring should focus on the maintenance or restoration of a stable tissue perfusion. Also, in non-surgical or postoperative children, balanced electrolyte solutions should be used instead of hypotonic solutions, both with 5% glucose, as recent clinical studies and reviews showed a lower incidence of hyponatremia.

Chapter 24. Obstetric, pulmonary, and geriatric surgery

Kathrine Holte

This chapter focuses on fluid management in obstetric, pulmonary, and geriatric surgery. In obstetrics, the fluid administration debate largely centers on the relevance of fluid infusions to counteract hypotension in conjunction with regional anesthesia administered for pain relief during labor or as anesthesia for Cesarean section, where both colloids and sympathomimetics reduce maternal hypotension. Particular to pulmonary surgery, a positive fluid balance is found to correlate with postoperative lung injury and should be strictly controlled. Elderly patients, while being at increased risk for postoperative complications, may also be more susceptible to perioperative fluid disturbances including preoperative dehydration.

In summary, evidence suggests that fluid management should be individualized and integrated into perioperative care programs. Both insufficient and excessive fluid administration may increase complications, and while determining fluid status is still a challenge, individualized fluid therapy to obtain certain hemodynamic goals may be recommended.

Chapter 25. Transplantations

Laurence Weinberg

Patients with end-stage liver disease have a hyperdynamic resting circulation with high cardiac output states and low systemic vascular resistance and tachycardia. During liver transplantation, this state is amplified. The potential for massive bleeding is common and can result in sudden and catastrophic hypovolemia. Massive blood transfusion results in large volumes of citrated blood being administered. With limited or no hepatic function to metabolize citrate, citrate intoxication can occur, and calcium chloride should be administered when appropriate. Mild to moderate acidosis can be safely tolerated. Albumin is the most common colloid used, while the use of lactate-based crystalloid solutions can result in hyperlactatemia as lactate anions are ineffectively metabolized. Acetate-buffered solutions should be preferred. The most common cause of death in fulminant liver failure is intractable intracranial hypertension from cerebral edema, present in approximately 50–80% of patients with fulminant liver failure. Therefore, permissive hypernatremia and use of hypertonic saline solutions are frequently treatment options in this setting.

Crystalloids are the mainstay and first choice of perioperative fluid intervention in renal transplantation. Conventionally, 0.9% saline is widely advocated because of concerns about hyperkalemia from the balanced/buffered solutions, which all contain potassium. However, this fear has not been confirmed in clinical trials. Hydroxyethyl starch should be avoided owing to increased risk of a delayed graft function.

Chapter 26. Neurosurgery

Hemanshu Prabhakar

Fluid administration is one of the basic components in the management of neurosurgical patients. Despite advances and extensive research in the field of neurosciences, there is still a debate on the ideal fluid. Issues related to adequate volume replacement and effects on the intracranial pressure persist. Studies have demonstrated the harmful effects of colloids over crystalloids. Normal saline has remained a fluid of choice, but there is now emerging evidence that it too is not free from its harmful effects. Hypertonic saline has also been accepted by many practitioners, but its use and administration requires close monitoring and vigilance. There is now growing evidence on the use of balanced solutions for neurosurgical patients. However, this evidence comes from a small number of studies. This chapter tries to briefly cover various clinical situations in neurosciences with respect to fluid administration.

Chapter 27. Intensive care

Alena Lira and Michael R. Pinsky

Fluid infusions are an essential part of the management of the critically ill, and include maintenance fluids to replace insensible loss and resuscitation efforts to restore blood volume. This chapter is on fluid resuscitation. Fluid administration is a vital component of resuscitation therapy, with the aim being to restore cardiovascular sufficiency. Initial resuscitation aims to restore a minimal mean arterial pressure and cardiac output compatible with immediate survival. This is often associated with emergency surgery and associated lifesaving procedures. Then, optimization aims to rapidly restore organ perfusion and oxygenation before irreversible ischemic damage occurs. Stabilization balances fluid infusion rate with risks of volume overload, and finally de-escalation promotes polyuria as excess interstitial fluid is refilled into the circulation. There is no apparent survival benefit of colloids over crystalloids. Hydroxyethyl starch solutions have deleterious effects in certain patient populations, for example in sepsis. Balanced salt solutions are superior to normal saline. Further fluid resuscitation should be guided by the patient's need for increased blood flow and by their volumeresponsiveness.

Chapter 28. Severe sepsis and septic shock

Palle Toft and Else Tønnesen

Sepsis is a systemic disorder with a protean clinical picture and a complex pathogenesis characterized by the release of both pro- and anti-inflammatory elements. The organ dysfunction and organ failure occurring in the early phase of severe sepsis are believed to result from an excessive inflammatory response. Degradation or destruction of the glycocalyx layer causes transudation of fluid from the vascular space into extravascular tissue. Such capillary leakage makes the patient hypovolemic and promotes a generalized edema in the lungs, heart, gut, brain, and other tissues, which impairs organ function and sometimes causes excessive weight gain. Early, aggressive goal-directed therapy (EGDT) based on the protocol by Rivers *et al.* from 2001 stresses that adequate volume replacement is a cornerstone in management, as restoration of flow is a key component in avoiding tissue ischemia or reperfusion injury. It is the speed with which septic patients are fluid resuscitated that makes the difference. Deep general anesthesia should be avoided and noradrenaline might be needed to prevent circulatory shock before sufficient amounts of fluid have been administered.

Survival improves from EGDT only if optimization is instituted before organ failure is manifested. Most patients require continuous aggressive fluid resuscitation during the first 24 hours of management. In the later course of the disease, between 2 and 7 days, a more restricted fluid management strategy should be instituted. Not all patients who are "fluid responders" should automatically receive fluids.

Chapter 29. Hypovolemic shock

Niels H. Secher and Johannes J. van Lieshout

Hypovolemic shock is a response to a reduced central blood volume (CBV) whatever its cause – hemorrhage, passive head-up tilt, or other cause – and follows three phases. The first comprises a reduction of CBV initially with reflex increase in heart rate (HR) to approximately 90 bpm and maintained blood pressure (BP) by increased vascular resistance. In the second phase, which corresponds to a reduction of the CBV by about 30%, a Bezold-Jarisch-like reflex ceases sympathetic activity, although plasma adrenaline continues to increase, and together with vagal activation enhances coagulation competence. At this stage of progressive CBV the HR decreases, eventually to extremely low values. In the third phase, BP remains low while HR increases to more than 100 bpm.

To treat hypovolemia, volume substitution can be directed to establish maximal values for stroke volume, cardiac output, or venous oxygen saturation. These variables do not increase when CBV is enhanced in supine healthy humans, and thereby define "normovolemia." The patient's bed can be tilted head-down, and if the mentioned variables then increase significantly, the patient is in need of volume. If not, a volume deficit does not explain the patient's condition. Plasma atrial natriuretic peptide (ANP) also decreases in response to a reduced CBV, and to maintain plasma ANP during major surgery requires a 2.5-liter surplus volume of lactated Ringer's solution. With recording of deviations in central cardiovascular variables, the blood volume can be maintained within 100 ml and provide a comfortable margin to the deficit that affects BP and regional blood flow.

Chapter 30. Uncontrolled hemorrhage

Robert G. Hahn

Fluid therapy in hemorrhage strives to restore hemodynamic function and tissue perfusion. However, these goals are not appropriate when there is an injury to a large blood vessel and the hemorrhage has not been stopped surgically (uncontrolled hemorrhage). Clinical situations in which this is the case include penetrating trauma, ruptured aortic aneurysm, and gastric bleeding. Numerous animal experiments in pigs and rats have shown that the low-flow, low-pressure state characterizing serious hemorrhage promotes coagulation, even if a large blood vessel is injured. An immature blood clot is easilywashedaway if the blood flow rate and the arterial pressure is normalized by infusion fluids. Vigorous fluid therapy then increases both the blood loss and the mortality. The road to optimal survival is to infuse less fluid at lower speed (half volume at half speed is suggested) and aim at a systolic arterial pressure of 90 mmHg. In this situation, the strategy is only to prevent progressive acidosis and irreversible shock. A deviation from normal hemodynamics should be accepted until the source of bleeding has been treated surgically. A sudden drop in arterial pressure during ongoing fluid resuscitation suggests that rebleeding is occurring, and the infusion rate should then be further reduced. There is an unfortunate lack of clinical studies showing that the fluid strategy that has been successful in animal experiments pertains also to humans. However, it is widely accepted in emergency departments and trauma hospitals to resuscitate trauma patients to a lower-than-usual systolic pressure (hypotensive resuscitation).

Chapter 31. Burns

Folke Sjöberg

The purpose of fluid treatment for burn-injured patients is to maintain organ perfusion despite major leakage of fluid from the intravascular space. The leakage is due to a sharp reduction of the pressure in the interstitial fluid space (negative imbibition pressure) and an increase of the vascular permeability. Most of the fluid loss due to the first factor takes place within the first 3–4 hours and the bulk of loss from the second factor within 12 hours after the burn.

The formula for plasma volume support most widely used today is the "Parkland" strategy, in which 2–4 ml of buffered Ringer's solution is administered per total body surface area % per kilogram body weight. Half of the calculated volume is given during the first 8 hours after the burn and the other half during the subsequent 16 hours. A colloid rescue strategy should come into play when the fluid volumes provided are very large, and is adequate after 8–12 hours post-burn.

The patient should be in a state of controlled hypovolemia. The combined use of urine output (aim 30–50 ml/h), mean arterial pressure, and the mental state of the patient is gold standard when guiding the fluid therapy. The use of central circulatory parameters increases the risk of fluid overload and does not improve the outcome. The maximal tissue edema reaches a maximum between the first 24 and 48 hours post-burn, and thereafter the added fluid volume is excreted as an ongoing process over 7–10 days.

Chapter 32. Trauma

Joshua D. Person and John B. Holcomb

In the United States, injury is the leading cause of death among individuals between the ages of 1 and 44 years, and the third leading cause of death overall. Approximately 20% to 40% of trauma deaths occurring after hospital admission are related to massive hemorrhage and are therefore potentially preventable with rapid hemorrhage control and improved resuscitation techniques. Over the past decade, the treatment of this population has transitioned into a damage control strategy with the development of resuscitation strategies that emphasize permissive hypotension, limited crystalloid administration, early balanced blood product transfusion, and rapid hemorrhage control. This resuscitation approach initially attempts to replicate whole blood transfusion, utilizing an empiric 1:1:1 ratio of plasma:platelets:red blood cells, and then transitions, when bleeding slows, to a goal-directed approach to reverse coagulopathy based on viscoelastic assays. Traditional resuscitation strategies with crystalloid fluids are appropriate for the minimally injured patient who presents without shock or ongoing bleeding. This chapter will focus on the assessment and resuscitation of seriously injured trauma patients who present with ongoing blood loss and hemorrhagic shock.

Chapter 33. Absorption of irrigating fluid

Robert G. Hahn

Absorption of irrigating fluid can occur in endoscopic surgeries. The complication is best known from transurethral prostatic resection and transcervical endometrial resection. When monopolar electrocautery is used, the irrigation is performed with electrolytefree fluid containing glycine, or mannitol or sorbitol. With bipolar electrocautery the irrigating fluid is usually isotonic saline. Incidence data on fluid absorption and associated adverse effects show great variation, but absorption in excess of 1 liter usually occurs in 5% to 10% of the operations and causes symptoms in 2–3 patients per 100 operations.

The pathophysiology of the complications arising from absorption of electrolyte-free irrigating fluids is complex. Symptoms can be related to metabolic toxicity, cerebral edema, and circulatory effects caused by rapid massive fluid overload. Available data on absorption of isotonic saline suggest that symptoms are likely when the volume exceeds 2 liters.

Ethanol monitoring is the most viable of the methods suggested for monitoring of fluid absorption in clinical practice. By using an irrigating fluid that contains 1% of ethanol, updated information about fluid absorption can be obtained at any time perioperatively by letting the patient breathe into a hand-held alcolmeter.

Treatment of massive fluid absorption is supportive with regard to ventilation, hemodynamics, and well-being. Hypertonic saline is indicated when electrolyte-free fluids are used, while diuretics should be withheld until the hemodynamic situation has been stabilized. In contrast, absorption of isotonic saline should (logically) be treated with diuretics as saline does not cause osmotic diuresis and is not distributed to the intracellular space.

Chapter 34. Adverse effects of infusion fluids

Robert G. Hahn

Adverse effects may arise if an infusion fluid diverges from the body fluids with respect to osmolality or temperature. Coagulation becomes impaired when the fluid induced hemodilution is approximately 40%. Infusion of 2–3 liters of crystalloid fluid prolongs the gastrointestinal recovery time, while 6–7 liters promotes poor wound healing, pulmonary edema, and pneumonia. In abdominal surgery, suture insufficiency and sepsis become more common. However, a liberal fluid program in the postoperative period probably does not increase the number of complications.

Isotonic saline probably shares these adverse effects with the balanced crystalloid fluids, but adds on a tendency to metabolic acidosis and slight impairment of the kidney function (-10%). Glucose solutions may induce hyperglycemia and post-infusion rebound hypoglycemia. Glucose 5% without electrolytes increases the risk of postoperative subacute hyponatremia.

Adverse effects associated with colloid fluids include anaphylactic reactions, which occur in approximately 1 out of 500 infusions. To reduce this problem when dextran is used, pretreatment with a hapten inhibitor (dextran 1 kDa) should be employed. Hyperoncotic colloid solutions may cause pre-renal anuria in dehydrated patients. The indications for hydroxyethyl starch have been limited, owing to impairment of kidney function in severely ill patients.

Edema from a colloid is most clearly associated with inflammation-induced acceleration of the capillary escape rate. A factor promoting peripheral edema from crystalloid fluids is that volume expansion negatively affects the viscoelastic properties of the interstitial fluid gel. The slow excretion of crystalloid fluid during anesthesia and surgery also contributes to the development of edema.

Chapter

1

The essentials

Robert G. Hahn

Fluid requirement

Minimum 1 ml/kg per hour, i.e. 2.4 liters daily for a person with a body weight of 100 kg and 1.2 liters for a person with body weight of 50 kg. In children add 50%.

Most common to provide 1.3–1.5 ml/kg per hour to those who can excrete fluid well.

Maintenance therapy

Provide fluid and nutrition intravenously for those who cannot eat and drink.

* Glucose 5% per 4–6 hours with electrolytes up to the daily fluid requirement. This provides a minimum of calories and can be used only for a few days.
* Electrolytes should be 1 mmol/kg each of sodium and potassium per 24 hours.
* Potassium should not be infused faster than 10 mmol/hour.

Preoperative fasting

Patients may drink clear fluids up to 2 hours before surgery.

Solid food up to 6 hours before surgery.

Contraindications may apply.

Induction of anesthesia

Common practice is to provide 500 ml of balanced crystalloid fluid during the induction to compensate for vasodilatation and as a safeguard against undetected hypovolemia. The fluid has no effect on the concomitant drop in arterial pressure.

Intraoperative fluid

Fluid elimination is slow. A restrictive program reduces the complications.

* 3–5 ml/kg per hour of a balanced crystalloid fluid (Ringer's lactate or Ringer's acetate, or Plasma-Lyte). This also covers minimal blood losses.
* Alternatively, 1–2 ml/kg per hour *and* volume optimization guided by stroke volume monitoring or equivalents. This option is of most obvious benefit in the sickest patients.
* Isotonic saline to be given only on special indications. These are vomiting, hyponatremia, trauma, and (especially) neurotrauma.
* Blood loss up to 500 ml is replaced by 3 times the bled volume of balanced fluid.
* Blood losses exceeding approximately 500 ml can be replaced by a colloid fluid before the target hematocrit, which depends on the preoperative blood hemoglobin (Hb) concentration and the patient's health status, is reached.

Postoperative care unit

Fluid elimination is normal or increased.

No evidence of benefit from fluid restriction, which increases the risk of nausea.

* 5–6 ml/kg per hour of a balanced crystalloid fluid.

Clinical Fluid Therapy in the Perioperative Setting, Second Edition, ed. Robert G. Hahn. Published by Cambridge University Press. © Cambridge University Press 2016.

Back at the surgical ward

(From 3–4 hours after the surgery)
  Normalization stage.

* Drink clear fluids, alone or combined with:
* Glucose 2.5% with electrolytes 1.5 ml/kg per hour (approximately 100 ml/hour in an adult). If necessary, add more electrolytes as guided from blood analysis. Use infusion pump.

Check for dehydration before you induce anesthesia

You must always evaluate the possibility of a preoperative fluid deficit.

* *Inability to drink* leads to **hypertonic dehydration** where serum osmolality >300 mosmol/kg. Slow correction with glucose solution is the cure. If you are in a hurry, restore extracellular volume with balanced Ringer's and then turn to glucose.

* *Vomiting* and *diarrhea* lead to **hypotonic dehydration**. Restore with isotonic saline.
* *Enteric lavage* should replaced 1:1 with balanced electrolyte solution.
* *Ileus* may result in very large fluid deficits (4–6 liters) resulting both from inability to drink and from vomiting. Estimate is 3 liters of loss for each day of complete ileus. Replace at least half the missing volume before inducing anesthesia under cardiovascular monitoring.

Two general guidelines for the use of fluid therapy in hospital patients have been published by British authors and can be downloaded free of charge from the Internet:

GIFTASUP (2007) – British Consensus Guidelines on Intravenous Fluid Therapy for Adult Surgical Patients; http://www.bapen_pubs/giftasup.pdf (last visited on 18 March 2016)

NICE (2013) – Intravenous fluid therapy in adults in hospital; http://www.nice.org.uk/guidance/cg174

Chapter

2

Crystalloid fluids

Robert G. Hahn

Summary

Crystalloid electrolyte solutions include isotonic saline, Ringer's lactate, Ringer's acetate, and Plasma-Lyte. In the perioperative period these fluids are used to compensate for anesthesia-induced vasodilatation, small to moderate blood losses, and urinary excretion. Although evaporation consists of electrolyte-free water, such fluid losses are relatively small during short-term surgery and may also be compensated by a crystalloid electrolyte solution.

These fluids expand the plasma volume to a lesser degree than colloid fluids as they hydrate both the plasma and the interstitial fluid space. However, the distribution to the interstitial fluid space takes 25–30 min to be completed, which is probably due to the restriction of fluid movement by the finer filaments in the interstitial gel. The slow distribution gives crystalloid electrolyte solutions a fairly good plasma volume-expanding effect as long as the infusion continues and shortly thereafter.

Isotonic saline is widely used, but has an electrolyte composition that deviates from that of the extracellular fluid ("unbalanced"). This fluid is best reserved for special indications, such as hyponatremia, hypochloremic metabolic alkalosis, and disease states associated with vomiting. Isotonic saline may also be considered in trauma and in children undergoing surgery. Hypertonic saline might be considered in neurosurgery and, possibly, in preoperative emergency care.

Ringer's lactate, Ringer's acetate, and Plasma-Lyte have been formulated to be more similar to the composition of the ECF ("balanced fluids"). They are the mainstay of fluid administration in the perioperative period and should be used in all situations where isotonic saline is not indicated.

The term *crystalloid fluid* refers to sterile water solutions that contain small molecules, such as salt and glucose, which are able to crystallize. These solutes easily pass through the capillary membrane, which is the thin fenestrated endothelium that divides the plasma volume from the interstitial fluid volume. This process of solute distribution brings water along with it. Hence, the volume of a crystalloid fluid is spread throughout the extracellular fluid (ECF) space.

Osmolality is the number of particles dissolved in the water solution. The osmolality of the body fluids is approximately 295 milliosmoles (mosmol) per kg and is a powerful driving force for water distribution. However, it is both the type of dissolved particles and the osmolality of the solution that determine the tonicity, i.e. to what degree the infusion fluid hydrates or dehydrates the intracellular fluid (ICF) space.[1]

If the solutes in the infusion fluid remain outside the cells, as is the case for sodium and chloride, the osmolality and the tonicity agree. An iso-osmotic infusion fluid (295 mosmol/kg) is then isotonic. In contrast, osmolality and tonicity are not equivalent in the case where the solutes easily penetrate the cell membrane, which separates the ECF from the ICF. An example is ethanol, which markedly raises the body osmolality but without redistributing water. Therefore, ethanol is said to have low tonicity.

The cell membrane regulates the distribution of many other solutes across the cell membrane in a finely graded manner via energy-consuming pump mechanisms, which then also modify the water distribution.

Table 2.1 Composition of plasma and the most common crystalloid solutions

	Osmolality (mosmol/kg)	pH	Na⁺ (mmol/l)	K⁺ (mmol/l)	HCO_3^- (mmol/l) equivalent	Cl⁻ (mmol/l)	Glucose (mmol/l)
Plasma	295	7.4	140	3.6–5.1	30	100	5
0.9% saline	308	5.0	154	0	0	154	0
7.5% saline	2400	3.5–7.0	1250	0	0	1250	0
Lactated Ringer's	274	6.5	130	4	30	110	0
Acetated Ringer's	270	6.0	130	4	30	110	0
Plasma-Lyte[a]	295	7.4	140	5	27	98	0
Glucose (5%)	278	5.0	0	0	0	0	278
Glucose (2.5%) + electrolytes	280	6.0	70	0	25	45	139

[a] Plasma-Lyte A also contains 23 mmol/l of gluconate.
The infusion fluids may contain small amounts of electrolytes such as magnesium and calcium.

These pumping mechanisms operate slowly (minutes to hours) whereas changes in osmolality redistribute water within seconds.

The marketed crystalloid infusion fluids are usually isotonic or nearly isotonic. Hence, they expand the ECF volume but not the ICF volume. Their main use in the perioperative period is to compensate for anesthesia-induced vasodilatation, small to moderate blood losses, and urinary excretion. Although evaporation consists of electrolyte-free water, such fluid losses are relatively small and can also be compensated by crystalloid electrolyte solutions.

Isotonic saline

A 0.9% solution of saline is isotonic and is therefore called physiological or "normal." However, the fluid can also be called "unbalanced" because no attempt has been made to mimic the electrolyte composition of the ECF. The fluid still contains a marked surplus of chloride ions and no buffer (Table 2.1) and, hence, infusion of >2 liters of the fluid causes hyperchloremic metabolic acidosis.[2]

Isotonic saline is the most widely used infusion fluid in Europe and probably worldwide, although the indications are limited. In adults, normal saline should be reserved for patients with hyponatremia and hypochloremic metabolic alkalosis, as in disease states associated with vomiting. The fluid has a more accepted role for perioperative fluid therapy in children where the risk of subacute postoperative hyponatremia is a more serious concern than in adults.

When infused in healthy volunteers, 2 liters of normal saline caused abdominal pain, which was not the case for lactated Ringer's.[3] The use of approximately 4 liters of isotonic saline during surgery caused more postoperative complications than the use of the same amount of Ringer's lactate.[4]

Normal saline is excreted more slowly than both lactated and acetated Ringer's solutions,[5] increasing the volume effect ("efficiency") of the fluid to be about 10% greater than for the Ringer's solutions (Figure 2.1). The reason for the slow elimination is probably that the surplus of chloride ions has a vasoconstrictive effect on the renal blood vessels.[6]

Small prospective [4] and large retrospective [7] studies have shown that surgical complications are more common after open abdominal operations where isotonic saline has been infused than for similar operations with Ringer's lactate. However, a difference in complication rate is unlikely if the infused volume is <2 liters. A more detailed comparison between isotonic saline and the buffered Ringer's solutions is given in Chapter 12, "Monitoring of the microcirculation."

Isotonic saline is devoid of calcium. This means that the fluid can be infused together with packed erythrocytes where citrate has been used as preservative without causing coagulation in the infusion line. Large volumes of saline dilute the plasma concentration of ionized calcium, which might be an untoward effect because hypocalcemia decreases myocardial contractility. Therefore, calcium needs to be substituted if large volumes of isotonic saline are provided. No

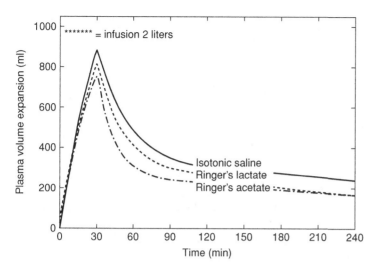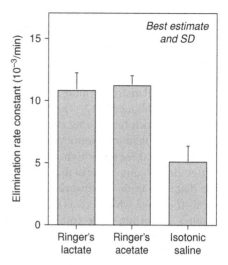

Figure 2.1 Left panel: Plasma volume expansion from infusion of 2 liters of isotonic saline, Ringer's lactate and Ringer's acetate over 30 min (asterisks) in 10 healthy volunteers. Each curve is based on the modeled average plasma dilution from experiments performed in 10 male volunteers multiplied by the plasma volume at baseline as estimated by anthropometry. Right panel: The rate of elimination of the three fluids. The half-life is the inverse of the shown elimination rate constant times 0.693. Hence, the half-life is about 60 min for the Ringer's solutions and 130 min for isotonic saline. Recalculations of data from Ref. [5] using a mixed-models analytical program (Phoenix NLME).

precise limit is given but it should be in the range of 4 liters in an adult.

Saline may also be marketed as hypertonic solutions at strengths of 3% and 7.5% solution. The first is mainly intended as a means of raising the serum sodium concentration in hospital in-patients and of reducing the intracranial pressure in neurotrauma patients. The latter is used for plasma volume expansion in emergency care, although the benefits have been questioned. In volunteers, 7.5% saline is four times as effective a plasma volume expander as normal saline.[5]

The Ringer's solutions

Ringer's solution is a composition created by Sydney Ringer in the 1880s to be as similar as possible to the ECF. Alexis Hartmann later added a lactate buffer to the fluid and made it Hartmann's solution, or "lactated" Ringer's solution.

Lactate and acetate

Today, Ringer's solution is used with the addition of buffer in the form of *lactate* or *acetate*, of which the former is more common. Both ions are metabolized to bicarbonate in the body, albeit with certain differences. Lactate is metabolized in the liver and the kidneys with the aid of oxygen and under production of bicarbonate

and carbon dioxide. Acetate is metabolized faster and in most tissues, and it consumes only half as much oxygen per mole of produced bicarbonate compared with lactate. Hence, lactate slightly increases the oxygen consumption [8] and might also raise plasma glucose, particularly in diabetic patients.[8,9] Large amounts of lactated Ringer's confuse assays used to monitor lactic acidosis.

Both lactate and acetate are vasodilatators. Rapid administration aggravates the reduction of the systemic vascular resistance that normally occurs in response to volume loading. Both lactate and acetate are also fuels, although the calorific content in 1 liter of any Ringer's solution is quite low (approximately 5 kcal).

Although the differences between lactate and acetate are usually negligible, several factors suggest that acetate is the better buffer in the presence of a compromised circulation and in shock. Lactate is metabolized in the liver and, therefore, Ringer's acetate is to be preferred in patients with impaired liver function. A more detailed comparison between lactate and acetate as buffers is given in Chapter 25, "Transplantations."

Pharmacokinetics

During intravenous infusion the Ringer's solutions distribute from the plasma to the interstitial fluid space in a process that requires 25–30 min for completion. The distribution half-life is approximately 8 min.[5,10]

Distribution. There is a difference in the pattern of distribution for small and large volumes of the Ringer's solutions. Infusing 300–400 ml at a rate of 10–20 ml/min will distribute fluid almost exclusively over the plasma volume.[11,12] This is rather due to the high compliance for volume expansion of the interstitial matrix than to a limiting effect of the capillary membrane. A three times higher rate of infusion overcomes the low compliance of the interstitial gel, but the fine filaments in the meshwork still retard the rate of the distribution, which explains why this process still requires 25–30 min to be completed. When the rate of infusion is further raised (50 ml/min and higher) the return of fluid from the interstitium to the plasma becomes progressively retarded, which is due to loss of stiffness in the matrix. Free fluid can even accumulate in the interstitium if an infusion is provided fast enough to overcome the normally negative interstitial fluid pressure.[1] This causes *pitting edema*, by which we can expect that the ratio of 1:2 for the fluid distribution between the plasma and interstitial fluid space has been abruptly reduced.

For the infusion rates normally used during surgery, the ratio of the plasma to the expandable parts of the interstitial fluid space is 1:2, which means that 33% of the infused fluid is retained in the plasma (if we disregard elimination).[13] However, slow distribution results in a stronger plasma volume expansion than offered by this relationship as long as the infusion continues (Figure 2.1).

Elimination. The elimination (by voiding) in volunteers is so rapid that the fluid may exhibit one-compartment kinetics, which has been interpreted to imply that the fluid is distributed only to the plasma and to areas of the interstitial fluid space with the highest compliance for volume expansion (half-life 20 min). In contrast, elimination is greatly retarded during surgery, where Ringer's always exhibits two-compartment kinetics.[10] Infusion of 2 liters of Ringer's in volunteers is followed by elimination of 50–80% of the fluid within 2 hours, whereas the corresponding figure in anesthetized patients is only 10–20%. This corresponds to a half-life of 200–400 min. Lowered blood pressure, vasodilatation and activation of the renin–aldosterone axis are factors thought to be responsible for the slow turnover of Ringer's during anesthesia and surgery.[14] The retarded elimination facilitates the development of edema as the retained fluid distributes both in the plasma and the interstitial fluid space.

Clinical use

The pharmacodynamics of the Ringer's solutions is strongly related to their capacity to expand the ECF volume.

These fluids may be used to replace preoperative losses of fluid due to diarrhea or bowel preparation. In contrast, vomiting should be replaced by normal saline.

The Ringer's solutions are commonly used (in a volume of approximately 500 ml) to compensate the blood volume for the expansion of the vascular tree that occurs from induction of both regional and general anesthesia.

The Ringer's solutions reverse the compensatory changes in blood pressure and sympathetic tone resulting from hypovolemia. There are numerous reports confirming that rapid infusion of Ringer's is a life-saving treatment in excessive hemorrhage, owing to the resulting expansion of the plasma volume.

In contrast, crystalloid fluid cannot reverse drug-induced hypotension.[14] If a crystalloid bolus has no effect in reversing hypotension during surgery, the anesthetist should change strategy and lighten the anesthesia, or else institute treatment with an adrenergic drug, rather than providing several liters of crystalloid fluid.

As crystalloids are inexpensive and carry no risk of allergic reactions, a Ringer's solution is often used to replace smaller blood losses while colloids are withheld until 10–15% of the blood volume has been lost. The commonly recommended dosage is to infuse three times as much Ringer's as the amount of blood lost (3:1 principle). If the patient's legs are placed in stirrups, a 2:1 replacement scheme can be used, with the last third given as a bolus infusion when the legs are lowered from the stirrups.[15]

There are concerns about the use of Ringer's in brain injury, because the fluid is slightly hypotonic (270 mosmol/kg) and increases brain cell mass when the central nervous system is traumatized. Normal saline is likely to be a better choice during neurosurgery and also in acute trauma. In volunteers, however, acetated Ringer's did not increase the ICF volume, as shown by the fact that the urinary sodium concentration was only half as high as that of the plasma.[16]

All Ringer's should be infused cautiously in patients with renal insufficiency, since these patients may not be able to excrete an excess amount of crystalloid fluid.

The buffered Ringer's solutions contain 2 mmol/l of calcium and therefore cause coagulation in the infusion line if given together with erythrocytes preserved with citrate. This agent operates as an anticoagulant by binding calcium, which is a co-factor in the coagulation process.

Dosing

The rate and volume of infused Ringer's solutions vary considerably during surgery. Overall, the volumes used in clinical practice today are lower than they were in the 1980s and 1990s. The most widely used basic rate of infusion to provide is 3–4 ml/kg per hour, i.e. about 300 ml per hour in an adult male. In major surgery, a widely advocated concept is to provide a basic rate of 2 ml/kg per hour of one of the buffered Ringer's solutions and then to increase the fluid administration whenever stroke volume decreases by >10% (goal-directed fluid therapy). To provide a Ringer's solution only at a rate of 2 ml/kg per hour or less with no additional infusions increases the risk of postoperative nausea.[17]

In healthy adult females, very rapid infusions of Ringer's (2 liters over 15 min) caused swelling sensations, dyspnea, and headache.[18] This rate (133 ml/min) should not be exceeded in the absence of severe hypovolemia. No symptoms were observed after infusing the same volume more slowly.

In elderly and debilitated patients, the rate of infusion of crystalloid fluid should be further reduced and adjusted according to the patient's cardiovascular status.

Too rapid volume loading might be complicated by instant pulmonary edema. Both the dilution of the plasma proteins and the increased cardiac pressures promote such edema, which should be treated with acute vasodilatation, administration of loop diuretics, and application of continuous positive airway pressure (or positive end-expiratory pressure if the patient is mechanically ventilated).

There is also a risk of pulmonary edema developing in the postoperative period if the total volume infused during the day of surgery amounts to 7 liters or more. Arieff [19] reported development of pulmonary edema in 7.6% of 8,195 patients who underwent major surgery. The mortality in this group was 11.9%.

Volume loading with 3 liters of lactated Ringer's in volunteers (mean age 63 years) reduced the forced expiratory capacity and the peak flow rate.[20]

Outcome studies using prospective registration of postoperative adverse events have demonstrated that crystalloid fluid administration during colonic surgery should be closer to 4 ml/kg per hour than 12 ml/kg per hour.[21] One of the earliest problems is that >2 liters prolongs the gastrointestinal recovery time after surgery, which has not been described after administration of hydroxyethyl starch.[22] Larger volumes of crystalloid electrolyte fluid promote a large number of postoperative complications, such as impaired wound healing and pneumonia.[23] Many similar outcome studies will be discussed later in this book that advise the anesthetist about the optimal infusion rates during various surgeries.

The restrictive protocol is best studied, and of undisputable value, in open abdominal surgery. Patients undergoing laparoscopic cholecystectomy and bariatric surgery seem to fare better with a more liberal program (7 ml/kg per hour or higher). There is little evidence that a restrictive fluid program is of value in the postoperative care unit, where the fluid turnover is normal, or rather slightly accelerated, owing to the surgical inflammatory response.

Plasma-Lyte

The infusion fluid Plasma-Lyte is constructed to further refine the "balanced" composition of acetated Ringer's solution. Here, the sodium and chloride concentrations are virtually identical to those of human plasma, and the osmolality is the same as that of the plasma (Table 2.1).

To make up for the increase in cation and decrease of anion concentration the solution also contains the negatively charged ion gluconate, which is also metabolized to carbon dioxide and water but still has only a weak alkalinizing effect. Gluconate has been used as a taste improver in the food industry during the past 150 years and is non-toxic. Gluconate is also a part of our intermediary metabolism, and an amount corresponding to the content of 4 liters of Plasma-Lyte is produced each day in the human body.

The Plasma-Lyte composition has been known for several decades and has only recently been marketed widely. Countries that are used to Ringer's lactate may show reluctance to use Plasma-Lyte because of the content of acetate, but the differences between the lactate and acetate buffers are indeed quite small. Clinicians may also hesitate to use the fluid owing to uncertainty caused by the presence of gluconate, which is not used in clinical medicine except perhaps as a chelate in oral calcium tablets.

Plasma-Lyte has no acidifying effect and is therefore more effective than isotonic saline to combat metabolic acidosis in diabetic ketosis [24] and trauma.[25] In kidney transplantation patients, infusion of Plasma-Lyte caused less aberration of the electrolyte balance than both isotonic saline and Ringer's lactate.[26] These differences are expected since the composition of Plasma-Lyte is more similar to the ECF than any of the other crystalloid electrolyte solutions are. Although Plasma-Lyte is intuitively the best of these fluids, a benefit with respect to clinical outcome might be difficult to demonstrate relative to the balanced Ringer's solutions as the composition-related problems associated with their use are few.

Plasma-Lyte is used on the same indications as the buffered Ringer's solutions. This fluid might also be considered in trauma patients and in children, given that it is iso-osmotic.

Similar to isotonic saline, Plasma-Lyte is devoid of calcium, which makes it possible to infuse the fluid in the same intravenous line as erythrocytes preserved with citrate. Calcium might need to be substituted when more than 4 liters of the fluid has been administered, owing to dilution of the plasma calcium concentration.

The SPLIT clinical trial did not disclose any difference in the incidence of acute kidney injury and mortality when isotonic saline or Plasma-Lyte was given in a mean volume of 2 liters on the first day of admission to intensive care.[27]

References

1. Guyton AC, Hall JE. *Textbook of Medical Physiology*, 9th edn. Philadelphia: WB Saunders Company, 1996; 185–6, 298–313.

2. Scheingraber S, Rehm M, Sehmisch C, Finisterer U. Rapid saline infusion produces hyperchloremic acidosis in patients undergoing gynecologic surgery. *Anesthesiology* 1999; 90: 1265–70.

3. Williams EL, Hildebrand KL, McCormick SA, Bedel MJ. The effect of intravenous lactated Ringer's solution vs. 0.9% sodium chloride solution on serum osmolality in human volunteers. *Anesth Analg* 1999; 88: 999–1003.

4. Wilkes NJ, Woolf R, Mutch M, *et al.* The effects of balanced versus saline-based hetastarch and crystalloid solutions on acid–base and electrolyte status and gastric mucosal perfusion in elderly surgical patients. *Anesth Analg* 2001; 93: 811–16.

5. Drobin D, Hahn RG. Kinetics of isotonic and hypertonic plasma volume expanders. *Anesthesiology* 2002; 96: 1371–80.

6. Chowdbury AH, Cox EF, Francis ST, Lobo DN. A randomized, controlled, double-blind crossover study on the effects of 2-L infusions of 0.9% saline and Plasma-Lyte 148 on renal blood flow velocity and renal cortical tissue perfusion in healthy volunteers. *Ann Surg* 2012; 256: 18–24.

7. Shaw AD, Bagshaw SM, Goldstein SL, *et al.* Major complications, mortality, and resource utilization after open abdominal surgery: 0.9% saline compared to Plasma-Lyte. *Ann Surg* 2012; 255: 821–9.

8. Ahlborg G, Hagenfeldt L, Wahren J. Influence of lactate infusion on glucose and FFA metabolism in man. *Scand J Clin Lab Invest* 1976; 36: 193–201.

9. Thomas DJB, Albertini KGMM. Hyperglycaemic effects of Hartmann's solution during surgery in patients with maturity onset diabetes. *Br J Anaesth* 1978; 50: 185–8.

10. Hahn RG. Volume kinetics of infusion fluids (review). *Anesthesiology* 2010; 113: 470–81.

11. Hahn RG, Bahlmann H, Nilsson L. Dehydration and fluid volume kinetics before major open abdominal surgery. *Acta Anaesthesiol Scand* 2014; 58: 1258–66.

12. Zdolsek J, Li Y, Hahn RG. Detection of dehydration by using volume kinetics. *Anesth Analg* 2012; 115: 814–22.

13. Hahn RG. Why crystalloids will do the job in the operating room. *Anaesthesiol Intensive Ther* 2014; 46: 342–9.

14. Norberg Å, Hahn RG, Husong Li, *et al.* Population volume kinetics predicts retention of 0.9% saline infused in awake and isoflurane-anesthetized volunteers. *Anesthesiology* 2007; 107: 24–32.

15. Hahn RG. Blood volume at the onset of hypotension in TURP performed during epidural anaesthesia. *Eur J Anaesth* 1993; 10: 219–25.

16. Hahn RG, Drobin D. Rapid water and slow sodium excretion of Ringer's solution dehydrates cells. *Anesth Analg* 2003; 97: 1590–4.

17. Apfel CC, Meyer A, Orphan-Sungur M, *et al.* Supplemental intravenous crystalloids for the prevention of postoperative nausea and vomiting. *Br J Anaesth* 2012; 108: 893–902.

18. Hahn RG, Drobin D, Ståhle L. Volume kinetics of Ringer's solution in female volunteers. *Br J Anaesth* 1997; 78: 144–8.

19. Arieff AI. Fatal postoperative pulmonary edema. Pathogenesis and literature review. *Chest* 1999; 115: 1371–7.

20. Holte K, Jensen P, Kehlet H. Physiologic effects of intravenous fluid administration in healthy volunteers. *Anesth Analg* 2003; 96: 1504–9.

21. Nisanevich V, Felsenstein I, Almogy G, *et al.* Effect of intraoperative fluid management on outcome after intraabdominal surgery. *Anesthesiology* 2005; 103: 25–32.

22. Li Y, He R, Ying X, Hahn RG. Ringer's lactate, but not hydroxyethyl starch, prolongs the food intolerance time after major abdominal surgery; an open-labelled clinical trial. *BMC Anesthesiol* 2015; 15: 72.

23. Brandstrup B, Tonnesen H, Beier-Holgersen R, *et al.* Effects of intravenous fluid restriction on postoperative complications: comparison of two perioperative fluid regimens. A randomized assessor-blinded multicenter trial. *Ann Surg* 2003; 238: 641–8.

24. Chua H-R, Venkatesh B, Stachowski E, *et al.* Plasma-Lyte 148 vs. 0.9% saline for fluid resuscitation in diabetic ketoacidosis. *J Crit Care* 2012; 27: 138–45.

25. Hasman H, Cinar O, Uzun A, *et al.* A randomized clinical trial comparing the effect of rapidly infused crystalloids on acid–base status in dehydrated patients in the emergency department. *Int J Med Sci* 2012; 9: 59–64.

26. Hadimioglu N, Saadawy I, Saglam T, Ertug Z, Dinckan A. The effect of different crystalloid solutions on acid–base balance and early kidney function after kidney transplantation. *Anesth Analg* 2008; 107: 264–9.

27. Young P, Bailey R, Beasley R, *et al.* Effect of buffered crystalloid solution vs. saline on acute kidney injury among patients in the intensive care unit. The SPLIT randomized clinical trial. *JAMA* 2015; 314: 1701–10. doi:10.1001/jama.2015.12334

Chapter

3

Colloid fluids

Robert G. Hahn

Summary

Colloid fluids are crystalloid electrolyte solutions with a macromolecule added that binds water by its colloid osmotic pressure. As macromolecules escape the plasma only with difficulty, the resulting plasma volume expansion is strong and has a duration of many hours. Clinically used colloid fluids include albumin, hydroxyethyl starch, gelatin, and dextran.

The plasma volume expansion shows one-compartment kinetics, which means that colloids, in contrast to crystalloids, have no detectable distribution phase. Marketed fluids are usually composed so that the infused volume expands the plasma volume by the infused amount. Exceptions include rarely used hyperoncotic variants and mixtures with hypertonic saline.

The main indication for colloid fluids is as second-line treatment of hemorrhage. Because of inherent allergenic properties, crystalloid electrolyte fluids should be used when the hemorrhage is small. A changeover to a colloid should be performed only when the crystalloid volume is so large that adverse effects may ensue (mild effects at 3 liters, severe at 6 liters). The only other clinical indication is that dextran can be prescribed to improve microcirculatory flow.

There has been lively debate about clinical use of colloid fluids after studies in septic patients have shown that hydroxyethyl starch increases the need for renal replacement therapy. This problem has not been found in the perioperative setting but the use of starch has still been restricted.

The colloids have defined maximum amounts that can be infused before adverse effects, usually arising from the coagulation system, become a problem.

The term *colloid fluid* refers to a sterile water solution with added macromolecules that pass through the capillary wall only with great difficulty. The osmotic strength of macromolecules is not great, so a colloid fluid must also contain electrolytes to be non-hemolytic. As long as macromolecules reside within the capillary walls their contribution to the total osmolality (the *colloid osmotic pressure*) is still sufficient to maintain a large proportion (or all) of the infused fluid volume inside the bloodstream.

Colloid fluids are used as plasma volume expanders and have a longer-lasting effect than crystalloid fluids. They carry a risk of allergic reactions not shared by crystalloid fluids. Therefore, one usually replaces smaller blood losses by crystalloid fluid, while colloids are withheld until 10–15% of the blood volume has been lost. The recommended use of colloid fluids in more specific clinical situations is further explained in many chapters in this book.

The colloids should be mixed in balanced electrolyte solutions instead of in normal saline. The reason for this is the metabolic acidosis induced by normal saline, but the changeover is important only if 2–3 liters of the colloid is administered. However, even minor acidosis from the saline in a colloid fluid adds to acidosis caused for other reasons.

Overall, the use of colloid solutions has declined in recent years. The change is due to the disclosure of

Clinical Fluid Therapy in the Perioperative Setting, Second Edition, ed. Robert G. Hahn. Published by Cambridge University Press. © Cambridge University Press 2016.

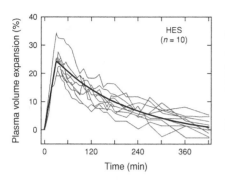
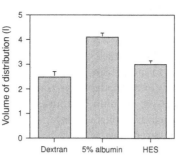
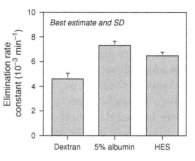

Figure 3.1 Left panel: Plasma volume expansion from infusion of 10 ml/kg of hydroxyethyl starch (HES) 130/0.4 (Voluven) in 10 male volunteers. The thick curve is the modeled average and the thin lines each of the underlying experiments. Middle and right panels: Kinetic parameters of 32 experiments where male volunteers received either 5 ml/kg of 6% dextran 70, 10 ml/kg 5% albumin, or 10 ml/kg hydroxyethyl starch 130/0.4 in saline. The half-life is the inverse of the elimination rate constant times 0.693, which becomes 160, 90, and 110 min, respectively. All calculations were performed in a single run with a mixed models analytical program, Phoenix NLME, without correction for evaporation. Based on data from Refs. [1], [17], and [49].

adverse renal effects on the kidneys from the use of artificial colloids in the intensive care setting. Moreover, there have been questions over whether the plasma volume-expanding effect is truly better than for crystalloids when fluid therapy is extended over several days in intensive care patients.

Albumin

Albumin is the most abundant protein in plasma and, therefore, has an important role in maintaining the intravascular colloid osmotic pressure. Albumin has a molecular weight of 70 kDa. Albumin solutions are prepared from blood donors and have a strength of 3.5%, 4%, or 5%, and are even available as a hyperoncotic 20% preparation.

Pharmacokinetics

Albumin 5% expands the plasma volume by 80% of the infused volume. In healthy volunteers, the plasma volume expansion fades away slowly according to a mono-exponential function, the half-life being almost 2 hours (Figure 3.1).

An infusion of 10 ml/kg of albumin 5% increases the serum albumin concentration by 10%, and this remains unchanged for more than 8 hours.[1] Restoration of normal blood volume is governed by translocation of albumin molecules from the plasma to the interstitial fluid space. Moreover, the plasma volume expansion *per se* has a diuretic effect. The albumin is gradually transported back to the plasma via lymphatic pathways, and the half-life of blood-derived albumin

in the body is much longer (16 hours) than the half-life of the accompanying plasma volume expansion.

Clinical use

Albumin is a "natural" colloid and remains an effective means of restoring the plasma volume and normal hemodynamics in hypovolemic shock.

Despite high cost and limited supply, the use of albumin in adults has undergone a revival in recent years. The main reason is that the adverse effects of the artificial colloids on kidney function do not seem to be shared by albumin.[2] Albumin also has a scavenger effect that is appreciated in intensive care. Acute reduction of serum albumin is a sign of capillary leak in inflammatory disorders, such as sepsis. The leakage rate is normally 5% per hour but can be raised to 20% per hour in septic patients.[3] The reason seems to be breakdown (shedding) of the glycocalyx layer of the endothelium, which binds the plasma proteins and other colloid particles more firmly to the vascular system.[4]

The use of albumin as a plasma volume expander in situations of increased capillary leak is a double-edged sword. The solution expands the plasma volume transiently, but the infused albumin creates peripheral edema later on, as the lymphatic drainage might not be able to catch up with the increased loss of protein from the plasma. In these situations, one should select colloids based on macromolecules that are eliminated from the blood by metabolism or renal excretion rather than by capillary leak, and that have a shorter half-life in the body than albumin (16 hours).

In intensive care, albumin infusions have been used to treat *hypoalbuminemia*. This therapy has gradually been taken out of practice as low serum albumin is a sign of severe disease rather than a problem in itself. The added albumin will soon be subject to catabolism and used in the same way as amino acids in the body. Albumin may be used to replace excessive albumin losses in special medical conditions, such as nephritis. Albumin is also the most commonly used plasma volume expander in children.

Hyperoncotic (20%) albumin does not improve survival in septic patients (ALBIOS study),[2] but both ALBIOS and the earlier SAFE study suggested a survival benefit for albumin treatment in patients with septic shock.[2,5]

The "albumin debate"

Treatment of the critically ill with albumin has been the subject of lively debate over the years.[6,7] In 1998, the Cochrane Library published a meta-analysis of 1,419 patients from 30 studies in which albumin was used. The results were surprising, since albumin treatment seemed to increase the mortality. The relative risk of death was 1.46 when albumin was given to treat hypovolemia, 1.69 if the indication was hypoalbuminemia, and 2.40 when albumin was given for burns.[8] In the United Kingdom, the use of albumin decreased by 40% during the months following publication of the meta-analysis.[9]

A later review of the same topic indicated that the risk of death associated with the use of albumin appeared to be lower the better the study was conducted. The best studies did not support that albumin increases the risk of death.[10]

These meta-analyses were followed by a randomized study (the SAFE study) that compared albumin 4% with normal saline.[5] No difference in outcome depending on the choice of infusion fluid was found in 7,000 intensive care patients. The mortality after 28 days was virtually identical in the groups (726 vs. 729).

However, a subgroup analysis of the SAFE study comprising the 460 patients with *head injury* showed that albumin 4% was followed by a higher mortality than normal saline (33% vs. 20%). The difference was greatest in the most severe cases.[11]

The research group of Marcus Rehm and Matthias Jacob of Munich has presented evidence that colloid solutions, and among them albumin 5%, only have an 80–100% volume effect when infused in normovolemic (bleeding) patients, while the volume effect is poorer in hypervolemic states. The reason is that marked hypervolemia raises the atrial natriuretic peptide (ANP) concentration, which negatively affects the glycocalyx layer.[12,13] They advocate the use of albumin as the colloid that helps to maintain the glycocalyx layer.

Starch

Hydroxyethyl starch (HES) consists of polysaccharides and is prepared from plants such as grain or maize.

HES is the only type of colloid preparation that has undergone a company-driven development to achieve refinement during the past 30 years. Several different formulations may be marketed, both old and new. They vary in concentration, usually being 6% or 10%. They also vary in chemical composition with respect to molecular weight, the number of hydroxyethyl groups per unit of glucose (substitution), and the placement of these hydroxyethyl groups on the carbon atoms of the glucose molecules (C2/C6 ratio).

The variability in chemical composition determines the differences in clinical effect between the solutions. Over the past decades, the trend has been to use molecules of smaller size to reduce the half-life and the risk of hemorrhagic complications. *Hetastarch* contains the largest molecules (450 kDa) and *pentastarch* contains intermediate-sized molecules (260 kDa). The most recently developed HES preparations have an even lower molecular size, on average 130 kDa. The degree of substitution may be low (0.45–0.60) or high (0.62–0.70), and the C2/C6 ratio is low if less than 8.

The preparations are usually described with the key characteristics of molecular size and substitution, which may or may not be followed by the C2/C6 ratio. Hence, currently the most widely promoted HES preparations are denoted HES 130/0.4/9:1 (Voluven from Fresenius-Kabi) and HES 130/0.62/6:1 (Venofundin from B. Braun). A modern adaptation is to mix the HES in balanced crystalloid solutions instead of in normal saline, which is to be preferred when several fluid bags are prescribed.

The degree of substitution is the key determinant for half-life. Higher molecular size increases risk of adverse effects in the form of anaphylactoid reactions, coagulopathy, and postoperative itching.

HES (6%) mixed in hypertonic (7.5%) saline is also marketed for emergency and trauma situations. Such a solution expands the plasma by much more than the infused volume, by virtue of osmotic volume transfer from the intracellular fluid space.

Pharmacokinetics

A 6% HES solution in iso-osmotic saline or balanced electrolytes expands the plasma volume by as much as the infused volume (Figure 3.1). Considerable variability in this respect may be encountered when administered to intensive care patients.[14]

The elimination of the HES molecules is a complex issue. They have a spectrum of sizes of which the smallest (<60–70 kDa) are quickly eliminated by renal excretion. Larger molecules first need to be cleaved by endogenous alpha-amylase into smaller fragments before being excreted, a process that increases the osmotic strength per gram of polysaccharide. The HES molecules are also subjected to phagocytosis by the reticuloendothelial system, and remnants may be found in the liver and spleen even after several years. Hence, the half-life of the HES molecules does not correspond closely with the plasma volume expansion over time.

The half-life of the HES molecules in Venofundin was 3.8 hours when administered to volunteers.[15] The half-life of the HES molecules of Voluven in plasma is said to be shorter, 1.4 hours, although the terminal half-life is 12 hours. After 72 hours, approximately 60% of the molecules can be recovered in the urine.[16]

The decay of the plasma volume expansion for HES 130/0.4 (Voluven) occurs with a half-life of 2 hours in volunteers [17] (Figure 3.1) and a similar duration of the intravascular persistence was found in laparoscopic cholecystectomy [18] and hip replacement surgery.[19] Hence, the intravascular persistence of the fluid volume is much shorter than the half-life of the HES molecules, which suggests that the molecules reside outside the circulation for many hours before being eliminated.

As for crystalloid fluids, the plasma volume expansion is greater if HES is infused during anesthesia-induced hypotension [20] and has a markedly longer duration when given to replace hemorrhage.[21]

The elimination of crystalloid fluid is known to be greatly retarded by anesthesia and surgery, but there are no data on the rate of elimination of colloid fluid volumes in the perioperative setting.

Clinical use

Hydroxyethyl starch is indicated solely for plasma volume expansion in bleeding patients. The colloid is not recommended for use in intensive care.

The first 10–20 ml should be infused slowly and the patient closely observed with respect to allergic reactions, which are rare and less severe than for dextran.

The highest recommended dose of Voluven to be given during 24 hours is 3.5 liters in an adult of 70 kg. Only half as much should be allowed for dextran and HES preparations that contain larger molecules.

Although small-sized HES (130 kDa) preparations have a shorter persistence in the blood, they have the same clinical efficacy as median-sized HES preparations while being safer.[22]

The "starch debate"

Europe has suffered a painful debate on the clinical use of HES in clinical medicine. In 2001, Schortgen et al. found a greater change in creatinine concentration in patients treated with 6% HES 200/0.60–0.66 (Elohes) as compared with 3% gelatin.[23] A second study, called VISEP, reported lactated Ringer's to be superior to 10% HES 200/0.5 (Hemohes).[24] In a small study of burn patients the latter hyperoncotic HES preparation also seemed to promote renal failure and even death.[25] These findings were initially thought to be because the tested HES solutions were of an older type and not of the most modern (molecular weight 130 type) HES, and also because the base solution was isotonic saline and not a balanced electrolyte preparation. However, a subsequent Scandinavian trial in septic patients, called the 6S study, found that HES 130/0.4 more often than Ringer's acetate is followed by renal replacement therapy and even death.[26]

Another study in 2012, the CHEST trial, also reported that HES 130/0.4 in saline (Voluven) was associated with more negative outcomes than isotonic saline in 7,000 patients treated for different diagnoses in the intensive care setting.[27] There was no difference in mortality, but serum creatinine rose more in the HES group. The fraction of the cohorts that fulfilled the criteria for kidney dysfunction (RIFLE-R) and kidney injury (RIFLE-I) was larger among those who received saline, but more patients who received HES fulfilled the criteria for kidney failure (10.5% versus 5.8%) and subsequently received renal replacement therapy (7.0% versus 5.8%). The adverse effect was more than twice as common after HES treatment (5.3% versus 2.8%), which is a more expected finding because colloids but not crystalloids have allergic properties.

These studies made it apparent that no type of HES solution should be used in septic patients. The existence of a negative influence on the clinical course and outcome in other patients is less clear. The only study with mixed diagnoses was the CHEST study, which is the least convincing of these trials. Critics of HES argue that this colloid has a dose-dependent toxic effect on the kidneys that had been demonstrated in several large trials. Defenders of HES pointed out that these trials never compared the fluids when used as first-line treatment, and that the administration often deviated from clinical practice.

In late 2013 the European Medicines Agency published a proposal that was later endorsed by the European Commission, and that put limitations on the use of HES. From then on, these colloids can only be used within the EU to combat hypovolemia in bleeding patients and not at all in the intensive care setting. Sepsis, burn injuries, and renal failure are contraindications. Treatment should be initiated only if crystalloids are insufficient. The lowest effective dose should be used, and treatment should be continued for the shortest period of time, and no longer than 24 hours. Serum creatinine must be monitored in the aftermath of the HES treatment.[28]

Three meta-analyses published during 2014 refuted a negative effect of HES on outcome when used in the operating theatre.[29–31] Naturally, these meta-analyses were mostly based on the same material.

The debate has been fueled by the CRISTAL study that compared the use of any colloid with any crystalloid fluid in the intensive care setting. There was no difference in 30-day mortality but there was a trend towards a survival benefit in the colloid group at 90 days.[32]

Gelatin

Gelatin solutions consist of polypeptides from bovine raw material. This colloid was already in use during World War I and since then has mostly been used in Great Britain and its former colonies. Gelatin is considered to have a fairly good plasma volume-expanding effect, similar to that of HES.[18] The

duration is shorter (approximately 2 hours) because of the relatively small size of the molecules (average 30 kDa), which makes them excretable by the kidneys. Mild anaphylactoid reactions occur at a frequency of 0.3%, which is relatively high, but severe reactions are rare.[33] The effect of gelatin on blood coagulation is small.

Gelatin had a bad reputation for some years because of the risk of spreading slow virus diseases such as "mad cow disease" (bovine spongiform encephalopathy). To prevent this problem, the gelatin preparations are now heated to high temperature before sale.

The two marketed solutions are Haemaccel, which contains 3.5% gelatin, and Gelofusine, which is a plasmion-succinylated gelatin mixed in isotonic saline. The latter is the most widely used gelatin today. The solution is slightly hypo-osmotic (274 mosmol/kg) and contains 154 mmol/l of sodium but only 120 mmol/l of chloride, whereby hyperchloremic acidosis will be less of a problem compared with Voluven and isotonic saline.

Dextran

Long chains of glucose molecules (polysaccharides) are synthesized by bacteria to serve as macromolecules in the group of infusion fluids called the *dextrans* (sometimes abbreviated to DEX). As with albumin, the osmolality of a water solution containing only the macromolecules is quite low and necessitates that electrolytes are added as well.

Commercially available dextran solutions have an average molecular weight of 70 kDa (dextran 70) or 40 kDa (dextran 40), and concentrations used are 3%, 6%, or 10%. The most widely used, 6% dextran 70, expands the plasma volume by the volume of the infused amount, although the initial volume expansion is slightly larger. The plasma volume expansion subsides with a half-life of almost 3 hours (Figure 3.1). A solution of 10% dextran 40 expands the plasma volume by twice the infused volume. The half-life is shorter than for dextran 70.

The dextran molecules are either excreted by the kidneys or metabolized by an endogenous hydrolase (dextranase) to carbon dioxide and water.

The dextrans decrease blood viscosity and improve microcirculatory blood flow. This can sometimes be noted by visual inspection of the cut surface in a surgical wound as small vessels seem to open up when dextran is infused, increasing the bleeding surface (oozing). This might be disturbing to the surgeon. However, it is debatable whether this oozing really increases the total blood loss, provided that the infused volume is limited to 500–1,000 ml.[34]

Dextran in hypertonic (7.5%) saline is available in some countries as an effective plasma volume expander in emergencies and prehospital trauma care. The dose is 4 ml/kg and should be provided as a fluid bolus. One unit of 250 ml is usually given. Studies performed in the 1980s showed a tendency toward reduced mortality, but more recent studies have not shown any benefit with regard to survival or neurological outcome in the prehospital setting.[35,36]

In volunteers, the effectiveness of this solution in expanding the plasma volume is six to seven times that of normal saline.[37]

Clinical use

Dextran 70 is used to expand the plasma volume and/or to prevent thromboembolism.

Dextran 40 is used to improve the microcirculation after vascular surgery.

The maximum dose is 1.5 g/(kg day), which corresponds to 1.5–2.0 l of 6% dextran 70 in an adult. Hemorrhagic complications may ensue if larger amounts are given.

There is a risk of *anaphylaxis* developing in patients who have irregular antibodies to dextran. This complication occurs in a frequency of 0.27% [33] but severe reactions can be prevented by dextran molecules of very small size (1 kDa). This pretreatment is performed by giving an intravenous injection of dextran 1, which blocks the irregular antibodies ("hapten binding"), just before dextran 40 or 70 is infused. The use of dextran 1 has reduced the number of allergic reactions by 95%.[38] Dextran 1 is less essential when treating prehospital trauma victims, as the associated stress response prevents anaphylaxis.

Plasma

Human plasma should be used to administer coagulation factors and only as a last resort as a plasma volume expander. However, plasma volume expansion is much more variable with plasma than with albumin 5%.[1] The difference is probably due to increased capillary leak caused by occasional cross-reactions with the recipient's immunological system.

Other drawbacks with the use of human plasma include the high occurrence of fever reactions (3–4%), the risk of anaphylaxis in patients with hereditary IgA deficiency, and the rare but dangerous complication called "transfusion-related acute lung injury" (TRALI).

Miscellaneous effects

Colloid fluids have a number of medical effects beyond their ability to expand the plasma volume. These include improvement of microcirculation, antioxidant effects (albumin), and suppression of trauma-induced immune activation (dextran, HES). Most of these characteristics are laboratory findings with unclear clinical relevance.

The only miscellaneous effect that is used clinically is the rheological effect of dextran, which effectively improves microcirculatory blood flow and also prevents thromboembolism.

All colloid fluids affect coagulation in a dose-dependent manner, although there are differences between the intensity of the changes. It is important to be aware of the maximum doses to limit the risk of hemorrhage. This limit is of particular importance when infusing dextran.

Crystalloid or colloid?

Whether crystalloid or colloid fluid should be preferred was much debated in the 1980s. The choice between crystalloid and colloid fluids should probably not be addressed as a general preference issue but rather governed by the specific clinical situation. Nevertheless, three meta-analyses have been performed to elucidate whether crystalloid or colloid fluids result in better survival.

The oldest of these meta-analyses, based on only eight studies, indicated that crystalloid fluid should be preferred in trauma as it was associated with a 12.3% lower mortality than colloids. When non-trauma patients were studied, however, there was a 7.8% difference in favor of *colloid* therapy. The overall result showed a 5.7% relative difference in mortality rate in favor of crystalloid therapy.[39]

A decade later, in 1998, a meta-analysis comprised 1,622 patients from 37 studies treated for surgery, trauma, or burns. The data showed an overall risk of death of 24% in the colloid group but only 20% in the crystalloid group, giving a relative risk of 1.29 for death by treatment with a colloid (95% confidence interval 0.94–1.77).[40]

Another meta-analysis evaluated 814 patients from 17 studies. Here, there was no difference in overall mortality between the two types of fluid, but the relative risk of death was only 0.39 when crystalloid fluid was used in trauma patients.[41]

The largest prospective evaluation of crystalloids versus a colloid was the SAFE trial from 2004, which demonstrated no difference in outcome between albumin and saline as the resuscitation fluid in intensive care patients.[5] A more recent randomized trial comparing any colloid with any crystalloid fluid, the CRISTAL study, showed that there is no difference in 30-day mortality between the two fluid types when used in intensive care.[32] At 90 days there was even a slightly higher mortality in the crystalloid group.

As death is rare in the operating theatre, there has been a strong trend towards using avoidable surgical complications as a more refined outcome measure. Survival is undoubtedly of great interest to the patient but, scientifically, it is a rough measure that is prone to be truly multifactorial. In contrast, the past decade has demonstrated that fluid therapy greatly affects the incidence of many surgical complications, and more clearly so in debilitated and poor-risk patients than in healthy youngsters.

A more negative attitude towards the use of colloid fluids in general has been adopted by intensivists after the data on adverse renal effects of HES began to be taken seriously (in 2012).

Therapeutic window for colloids

When to use a colloid fluid has always been a matter of opinion, but using exclusively crystalloids or colloids does not seem to be rational. Both types of fluid have important downsides that mostly can be avoided by judicious combination of the two types of fluid.

The use of colloids is always hampered by a risk of anaphylaxis, which occurs even from very small doses, and a risk of coagulopathy from infusion of 1 liter or more of colloid. Crystalloids prolong the gastrointestinal recovery time when more than 2 liters has been infused [42] and there is a statistically increased risk of complications when the volume exceeds 3 liters.[43] Hence, the anesthetist should avoid providing more than 3 liters of crystalloid fluid, owing to the increased

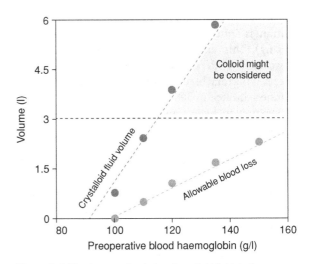

Figure 3.2 The therapeutic window for colloid fluid during surgery. Calculations were based on the assumption that the blood loss is replaced by 3 times the surgical hemorrhage. The gastrointestinal recovery time is prolonged when the crystalloid fluid volume exceeds 2–3 liters, and adverse effects become worse when 6 liters is given (from Ref. [46]. Used with permission from *Anesthesiology Intensive Therapy*).

risk of adverse effect. The risk scenario becomes aggravated if 6–7 liters are infused.[44,45]

Crystalloid fluid is the first-line treatment because of the allergic risks associated with colloids. These risks can only be accepted when the administered amount of crystalloid is so large that their adverse effects appear in a statistically increased frequency.

Figure 3.2 shows how the "therapeutic window" for colloids looks when following this reasoning. In the example a patient weighing 75 kg is operated on.[46] A bolus of 500 ml of buffered Ringer's solution is given during induction of anesthesia to compensate for vasodilatation, which is expected to reduce the hemoglobin (Hb) concentration by 10%. During surgery, buffered Ringer's was infused at the rate of 2 ml/kg per hour to replace evaporation and basal diuresis.

Surgical hemorrhage could then be replaced with clear fluids until the predetermined target Hb concentration (Hb_n) of 90 g/l was reached. The blood loss that could then be allowed before this target was reached differs depending on the preoperative Hb level (Hb_o) according to the following equation: [47]

$$\text{Allowable blood loss} = BV_o \left[\ln Hb_o - \ln(Hb_n) \right]$$

This equation depicts how much blood can be lost before the blood Hb level has decreased from Hb_o to

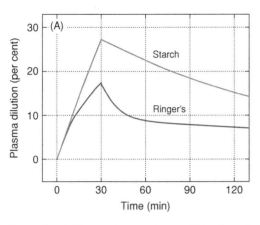
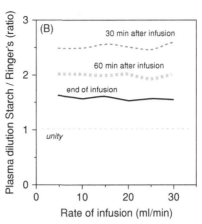

Figure 3.3 A: Dilution of venous plasma, which reflects the plasma volume expansion, following infusion of 30 ml/min over 30 min (900 ml) of Ringer's acetate and hydroxyethyl starch 130/0.4 in adult males with a body weight of 80 kg undergoing thyroid surgery under propofol anesthesia. The Ringer's curve is corrected for a volume-dependent disappearance of fluid to a "non-functional fluid space" as suggested by Ref. [48]. **B**: How much greater the plasma dilution would be if starch were infused instead of Ringer's acetate during surgery. Simulations based on data from Refs. [17] and [48].

Hb_n provided that the blood volume is unchanged. Here, the initial blood volume BV_o was set to 7% of the body weight. The calculation further assumes that buffered Ringer's is replaced by 3 times the bled volume.

The window for colloids shown in Figure 3.2 is quite small. Colloid fluid has no indication if the preoperative Hb concentration is on the low side because the preoperative blood Hb concentration soon reaches the target Hb level and the crystalloid administration is still below the 3-liter limit, which assures a low incidence of adverse effects. The limit of 6 liters of crystalloid can be hit only when the preoperative Hb exceeds 130 g/l.

Figure 3.2 does not consider the effect of distribution on the hemodilution. As stated previously, the volume effect will be greater (and the hemodilution more pronounced) during the infusion and for 25–30 min thereafter than indicated here.

Volume equivalents between colloids and crystalloids

The potency of colloid and crystalloid fluids can be compared by using volume kinetics (for details, see Chapter 7, "Body volumes and fluid kinetics"). The situation during anesthesia and surgery is characterized by marked inhibition of the excretion of crystalloid fluid and, as always, a "boosting" effect on the plasma volume expansion caused by the distribution function during infusion and for 30 min after it has

ended. There is no evidence that the plasma volume expansion from colloid fluids differs between the anesthetized and the conscious state; however, exceptions are an exaggeration of the volume expansion just after anesthesia has been induced,[20] and the acceleration of the plasma volume decay that is due to inflammatory response and occurs late during lengthy surgery.

In the example shown in Figure 3.3, HES 130/0.4 (Voluven) has a potency of between 2.5 and 1.6 times that of Ringer's acetate depending on the phase in which we assess the difference. At the end of the 30-min infusion, starch has diluted the plasma 60% more than the same amount of Ringer's acetate.[48] The difference has increased to 150% at 30 min after the infusion has been turned off. If we assess the situation 60 min after the end of the infusion the difference has decreased to 100% (Figure 3.3B).

Colloid fluids are even more potent as compared with crystalloids in conscious subjects than they are during anesthesia and surgery, the reason being a larger central volume of distribution (4–5 liters, in contrast to 3 liters or less during anesthesia) and much faster excretion. The difference can be estimated at 3–4 times, which is twice as much as during anesthesia and surgery.

In the example in Figure 3.3, a correction for dose-dependent deposition of fluid crystalloid fluid in "non-functional spaces" was made. Such deposition more clearly affects the urine flow rate than the plasma volume expansion. Currently there is no evidence for hysteresis in the kinetics of the fluids within the limits simulated here, except that the plasma volume effect of Ringer's acetate is probably stronger than indicated owing to the low compliance for volume expansion in the interstitial fluid space.

References

1. Hedin A, Hahn RG. Volume expansion and plasma protein clearance during intravenous infusion of 5% albumin and autologous plasma. *Clin Sci* 2005; 106: 217–24.

2. Caironi P, Tognoni G, Masson S, *et al.* Albumin replacement in patients with severe sepsis or septic shock. *N J Engl Med* 2014; 370: 1412–21.

3. Fleck A, Raines G, Hawker F, *et al.* Increased vascular permeability: a major cause of hypoalbuminaemia in disease and injury. *Lancet* 1985; 325: 781–4.

4. Woodcock TE, Woodcock TM. Revised Starling equation and the glycocalyx model of transvascular fluid exchange: an improved paradigm for prescribing intravenous fluid therapy. *Br J Anaesth* 2012; 108: 384–94.

5. The SAFE Study Investigators. A comparison of albumin and saline for fluid resuscitation in the intensive care unit. *N Engl J Med* 2004; 350: 2247–56.

6. Guthrie RD, Hines C. Use of intravenous albumin in the critically ill patient. *Am J Gastroenterol* 1991; 86: 255–63.

7. Marik PE. The treatment of hypoalbuminemia in the critically ill patient. *Heart Lung* 1993; 22: 166–70.

8. Cochrane Injuries Group Albumin Reviewers. Human albumin administration in critically ill patients: systematic review of randomised trials. *BMJ* 1998; 317: 235–40.

9. Roberts I, Edwards P, McLelland B. More on albumin. Use of human albumin in UK fell substantially when systematic review was published (letter). *BMJ* 1999; 318: 1214–15.

10. Wilkes MM, Navickis RJ. Patient survival after human albumin administration. A meta-analysis of randomized, controlled trials. *Ann Intern Med* 2001; 135: 149–64.

11. The SAFE Study Investigators. Saline or albumin for fluid resuscitation in patients with traumatic brain injury. *N Engl J Med* 2007; 357: 874–84.

12. Rehm M, Haller M, Orth V, *et al.* Changes in blood volume and hematocrit during acute perioperative volume loading with 5% albumin or 6% hetastarch solutions in patients before radical hysterectomy. *Anesthesiology* 2001; 95: 849–56.

13. Jacob M, Chappell D, Rehm M. Clinical update: perioperative fluid management. *Lancet* 2007; 369: 1984–6.

14. Christensen P, Andersson J, Rasmussen SE, Andersen PK, Henneberg SW. Changes in circulating blood volume after infusion of hydroxyethyl starch 6% in critically ill patients. *Acta Anaesthesiol Scand* 2001; 45: 414–20.

15. Lehmann GB, Asskali F, Boll M, *et al.* HES 130/0.42 shows less alteration of pharmacokinetics than HES 200/0.5 when dosed repeatedly. *Br J Anaesth* 2007; 98: 635–44.

16. Voluven 6% hydroxyethyl starch 130/0.4 product monograph. Bad Homburg (Germany): Fresenius Kabi, 2007.

17. Hahn RG, Bergek C, Gebäck T, Zdolsek J. Interactions between the volume effects of hydroxyethyl starch 130/0.4 and Ringer's acetate. *Crit Care* 2013; 17: R104.

18. Awad S, Dharmavaram S, Wearn CS, Dube MG, Lobo DN. Effects of an intraoperative infusion of 4% succinylated gelatine (Gelofusine®) and 6% hydroxyethyl starch (Voluven®) on blood volume. *Br J Anaesth* 2012; 109: 168–76.

19. Zdolsek HJ, Vegfors M, Lindahl TL, *et al.* Hydroxyethyl starches and dextran during hip replacement surgery: effects on blood volume and coagulation. *Acta Anaesthesiol Scand* 2011; 55: 677–85.

20. Li Y, He R, Ying X, Hahn RG. Dehydration, haemodynamics and fluid volume optimization after induction of general anaesthesia. *Clinics* 2014; 69: 809–16.

21. James MF, Latoo MY, Mythen MG, *et al.* Plasma volume changes associated with two hydroxy ethyl starch colloids following acute hypovolaemia in volunteers. *Anaesthesia* 2004; 59: 738–42.

22. Ickx BE, Bepperling F, Melot C, Schulman C, van der Linden PJ. Plasma substitution effects of a new hydroxyethyl starch HES 130/0.4 compared with HES 200/0.5 during and after extended acute normovolaemic haemodilution. *Br J Anaesth* 2003; 91: 196–202.

23. Schortgen F, Lacherade LC, Bruneel F, *et al.* Effects of hydroxyethyl starch and gelatine on renal function in severe sepsis: a multicentre randomised study. *Lancet* 2001; 357: 911–16.

24. Brunkhorst FM, Engel C, Bloos F, *et al.* Intensive insulin therapy and pentastarch resuscitation in severe sepsis. *N Engl J Med* 2008; 358: 125–38.

25. Béchir M, Puhan MA, Neff SB, *et al.* Early fluid resuscitation with hyperoncotic hydroxyethyl starch 200/0.5 (10%) in severe burn injury. *Crit Care* 2010; 14: R123.

26. Perner A, Haase N, Guttormsen AB, *et al.* Hydroxyethyl starch 130/0.42 versus Ringer's acetate in severe sepsis. *N Engl J Med* 2012; 367: 124–34.

27. Myburgh JA, Finfer S, Bellomo R, *et al.* Hydroxyethyl starch or saline for fluid on intraoperative oliguria resuscitation in intensive care. *N Engl J Med* 2012; 367: 1901–11.

28. European Medicines Agency. Hydroxyethyl starch for infusion. http://www.ema.europa.eu/ Published on the Internet 06/03/2014.

29. Martin C, Jacob M, Vicaut E, *et al.* Effect of waxy maize-derived hydroxyethyl starch 130/0.4 on renal function in surgical patients. *Anesthesiology* 2013; 118: 387–94.

30. van der Linden P, James M, Mythen M, Weiskopf RB. Safety of modern starches used during surgery. *Anesth Analg* 2013; 116: 35–48.

31. Gilles MA, Habicher M, Jhanji S, *et al.* Incidence of postoperative death and acute kidney injury associated with i.v. 6% hydroxyethyl starch use: systematic review and meta-analysis. *Br J Anaesth* 2014; 112: 25–34.

32. Annane D, Siami S, Jaber S, *et al.* Effects of fluid resuscitation with colloids vs. crystalloids on mortality in critically ill patients presenting with hypovolemic shock: the CRISTAL randomized trial. *JAMA* 2013; 310: 1809–17.

33. Laxenaire MC, Charpentier C, Feldman L. Anaphylactoid reactions to colloid plasma substitutes: incidence risk factor mechanisms. A French multicenter prospective study. *Ann Fr Anesth Reanimat* 1994; 13: 301–10.

34. Hahn RG. Dextran70 and the blood loss during transurethral resection of the prostate. *Acta Anaesthesiol Scand* 1996; 40: 820–4.

35. Bulger EM, May S, Kerby J, *et al.* Out-of-hospital hypertonic resuscitation following traumatic hypovolemic shock: a randomized, placebo controlled trial. *Ann Surg* 2011; 253: 431–41.

36. Bulger EM, May S, Brasel KJ, *et al.* Out-of-hospital hypertonic resuscitation following severe traumatic brain injury: a randomized controlled trial. *JAMA* 2010; 304: 1455–64.

37. Drobin D, Hahn RG. Kinetics of isotonic and hypertonic plasma volume expanders. *Anesthesiology* 2002; 96: 1371–40.

38. Ljungström K-G. Safety of dextran in relation to other colloids – ten years experience with hapten inhibition. *Infusionsther Transfusionsmed* 1993; 20: 206–10.

39. Velanovich V. Crystalloid versus colloid fluid resuscitation: a meta-analysis of mortality. *Surgery* 1989; 105: 65–71.

40. Schierhout G, Roberts I. Fluid resuscitation with colloid or crystalloid solutions in critically ill patients: a systematic review of randomised trials. *BMJ* 1998; 316: 961–4.

41. Choi PT, Yip G, Quinonez LG, Cook DJ. Crystalloids vs. colloids in fluid resuscitation: a systematic review. *Crit Care Med* 1999; 27: 200–10.

42. Li Y, He R, Ying X, Hahn RG. Ringer's lactate, but not hydroxyethyl starch, prolongs the food intolerance time after major abdominal surgery; an open-labelled clinical trial. *BMC Anesthesiol* 2015; 15: 72.

43. Varadhan KK, Lobo DN. Symposium 3: A meta-analysis of randomised controlled trials of intravenous fluid therapy in major elective open abdominal surgery: getting the balance right. *Proc Nutr Soc* 2010; 69: 488–98.

44. Brandstrup B, Tonnesen H, Beier-Holgersen R, *et al.* Effects of intravenous fluid restriction on postoperative complications: comparison of two perioperative fluid regimens. A randomized assessor-blinded multicenter trial. *Ann Surg* 2003; 238: 641–8.

45. Arieff AI. Fatal postoperative pulmonary edema. Pathogenesis and literature review. *Chest* 1999; 115: 1371–7.

46. Hahn RG. Why crystalloids will do the job in the operating room. *Anaesthesiol Intensive Ther* 2014; 46: 342–9.

47. Bourke DL, Smith TC. Estimating allowable hemodilution. *Anesthesiology* 1974; 41: 609–12.

48. Ewaldsson C-A, Hahn RG. Kinetics and extravascular retention of acetated Ringer's solution during isoflurane and propofol anesthesia for thyroid surgery. *Anesthesiology* 2005; 103: 460–9.

49. Svensén C, Hahn RG. Volume kinetics of Ringer solution, dextran 70 and hypertonic saline in male volunteers. *Anesthesiology* 1997; 87: 204–12.

Chapter

4

Glucose solutions

Robert G. Hahn

Summary

Glucose 5% is given after surgery to prevent starvation and to provide free water for hydration of the intracellular fluid space. Glucose is sometimes infused before surgery as well, in particular when surgery is started late during the day, and, in some hospitals, also as a 2.5% solution during the surgical procedure. Glucose infusion has also been used together with insulin to improve outcome in cardiac surgery and in intensive care.

Because of the risk of hyperglycemia, intravenous glucose infusions need to be managed with knowledge, attention, and responsibility. Hyperglycemia promotes wound infection and osmotic diuresis, by which the kidneys lose control of the urine composition. The anesthetist has to consider a four-fold modification in infusion rate of glucose to account for the perioperative change in glucose tolerance. The suitable rate of infusion when a glucose infusion is initiated can be predicted by pharmacokinetic simulation. A control plasma sample taken one hour later shows whether the prediction was correct, and also that plasma glucose will only rise by another 25% if no adjustment of the infusion rate is made.

Glucose solution is contraindicated in acute stroke and not recommended in operations associated with a high risk of perioperative cerebral ischemia, such as carotid artery and cardiopulmonary bypass surgery. Subacute hyponatremia is a postoperative complication that is promoted by infusing >1 liter of plain 5% glucose in the perioperative setting.

Glucose (dextrose) solutions are used to administer calories to prevent starvation, and also to provide body water. They are the only available infusion fluids that add volume to both the extracellular fluid (ECF) and the intracellular fluid (ICF) volumes.

There is a two-fold purpose to infusing glucose solutions. The first is to prevent starvation, which aids wound healing, well-being, and recovery. The second purpose is to provide free water to hydrate the ICF. The endogenous production of water in humans is only 0.2 ml/kg per hour while the baseline fluid losses amount to at least 1 ml/kg per hour, half of which is due to evaporation and the other half to urinary excretion. Therefore, free water needs to be supplied to prevent dehydration. Glucose solutions are the mainstay of such treatment in debilitated patients who cannot be fed orally. However, glucose treatment in the perioperative period is a challenge to carry out well, owing to the risk of inducing hyperglycemia.

Pharmacokinetics

Infused glucose distributes rapidly over two-thirds of the ECF space. Elimination occurs by insulin-dependent uptake by the body cells. The half-life is approximately 15 min in healthy volunteers [1] but twice as long during laparoscopic cholecystectomy.[2] Elimination apparently occurs even more slowly in the presence of diabetes.

The *volume* component of isotonic glucose 2.5% with electrolytes and plain glucose 5% (the latter fluid is sometimes abbreviated to D5W) initially expands the plasma volume as effectively as acetated Ringer's solution.[1] The fact that glucose solutions have a relatively strong initial plasma volume-expanding effect is contrary to common belief, and one of the most widely spread misunderstandings about their behavior in the body. The fluids show no distribution phase if we assume that uptake of glucose to the cells brings along water in proportion to their osmotic strength. However, the infused fluid volume later redistributes throughout the total body water because the osmotic strength of glucose fades away when being incorporated into large glycogen molecules and ultimately metabolized.

Glucose 2.5% with electrolytes and plain glucose 5% are almost entirely eliminated within 2.5 hours in volunteers (which is faster than for Ringer's).[1] However, some of the volume component of glucose 5% might still reside in the ICF space at that time.

Glucose solutions of 10% and 20% are hypertonic and withdraw fluid from the ICF to the ECF by virtue of osmosis. This volume returns to the cells when the glucose is metabolized.

How to avoid hyperglycemia

Providing intravenous glucose always carries the risk of inducing hyperglycemia.[3,4] Plasma glucose >10 mmol/l increases the risk of postoperative infection,[5–7] and osmotic diuresis develops when plasma glucose is 12–15 mmol/l, which implies that the kidneys lose control of the fluid and electrolyte excretion. Moreover, more pronounced cerebral damage occurs in the event of cardiac arrest.[8,9] Therefore, the management of glucose infusions requires knowledge, attention, and responsibility.

Infusion rates that provide effective fluid and nutritional support therapy while avoiding hyperglycemia might be difficult to determine in the perioperative setting, as glucose turnover becomes impaired as part of the trauma response. The anesthetist has to consider a four-fold modification in infusion rate of glucose to account for the perioperative change in glucose tolerance.

Based on six studies of glucose kinetics, Figure 4.1 shows the plasma glucose concentrations that can be expected from various rates of infusion of glucose 5% before, during, and after surgery in relatively healthy non-diabetic subjects, standardized to a body weight of 70 kg.[2,10–14]. Anesthetists wishing to use this figure to find the optimal infusion rate for glucose 2.5% (which can be considered as first choice when starting an infusion) should simply double the indicated rates.

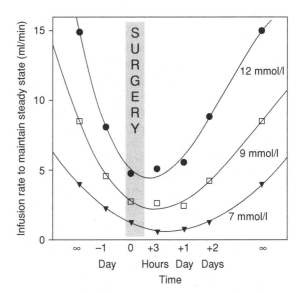

Figure 4.1 Plasma steady-state glucose concentrations (isobars) resulting from various rates of infusion of glucose 5% (y-axis) for various points in time during the perioperative period. The rates are standardized for a patient having a body weight of 70 kg. Computer simulation based on kinetic data from Refs. [2,10–14].

A practical question is at which point in time a control blood sample should be taken when a check for hyperglycemia is desired in an individual patient. The time at which the steady state level for plasma glucose is attained during a continuous infusion of glucose is determined by the half-life, which is usually between 30 and 40 min before, during, and after surgery. A useful approach would be to take a control sample after one hour, which roughly corresponds to two half-lives, and to consider that the plasma glucose will then increase by another 25% if no adjustment to the infusion rate is made.

Insulin resistance is the key mechanism for the slowing of glucose turnover one day after surgery.[15,16] When tested in the postoperative care unit, the mechanism for the impaired glucose tolerance is not insulin resistance, but an impaired insulin response to glucose stimulation.[14]

Clinical use

Glucose 5% is routinely given after surgery to provide free water for hydration of the ICF space and to prevent starvation. Glucose is sometimes infused before surgery as well, in particular when surgery is started late during the day, and, in some hospitals, also as a 2.5% solution during the surgical procedure.

In the perioperative period, infusing a glucose solution with little or no electrolyte content is the most logical way to provide free water to compensate for vaporization from airways and surgical wounds. The glucose component of the fluid is indicated in patients at risk of developing hypoglycemia, such as in diabetes, alcohol dependency, hepatomas, and pancreatic islet cell tumors. Certain drugs, such as propranolol, increase the risk of hypoglycemia.

There seems to be little reason to routinely administer glucose intraoperatively. In the vast majority of patients, hormonal changes associated with surgery raise the blood glucose level sufficiently (by stimulating glycogenolysis and gluconeogenesis) to maintain normoglycemia, or even to reach mild hyperglycemia. The stress response, in turn, makes it difficult for the body to adequately use exogenous glucose to limit gluconeogenesis and protein catabolism ("protein-sparing effect").

Another argument to refrain from glucose administration intraoperatively is that a very high glucose concentration worsens the *cerebral damage* that develops in association with cardiac arrest.[8,9] Therefore, glucose solution is contraindicated in acute stroke and not recommended in operations associated with a high risk of perioperative cerebral ischemia, such as carotid artery and cardiopulmonary bypass surgery.

Overall, shorter preoperative fasting and fast-track surgery with early postoperative mobilization have limited the use of intravenous glucose treatment in routine surgery.

Modifying the plasma glucose level by glucose infusions and insulin is a tool to reduce complications and improve survival in intensive care and after cardiac surgery.[17–19] Cardiac function may even be improved in patients undergoing cardiac surgery by infusing a solution containing glucose, insulin, and potassium.[20] These special treatments can only be performed if rigorous control of the blood glucose concentration is undertaken. Likewise, glucose infusions in diabetic patients should be monitored with frequent measurements of the blood glucose level.

In Europe, "carbohydrate loading" by mouth is sometimes performed in the evening and morning before abdominal operations. The treatment reduces thirst and hunger sensations and might improve the way the patient copes with hemorrhage. A proposed benefit is that carbohydrate loading reduces the surgery-induced insulin resistance,[21] but this has not been confirmed in more recent work.[14,15]

Electrolytes are often added to the glucose solutions used for maintenance fluid therapy during the postoperative phase. Many preparations already contain half the electrolyte content of a balanced Ringer's solution. In other cases, sodium and potassium are added based on measurements of the plasma concentrations of these ions.

Patients with postoperative complications impairing gastrointestinal function, who are not able to feed themselves or receive oral nutrition, should be given intravenous 5% glucose solution with electrolytes as maintenance therapy. If no improvement occurs within 7 days the glucose administration should be replaced with full parenteral nutrition containing protein, glucose, and lipids.

Dosing

The basic need for glucose in an adult corresponds to 4 liters of glucose 5% per 24 hours (800 kcal, 2.8 ml/min), which prevents straightforward starvation while not providing adequate nutrition. However, the amount administered to hospital patients is more often guided by the need for "free" body water, which is 2–3 liters per 24 hours. Although the commonly infused amount provides less glucose than the body utilizes, the glucose supplementation reduces muscle wasting.[3] This "nitrogen-sparing effect" of glucose is poorer in association with surgery owing to the accompanying physiological stress response.

The rate of glucose infusion should not increase plasma glucose concentrations above the *renal threshold*, which is 12–15 mmol/l. Higher levels induce *osmotic diuresis* in which water and electrolytes losses are poorly controlled. This limit is reached by infusing 1 liter of glucose 5% over 45 min in healthy volunteers.[1]

Because of the ease with which plasma glucose becomes elevated during surgery, most anesthetists prefer to use glucose 2.5% with electrolytes in the perioperative setting. During laparoscopic cholecystectomy 1.4 liters of glucose 2.5% with electrolytes over 60 min raised plasma glucose from normal to the renal threshold for osmotic diuresis (16 mmol/l).[2] The limitations set on the infusion rate owing to the risk of hyperglycemia make both glucose 2.5% and 5% unsuitable for use as plasma volume expanders.

Hypertonic glucose solutions (10% and 20%) must be monitored by measurements of the plasma glucose concentration and frequently need to be supplemented by exogenous insulin. These fluids are used for more ambitious supplementation of calories in postoperative care and also in the intensive care unit.[18]

Glucose metabolism yields CO_2, and the accompanying increased breathing might be a problem in debilitated patients with impaired lung function.

Electrolytes

When used for maintenance therapy, a glucose solution should provide the basic need of electrolytes. The NICE guideline recommends 1 mmol of sodium and 1 mmol of potassium per kilo body weight per 24 hours. The need varies, and it is common to guide the administration by measurements of the serum sodium and potassium concentrations 1–2 times daily.

An infusion containing potassium cannot be given at a high rate because of a risk of cardiac arrhythmias. This means that, in addition to the limitations of the infusion rate given by the risk of hyperglycemia, another risk factor has to be considered. A safe rate of administration is 10 mmol of potassium per hour, which can be increased to 20 mmol per hour if the electrocardiogram is monitored. Therefore, one liter of glucose with 40 mmol/l of sodium and potassium added cannot be infused during a shorter period of time than 4 hours. Owing to the dangers inherent in this therapy, the anesthetist should personally monitor the infusion or else let the fluid be administered via an infusion pump.

Potassium supplementation exceeding the content of a Ringer's solution is not advisable during the intraoperative period. The reason is that surgery always carries a risk of postoperative kidney failure, which can greatly raise serum potassium. The anesthetist should be aware of the trauma and surgery redistributes potassium to the ICF space owing to stimulation of the adrenergic beta-2-receptors. Hence, the plasma concentration is usually falsely low in the postoperative care unit. The hypokalemia resolves spontaneously within a few hours and should not lead to extreme measures to raise serum potassium, at least not as long as cardiac arrhythmias are absent.

Hyponatremia

Repeated infusion of electrolyte-free glucose solution (usually plain 5%) might induce *subacute hyponatremia*.[22,23] This complication usually develops 2–3 days after surgery and is characterized by neurological disturbances, nausea, and vomiting.[24] When symptoms appear, serum sodium is usually between 120 and 130 mmol/l (normal level 138–142 mmol/l).

Hyponatremia might cause permanent brain damage if left untreated. Menstruating women are most prone to develop such sequelae.[25] The surgery might be trivial but has often (at some stage) been complicated by sudden hypotension, which boosts the vasopressin concentration. Impaired renal function and liberal postoperative ingestion of soft juice drinks devoid of salt are other risk factors.[22,23]

Treatment in symptomatic patients consists of hypertonic saline, which should be monitored so as to increase serum sodium no faster than 1–2 mmol/l per hour. If hyponatremia has not appeared after surgery the development has probably been more gradual, and serum sodium in such *chronic hyponatremia* should be raised even more slowly, at 0.5 mmol/l per hour. The reason for the caution is that the brain gradually adapts to the lower osmolality, and damage might occur if the normal concentration is attained rapidly.

The risk of subacute hyponatremia is reduced by limiting the amount of plain glucose 5% to 1 liter only. All other glucose solutions should contain sodium.

Rebound hypoglycemia

Moderate hypoglycemia and hypovolemia are likely to develop 30 min after a glucose infusion has been stopped abruptly in subjects with a strong insulin response to glucose, or when glucose is infused together with insulin.[26] This complication is called "rebound hypoglycemia" and is an issue when, for example, parenteral nutrition is turned off. This complication might occur during minor surgery but is unlikely during extensive surgery owing to the insulin resistance.

This complication may also occur during labor. Glucose from the mother crosses the placenta and induces an insulin response in the fetus. At birth, a strong insulin effect remains in the newborn, whose capacity to increase endogenous glucose production is limited.[27] Dangerous hypoglycemia develops, which might result in convulsions and brain damage. The "rebound" effect can be avoided by infusing the glucose no faster than required to prevent starvation, which is 1 liter glucose 5% over 6 hours. A practical rule is to slow the rate of infusion of the glucose solution at the end of delivery.

The same critical situation for the newborn might develop if maternal volume loading is provided with glucose-containing fluid just before Cesarean section.[28]

Mannitol

Mannitol is an isomer of glucose that is not metabolized in the body but is eliminated by renal excretion. The molecule remains essentially in the ECF. The half-life is approximately 130 min but can be twice as long in the presence of impaired kidney function.[29]

The isotonic concentration of mannitol is the same as for 5% glucose, which is sometimes used as an irrigating solution in endoscopic surgery. The clinical use of mannitol for intravenous administration is restricted to a plain 10% or 20% solution (in some countries only 15%), which induces diuresis in failing, oliguric kidneys. The mechanism is that the renal excretion of mannitol occurs by virtue of osmotic diuresis, by which the body loses water.

The hypertonic nature of 15% mannitol has made it a means of acutely reducing the intracranial pressure in patients with head trauma. The volume used is then 500–750 ml, of which half is given as a bolus infusion. Despite a long history, mannitol treatment remains poorly evaluated in outcome studies. As the fluid contains no electrolytes, users should be aware the osmotic diuresis creates an absolute loss of sodium and other electrolytes from the body that may need to be replaced. If not, the ICF volume will increase in the aftermath of the treatment, which is a dreaded adverse effect unlikely to be shared by hypertonic saline.

The marked increase in ECF volume makes infusion of hypertonic mannitol contraindicated in congestive heart failure.

Like all hypertonic fluids, mannitol 15% should not be administered together with erythrocyte transfusions.

References

1. Sjöstrand F, Edsberg L, Hahn RG. Volume kinetics of glucose solutions given by intravenous infusion. *Br J Anaesth* 2001; 87: 834–43.

2. Sjöstrand F, Hahn RG. Volume kinetics of 2.5% glucose solution during laparoscopic cholecystectomy. *Br J Anaesth* 2004; 92: 485–92.

3. Sieber FE, Smith DS, Traystman RJ, Wollman H. Glucose: a reevaluation of its intraoperative use (review). *Anesthesiology* 1987; 67: 72–81.

4. Doze VA, White PF. Effects of fluid therapy on serum glucose levels in fasted outpatients. *Anesthesiology* 1987; 66: 223–6.

5. Hanazaki K, Maeda H, Okabayashi T. Relationship between perioperative glycemic control and postoperative infections. *World J Gastroenterol* 2009; 15: 4122–5.

6. Kwon S, Thompson R, Dellinger P, et al. Importance of perioperative glycemic control in general surgery: a report from the Surgical Care and Outcomes Assessment program. *Ann Surg* 2013; 257: 8–14.

7. Frisch A, Hudson M, Chandra P, et al. Prevalence and clinical outcome of hyperglycemia in the perioperative period in non-cardiac surgery. *Diabetes Care* 2010; 33: 1783–8.

8. Myers RE, Yamaguchi S. Nervous system effects of cardiac arrest in monkeys. *Arch Neurol* 1977; 34: 65–74.

9. Siemkowicz E. The effect of glucose upon restitution after transient cerebral ischemia: a summary. *Acta Neurol Scand* 1985; 71: 417–27.

10. Sjöstrand F, Hahn RG. Validation of volume kinetic analysis of glucose 2.5% solution given by intravenous infusion. *Br J Anaesth* 2003; 90: 600–7.

11. Hahn RG, Ljunggren S, Larsen F, Nyström T. A simple intravenous glucose tolerance test for assessment of insulin sensitivity. *Theor Biol Med Model* 2011; 8: 12.

12. Hahn RG, Nyström T, Ljunggren S. Plasma volume expansion from the intravenous glucose tolerance test before and after hip replacement surgery. *Theor Biol Med Model* 2013; 10: 48.

13. Strandberg P, Hahn RG. Volume kinetics of glucose 2.5% solution and insulin resistance after abdominal hysterectomy. *Br J Anaesth* 2005; 94: 30–8.

14. Ljunggren S, Hahn RG. Oral nutrition or water loading before hip replacement surgery; a randomized clinical trial. *Trials* 2012; 13: 97.

15. Ljungqvist O, Thorell A, Gutniak M, Häggmark T, Efendic S. Glucose infusion instead of preoperative fasting reduces postoperative insulin resistance. *J Am Coll Surg* 1994; 178: 329–36.

16. Ljunggren S, Hahn RG, Nyström T. Insulin sensitivity and beta-cell function after carbohydrate oral loading in hip replacement surgery: a double-blind, randomised controlled clinical trial. *Clin Nutr* 2014; 33: 392–8.

17. Svedjeholm, R, Håkanson, E, Vanhanen I. Rationale for metabolic support with amino acids and

glucose-insulin-potassium (GIK) in cardiac surgery. *Ann Thorac Surg* 1995; 59: S15–22.

18. Van der Berghe G, Wouters P, Weekers F, *et al.* Intensive insulin therapy in critically ill patients. *N Engl J Med* 2001; 345: 1359–67.

19. Lebowitz G, Raizman E, Brezis M, *et al.* Effects of moderate intensity glycemic control after cardiac surgery. *Ann Thorac Surg* 2010; 90: 1825–32.

20. Gradinac S, Coleman GM, Taegtmeyer H, Sweeney MS, Frazier OH. Improved cardiac function with glucose-insulin-potassium after aortocoronary bypass grafting. *Ann Thorac Surg* 1989; 48: 484–9.

21. Nygren J, Soop M, Thorell A, *et al.* Preoperative oral carbohydrate administration reduces postoperative insulin resistance. *Clin Nutr* 1998; 17: 65–71.

22. Chung HM, Kluge R, Schrier RH, Anderson RJ. Postoperative hyponatremia: a prospective study. *Arch Intern Med* 1986; 146: 333–6.

23. Häggström J, Hedlund M, Hahn RG. Subacute hyponatraemia after transurethral resection of the prostate. *Scand J Urol Nephrol* 2001; 35: 250–1.

24. Arieff AI. Hyponatremia, convulsions, respiratory arrest, and permanent brain damage after elective surgery in healthy women. *N Engl J Med* 1986; 314: 1529–35.

25. Ayus JC, Wheeler JM, Arieff AI. Postoperative hyponatremic encephalopathy in menstruant women. *Ann Intern Med* 1992; 117: 891–7.

26. Berndtson D, Olsson J, Hahn RG. Hypovolaemia after glucose-insulin infusions in volunteers. *Clin Sci* 2008; 115: 371–8.

27. Philipson EH, Kalham SC, Riha MM, Pimentel R. Effects of maternal glucose infusion on fetal acid–base status in human pregnancy. *Am J Obstet Gynecol* 1987; 157: 866–73.

28. Kenepp NB, Shelley WC, Gabbe SG, *et al.* Neonatal hazards of maternal hydration with 5% dextrose before caesarean section. *Lancet* 1982; 1: 1150–2.

29. Anderson P, Boréus L, Gordon E, *et al.* Use of mannitol during neurosurgery: interpatient variability in the plasma and CSF levels. *Eur J Clin Pharmacol* 1988; 35: 643–9.

Chapter

5

Hypertonic fluids

Eileen M. Bulger

Summary

Hypertonic fluids have an osmotic content that is higher than in the body fluids. When this content remains in the extracellular fluid space, such as with saline, the volume effect becomes very powerful owing to osmotic allocation of fluid from the intracellular to the extracellular fluid space. These fluids have also been found to favorably modulate the inflammatory response. The most studied preparations are saline 7.5% with and without a colloid (dextran or hydroxyethyl starch) added.

This chapter reviews the current clinical evidence regarding the use of hypertonic fluids for the early resuscitation of injured patients and for perioperative indications for a variety of procedures. While there is a wealth of preclinical data suggesting potential benefit from this resuscitation strategy, the clinical trial data have failed to show any clear benefit to the prehospital administration of these fluids in trauma patients, and the data for perioperative use is limited. More study is needed to define the best use of these fluids in a variety of patient populations and surgical procedures.*

Hypertonic fluids have been under investigation for the resuscitation of injured patients for over 30 years. Several studies have suggested that the use of these fluids is of potential benefit in the resuscitation of patients with hypovolemic shock and traumatic brain injury.[1–3] More recent studies, however, have failed to show a mortality benefit for early treatment in these patient cohorts.[4–6] In addition, there have been a

---

* First half of Summary added by the Editor.

number of reports describing the use of hypertonic fluids in the perioperative setting, including aortic surgery, cardiac surgery, transplant surgery, and spinal surgery.[7,8]

Hypertonic fluids include a wide spectrum of products with a range of hypertonic saline (HTS) solutions varying from 1.6% to 23.4% sodium chloride. In addition, HTS is also available coupled with a variety of colloid solutions including dextran 70 and hetastarch.

This review seeks to describe the mechanisms of action of hypertonic fluids that may offer benefits for acute resuscitation and perioperative management of patients undergoing major surgery, and to review the current clinical trial evidence in this regard.

Mechanism of action

Hypertonic fluids have several physiological and immunological effects that suggest potential benefit in management of severely injured patients. Because these agents have an osmotic effect, when administered intravenously they draw interstitial fluid into the intravascular space, thus restoring tissue perfusion in the setting of hypovolemic shock. This allows improvement in blood pressure with a smaller volume of fluid than traditional isotonic crystalloid solutions. Furthermore, several *in vitro* and animal studies suggest that these fluids reduce endothelial cell edema and enhance microcirculatory flow following hemorrhagic shock.

In addition to these physiological changes, a wide body of literature describes the significant impact of hypertonic solutions on the inflammatory response. Several animal studies have demonstrated that resuscitation with hypertonic solutions attenuates the activation of neutrophils after injury and reduces remote inflammatory lung injury. This effect appears to be due

---

Clinical Fluid Therapy in the Perioperative Setting, Second Edition, ed. Robert G. Hahn. Published by Cambridge University Press. © Cambridge University Press 2016.

to down-regulation of the adhesion molecule CD 11b and enhanced shedding of L-selectin.

These observations have also been made in humans receiving HTS early after severe injury.[9,10] Modulation of circulating monocyte function has also been described, which may down-regulate the production of pro-inflammatory cytokines and enhance production of anti-inflammatory cytokines such as interleukin (IL)-10. This suppression of the innate immune response appears to be transient and resolves once the serum osmolarity returns to normal. While the innate immune response appears to be inhibited, the cellular response, as manifested by changes in T-cell function, appears to be enhanced. Extensive work by Junger *et al.* has demonstrated that hypertonicity increases T-cell proliferation, enhances mitogen-stimulated IL-2 production, and rescues T-cells from suppressive cytokines.[11–13] Taken together, these studies suggest a potential role for hypertonic fluids in modulating the immunosuppressive response observed after severe injury or insult.

Finally, a large body of research has focused on the mechanism of action of hypertonic fluids to reduce cerebral edema and improve cerebral perfusion after brain injury. In addition to the obvious physiological effects, hypertonic fluids have been associated with improved cerebral vasoregulation resulting in reduced vasospasm, modulation of cerebral leukocytes, and inhibition of the sodium glutamate exchanger, leading to reduced extracellular accumulation of glutamate, which is neurotoxic.[14] These studies, coupled with animal models showing reduction of intracranial pressure (ICP) in brain-injured animals, have led to a number of clinical studies of these fluids for the management of patients with severe traumatic brain injury.

In summary, there is compelling preclinical scientific evidence that hypertonic fluids have physiological and anti-inflammatory effects that may prove beneficial for the management of a number of perioperative concerns including resuscitation of hypovolemic shock, management of traumatic brain injury, and management of ischemia and reperfusion injury such as occurs following cardiopulmonary bypass or transplant surgery. This has led to numerous clinical reports.

Clinical trial experience

Clinical studies of hypertonic solutions have largely been focused on three areas: early resuscitation of hemorrhagic shock in the prehospital or emergency department setting, management of increased ICP largely in the intensive care unit setting, and operative reports in a variety of major surgical interventions. Each of these areas is addressed separately.

Hemorrhagic shock

There have been 10 clinical trials of hypertonic fluids for the management of hemorrhagic shock following injury (Table 5.1). These studies were conducted in the prehospital or early hospital setting. It was hypothesized that the earlier the fluid is given after injury the more likely one would be to observe a significant effect. These studies used a 7.5% saline solution with or without the addition of 6% dextran 70. The early investigations were largely too small to demonstrate a definitive difference in outcome. However, meta-analysis of the studies conducted before 1997 suggested an overall survival benefit from HTS with dextran (HSD), with an odds ratio of 1.47 (95% confidence interval 1.04–2.08).[3]

These early studies led to the regulatory approval of HSD in several European countries, but did not afford approval by the US Food and Drug Administration. Two subsequent studies have been conducted. The first was a study by Bulger *et al.*, which focused on the impact of HSD on the development of acute respiratory distress syndrome (ARDS) in a blunt trauma population with evidence of hypovolemic shock.[15] This study closed after enrollment of 209 patients because of futility, with no overall difference in the rate of 28-day ARDS-free survival between the treatment groups.

A predefined subgroup analysis suggested a potential benefit in those patients at highest risk for ARDS as defined by the need for >10 units of blood transfusion in the first 24 hours. This led to a subsequent trial conducted by the Resuscitation Outcomes Consortium, a clinical trial network in the USA and Canada. This trial sought to enroll injured patients with more severe shock based on a prehospital systolic blood pressure of <70 mmHg or 70–90 mmHg with a heart rate >108 beats/min. This study was also closed before reaching its full proposed sample size after enrolling 895 patients randomized to either 7.5% saline (HS), HSD, or normal saline (NS). The results of this study show no difference in overall 28-day survival (HSD 74.5%, HS 73.0%, NS 74.4%, $p = 0.91$).[4]

In addition, there was a concern raised by the Data Safety Monitoring Board regarding a higher

Table 5.1 Human trials of hypertonic saline as a resuscitation fluid for hemorrhagic shock

Reference	Population	Design	n	Hypertonic fluid	Outcome
Holcroft et al. (1987) [36]	Prehospital trauma pts	Prospective, randomized	49	7.5% NaCl/6% dextran 70	Improved SBP and overall survival
Holcroft et al. (1989) [37]	Hypotensive trauma pts in ED (SBP < 80)	Prospective, randomized	32	7.5% NaCl/6% dextran 70	No difference in survival
Vassar et al. (1991) [38]	Prehospital trauma pts (SBP < 100)	Prospective, randomized	166	7.5% NaCl/6% dextran 70	Improved SBP and improved survival for pts with traumatic brain injury
Mattox et al. (1991) [39]	Prehospital trauma pts (SBP < 90) 72% penetrating	Prospective, randomized	359	7.5% NaCl/6% dextran 70	Improved SBP, trend toward improved survival
Younes et al. (1992) [40]	Hypovolemic shock in ED (SBP < 80)	Prospective, randomized	105	7.5% NaCl and 7.5% NaCl/6% dextran 70	Improved SBP, no difference in survival
Vassar et al. (1993a) [41]	Prehospital trauma pts (SBP < 90)	Prospective, randomized	258	7.5% NaCl and 7.5% NaCl/6% dextran 70	Improved survival vs. predicted historical controls
Vassar et al. (1993b) [42]	Prehospital trauma pts (SBP < 90)	Prospective, randomized	194	7.5% NaCl and 7.5% NaCl/6% dextran 70	Improved survival vs. historical controls and for pts with traumatic brain injury
Younes et al. (1997) [43]	Hypovolemic shock in ED	Prospective, randomized	212	7.5% NaCl/6% dextran 70	Improved survival for pts with SBP < 70
Bulger et al. (2008) [15]	Prehospital blunt trauma pts (SBP < 90)	Prospective, randomized	209	7.5%NaCl/6% dextran 70	No difference in ARDS-free survival
Bulger et al. (2011) [4]	Prehospital trauma pts (SBP < 70 or SBP 70–90, HR > 108)	Prospective, randomized	895	7.5% NaCl and 7.5% NaCl/6% dextran 70	No difference in 28-day mortality

ARDS, acute respiratory distress syndrome; ED, emergency department; HR, heart rate; pts, patients; SBP, systolic blood pressure.

mortality seen among the post-randomization subgroup of patients who did not receive any blood transfusions in the first 24 hours. Subsequent analysis suggested a higher proportion of early deaths: some patients in the hypertonic groups died before blood products became available or were administered. This difference was no longer evident 6 hours after injury. A subsequent systematic review of the safety data demonstrated that HSD administration delayed the administration of blood products by altering standard transfusion triggers, such as systolic blood pressure, with no effect on survival.[16] Thus, despite a large number of clinical trials in this patient population, there remains no compelling evidence to support the routine use of hypertonic fluids in the early management of these patients in the civilian (non-military) community.

Traumatic brain injury

There have been a number of studies examining the use of hypertonic fluids ranging in concentration from 1.6% to 23.4%, given as both bolus and continuous infusions for the management of patients with intracranial hypertension. Most of these studies are case series or descriptive studies, which describe improved ICP with the use of hypertonic fluids in patients who have been refractory to conventional therapy. There have been few randomized controlled trials.

The first trial, by Shackford et al., randomized patients to HTS vs. lactated Ringer's along with conventional therapies for increased ICP.[17] They were unable to demonstrate any major differences between the treatment groups but were hampered by the randomization of more severely injured patients into the HTS group.

Francony et al. compared equimolar doses of 20% mannitol and 7.45% HTS for management of patients with sustained elevations in ICP and found them to be equally effective.[18] Despite the lack of definitive data in this area, many neurosurgeons are now using HTS routinely for management of elevated ICP.

Three randomized controlled trials have specifically focused on the *prehospital administration* of HTS to patients with suspected traumatic brain injury. All of these studies utilized the Glasgow Outcome Score (GOS) as a measure of the long-term neurological outcome for these patients.

The first of these studies, by Cooper *et al.*, enrolled injured patients with a prehospital Glasgow Coma Scale (GCS) value <8 and systolic blood pressure <100 mmHg.[6] This trial, which compared 7.5% saline with normal saline, was closed for futility ($n =$ 229) with no difference in extended GOS between the treatment groups 6 months after injury. Because this study included patients who had both severe traumatic brain injury and shock, it was limited by a 50% mortality in the study cohort.

A second trial recently completed in Toronto, Canada was also closed with limitations in obtaining long-term outcome data.[19]

The largest trial in this patient population was recently completed by the Resuscitation Outcomes Consortium. The study was closed early for futility after enrolling 1,331 patients with no difference in the GOS at 6 months after injury.[5] Importantly, this trial enrolled patients with a GCS value <8 but no prehospital hypotension. Thus, like the hypovolemic shock studies, despite a large body of preclinical evidence supporting these resuscitation strategies, clinical trials have been unable to show convincing evidence of improved outcome.

Intraoperative and postoperative studies

A number of small studies have been reported regarding the use of hypertonic solutions in *operative cases*. Most of these have been conducted during either cardiac or aortic surgery. For patients undergoing cardiopulmonary bypass surgery, the most consistent finding has been a significant decrease in the positive fluid balance with the use of hypertonic fluids.[7] This finding was also noted in a recent Cochrane review of this literature.[8]

Many of these studies have also demonstrated improvement in *cardiac index* (CI) with hypertonic fluids, but the duration of this effect has been variable. Two studies noted improved CI up to 48 hours after surgery,[20,21] while others suggested a transient effect as short as 1–3 hours.[22,23] This variability may be due to variations in the dose of hypertonic fluids

used and additional fluid given. These studies have been too small to identify any significant improvement in outcome.

Nine studies have examined the use of hypertonic solutions during *aortic surgery*. Like the studies in cardiac surgery, these studies also supported a lower overall fluid requirement in patients receiving hypertonic fluids. Auler *et al.* reported a small case series ($n = 10$) describing the administration of HTS vs. isotonic saline at the time of removal of the aortic clamp.[24] These authors report improved physiological endpoints and lower overall volumes of fluid required in the patients given HTS.

In another study, Shackford *et al.* randomized 58 patients undergoing elective aortic reconstruction to lactated Ringer's vs. HTS (250 mEq sodium per liter) solution during operative repair.[25] The hypertonic group required on average half the amount of intraoperative fluid as the lactated Ringer's group but there was no difference in clinical outcomes.

The most recent study by Bruegger *et al.* ($n = 28$) compared HTS with hydroxyethyl starch in normal saline for administration during the period of aortic clamping and found no difference between the groups.[26] Several other studies have also shown improved hemodynamic parameters (for review, see Azoubel *et al.* [7]), but none were large enough to demonstrate improved outcome.

Other operative scenarios explored have included transplantation, elective hysterectomy, and spinal surgery. One case series has been reported describing the use of 7.5% saline for patients with fulminant hepatic failure and Grade IV encephalopathy while undergoing orthotopic liver transplant.[27] These authors compare these patients with historical controls, and suggest that patients receiving HTS had more favorable hemodynamics and improved ICP. Another study examined the immune effect of HTS administration for patients undergoing elective hysterectomy and did not find any significant changes.[28]

One recent study examined the use of 3% saline infusions (30 cc/hour) in trauma patients following damage control surgery with open abdomens.[29] This was not a randomized trial, but patients receiving the hypertonic fluids demonstrated a shorter time to abdominal wall closure and higher rates of primary fascial closure, suggesting better management of postoperative tissue edema.

A recent meta-analysis also explored the intraoperative use of hypertonic solutions for elective neurosurgical procedures. These authors suggest that HTS may be superior to mannitol for brain relaxation during tumor resection.[30] A recent review highlights the many limitations in interpreting this literature.[31]

Finally, a retrospective, case-controlled study compared outcomes for patients undergoing major spinal surgery who received intraoperative HTS with those that did not, and suggested an association with lower postoperative infection rates.[32] A few studies have also examined the role of preloading patients undergoing spinal anesthesia with hypertonic fluids.[33–35] These studies have had mixed results, with some demonstrating improved hemodynamic parameters while others did not. All of these studies are limited by very small sample size.

Conclusion

In conclusion, despite a wide body of supportive preclinical data suggesting that hypertonic fluids are associated with improved hemodynamic response, reduction in cerebral edema, reduced fluid requirements, and modulation of the inflammatory response, clinical trials have been disappointing in the lack of definitive improvement in overall patient outcome with this resuscitation strategy. In particular, studies of the intraoperative use of these fluids are very limited. Future studies need to focus carefully on selection of patients, and ensure a randomized, placebo-controlled design and adequate sample size to observe a meaningful difference in clinical outcome.

References

1. Wade CE, Kramer GC, Grady JJ, Fabian TC, Younes RN. Efficacy of hypertonic 7.5% saline and 6% dextran-70 in treating trauma: a meta-analysis of controlled clinical studies. *Surgery* 1997; 122: 609–16.

2. Wade C, Grady J, Kramer G. Efficacy of hypertonic saline dextran (HSD) in patients with traumatic hypotension: meta-analysis of individual patient data. *Acta Anaesthesiol Scand Suppl* 1997; 110: 77–9.

3. Wade CE, Grady JJ, Kramer GC, *et al.* Individual patient cohort analysis of the efficacy of hypertonic saline/dextran in patients with traumatic brain injury and hypotension. *J Trauma* 1997; 42(5 Suppl): S61–5.

4. Bulger EM, May S, Kerby JD, *et al.* Out-of-hospital hypertonic resuscitation after traumatic hypovolemic shock: a randomized, placebo controlled trial. *Ann Surg* 2011; 253: 431–41.

5. Bulger EM, May S, Brasel KJ, *et al.* Out-of-hospital hypertonic resuscitation following severe traumatic brain injury: a randomized controlled trial. *JAMA* 2010; 304: 1455–64.

6. Cooper DJ, Myles PS, McDermott FT, *et al.* Prehospital hypertonic saline resuscitation of patients with hypotension and severe traumatic brain injury: a randomized controlled trial. *JAMA* 2004; 291: 1350–7.

7. Azoubel G, Nascimento B, Ferri M, Rizoli S. Operating room use of hypertonic solutions: a clinical review. *Clinics* 2008; 63: 833–40.

8. McAlister V, Burns KE, Znajda T, Church B. Hypertonic saline for peri-operative fluid management. *Cochrane Database Syst Rev* 1: CD005576. doi:10.1002/14651858.CD005576.pub2.

9. Rizoli SB, Rhind SG, Shek PN, *et al.* The immunomodulatory effects of hypertonic saline resuscitation in patients sustaining traumatic hemorrhagic shock: a randomized, controlled, double-blinded trial. *Ann Surg* 2006; 243: 47–57.

10. Bulger EM, Cuschieri J, Warner K, Maier RV. Hypertonic resuscitation modulates the inflammatory response in patients with traumatic hemorrhagic shock. *Ann Surg* 2007; 245: 635–41.

11. Junger WG, Coimbra R, Liu FC, *et al.* Hypertonic saline resuscitation: a tool to modulate immune function in trauma patients? *Shock* 1997; 8: 235–41.

12. Junger WG, Rhind SG, Rizoli SB, *et al.* Prehospital hypertonic saline resuscitation attenuates the activation and promotes apoptosis of neutrophils in patients with severe traumatic brain injury. *Shock* 2013; 40: 366–74.

13. Junger WG, Rhind SG, Rizoli SB, *et al.* Resuscitation of traumatic hemorrhagic shock patients with hypertonic saline – without dextran – inhibits neutrophil and endothelial cell activation. *Shock* 2012; 38: 341–50.

14. Doyle JA, Davis DP, Hoyt DB. The use of hypertonic saline in the treatment of traumatic brain injury. *J Trauma* 2001; 50: 367–83.

15. Bulger EM, Jurkovich GJ, Nathens AB, *et al.* Hypertonic resuscitation of hypovolemic shock after blunt trauma: a randomized controlled trial. *Arch Surg* 2008; 143: 139–48.

16. Del Junco DJ, Bulger EM, Fox EE, *et al.* Collider bias in trauma comparative effectiveness research: the stratification blues for systematic reviews. *Injury* 2015; 46: 775–80.

17. Shackford SR, Bourguignon PR, Wald SL, *et al.* Hypertonic saline resuscitation of patients with head

injury: a prospective, randomized clinical trial. *J Trauma* 1998; 44: 50–8.

18. Francony G, Fauvage B, Falcon D, *et al.* Equimolar doses of mannitol and hypertonic saline in the treatment of increased intracranial pressure. *Crit Care Med* 2008; 36: 795–800.

19. Morrison LJ, Rizoli SB, Schwartz B, *et al.* The Toronto prehospital hypertonic resuscitation-head injury and multi organ dysfunction trial (TOPHR HIT) – methods and data collection tools. *Trials* 2009; 10: 105.

20. Bueno R, Resende AC, Melo R, Neto VA, Stolf NA. Effects of hypertonic saline-dextran solution in cardiac valve surgery with cardiopulmonary bypass. *Ann Thorac Surg* 2004; 77: 604–11.

21. Boldt J, Zickmann B, Ballesteros M, *et al.* Cardiorespiratory responses to hypertonic saline solution in cardiac operations. *Ann Thorac Surg* 1991; 51: 610–15.

22. Jarvela K, Kaukinen S. Hypertonic saline (7.5%) after coronary artery bypass grafting. *Eur J Anaesthesiol* 2001; 18: 100–7.

23. Sirieix D, Hongnat JM, Delayance S, *et al.* Comparison of the acute hemodynamic effects of hypertonic or colloid infusions immediately after mitral valve repair. *Crit Care Med* 1999; 27: 2159–65.

24. Auler JOJ, Pereira MH, Gomide-Amaral RV, *et al.* Hemodynamic effects of hypertonic sodium chloride during surgical treatment of aortic aneurysms. *Surgery* 1987; 101: 594–601.

25. Shackford SR, Sise MJ, Fridlund PH, *et al.* Hypertonic sodium lactate versus lactated ringer's solution for intravenous fluid therapy in operations on the abdominal aorta. *Surgery* 1983; 94(1): 41–51.

26. Bruegger D, Bauer A, Rehm M, *et al.* Effect of hypertonic saline dextran on acid–base balance in patients undergoing surgery of abdominal aortic aneurysm. *Crit Care Med* 2005; 33: 556–63.

27. Filho JA, Machado MA, Nani RS, *et al.* Hypertonic saline solution increases cerebral perfusion pressure during clinical orthotopic liver transplantation for fulminant hepatic failure: preliminary results. *Clinics* 2006; 61: 231–8.

28. Kolsen-Petersen JA, Nielsen JO, Tonnesen EM. Effect of hypertonic saline infusion on postoperative cellular immune function: a randomized controlled clinical trial. *Anesthesiology* 2004; 100: 1108–18.

29. Harvin JA, Mims MM, Duchesne JC, *et al.* Chasing 100%: the use of hypertonic saline to improve early, primary fascial closure after damage control laparotomy. *J Trauma Acute Care Surg* 2013; 74: 426–30.

30. Prabhakar H, Singh GP, Anand V, Kalaivani M. Mannitol versus hypertonic saline for brain relaxation in patients undergoing craniotomy. *Cochrane Database Syst Rev* 2014; 7: CD010026.

31. Thongrong C, Kong N, Govindarajan B, *et al.* Current purpose and practice of hypertonic saline in neurosurgery: a review of the literature. *World Neurosurg* 2014; 82: 1307–18.

32. Charalambous MP, Swoboda SM, Lipsett PA. Perioperative hypertonic saline may reduce postoperative infections and lower mortality rates. *Surg Infect (Larchmt)* 2008; 9: 67–74.

33. Jarvela K, Honkonen SE, Jarvela T, Koobi T, Kaukinen S. The comparison of hypertonic saline (7.5%) and normal saline (0.9%) for initial fluid administration before spinal anesthesia. *Anesth Analg* 2000; 91: 1461–5.

34. Jarvela K, Koobi T, Kauppinen P, Kaukinen S. Effects of hypertonic 75 mg/ml (7.5%) saline on extracellular water volume when used for preloading before spinal anaesthesia. *Acta Anaesthesiol Scand* 2001; 45: 776–81.

35. Durasnel P, Cresci L, Madougou M, *et al.* Practice of spinal anesthesia in a developing country: usefulness of vascular preloading with a 7.5% hypertonic saline solution. *Ann Fr Anesth Reanim* 1999; 18: 631–5.

36. Holcroft JW, Vassar MJ, Turner JE, Derlet RW, Kramer GC. 3% NaCl and 7.5% NaCl/dextran 70 in the resuscitation of severely injured patients. *Ann Surg* 1987; 206: 279–88.

37. Holcroft JW, Vassar MJ, Perry CA, Gannaway WL, Kramer GC. Use of a 7.5% NaCl/6% Dextran 70 solution in the resuscitation of injured patients in the emergency room. *Prog Clin Biol Res* 1989; 299: 331–8.

38. Vassar MJ, Perry CA, Gannaway WL, Holcroft JW. 7.5% sodium chloride/dextran for resuscitation of trauma patients undergoing helicopter transport. *Arch Surg* 1991; 126: 1065–72.

39. Mattox KL, Maningas PA, Moore EE, *et al.* Prehospital hypertonic saline/dextran infusion for post-traumatic hypotension. The U.S.A. Multicenter Trial. *Ann Surg* 1991; 213: 482–91.

40. Younes RN, Aun F, Accioly CQ, *et al.* Hypertonic solutions in the treatment of hypovolemic shock: a prospective, randomized study in patients admitted to the emergency room. *Surgery* 1992; 11: 380–5.

41. Vassar MJ, Perry CA, Holcroft JW. Prehospital resuscitation of hypotensive trauma patients with 7.5% NaCl versus 7.5% NaCl with added dextran: a controlled trial. *J Trauma* 1993a; 34: 622–32.

42. Vassar MJ, Fischer RP, O'Brien PE, *et al.* A multicenter trial for resuscitation of injured patients with 7.5%

sodium chloride. The effect of added dextran 70. The Multicenter Group for the Study of Hypertonic Saline in Trauma Patients. *Arch Surg* 1993b; 128: 1003–11.

43. Younes RN, Aun F, Ching CT, *et al*. Prognostic factors to predict outcome following the administration of hypertonic/hyperoncotic solution in hypovolemic patients. *Shock* 1997; 7: 79–83.

Chapter

6

Fluids or blood products?

Oliver Habler

Summary

Thanks to the impressive anemia tolerance of the human body, red blood cell (RBC) transfusion may often be avoided despite even important blood losses – provided that normovolemia is maintained. While a hemoglobin (Hb) concentration of 60–70 g/l can be considered safe in young, healthy patients, older patients with preexisting cardiopulmonary morbidity should be transfused at Hb 80–100 g/l. Physiological transfusion triggers (e.g. decrease of VO_2, ST-segment depression in the ECG, arrhythmia, continuous increase in catecholamine needs, echocardiographic wall motion disturbancies, lactacidosis) appearing prior to the aforementioned Hb concentrations necessitate immediate RBC transfusion. In the case of unexpected massive blood losses and/or logistic difficulties impeding an immediate start of transfusion, the anemia tolerance of the patient can be effectively increased by several measures (e.g. hyperoxic ventilation, muscular relaxation, or adequate depth of anesthesia).

In cases of dilutional coagulopathy – often reflected by an intraoperatively diffuse bleeding tendency – a differentiated coagulation therapy can either be directed on the basis of viscoelastic coagulation tests (e.g. thromboelastometry/-graphy) or directed empirically by replacing the different components in the order of their developing deficiency (i.e. starting with fibrinogen, followed by factors of the prothrombin complex and platelets). The "global" stabilization of coagulation with fresh frozen plasma requires the application of high volumes and bears the risk
of cardiac overload (TACO) and immunological alterations (TRIM).

The transfusion dilemma and the concept of "patient blood management" (PBM)

Although safer than ever, allogeneic transfusion is still associated with risks for the recipient and has been identified in numerous investigations as an "independent risk factor" for survival.[1–3] While the key problems, i.e. lethal incompatible transfusion and transfusion-associated infection, are well controlled today, transfusion-related immunomodulation (TRIM) – although not yet understood in detail – seems to be at least partly responsible for this increase in mortality. Via the pathomechanism of TRIM, allogeneic transfusion is implicated in an increased rate of nosocomial infections [4] and an increased recurrence rate after oncological surgery for malignancy.[5] Moreover, the costs for allogeneic blood products are expected to rise in the future [6] owing to an increasing imbalance between blood donors and potential recipients, particularly older patients undergoing major surgery.

To control both the risks and the increasing costs, allogeneic transfusion should be either avoided or at least minimized during surgical procedures. The precondition for this is "patient blood management" (PBM), including (1) the optimization of the patient's preoperative hematocrit (hct), (2) the perioperative collection and retransfusion of autologous blood, (3) the control of perioperative blood losses, and (4) the tolerance of low perioperative hemoglobin (Hb)

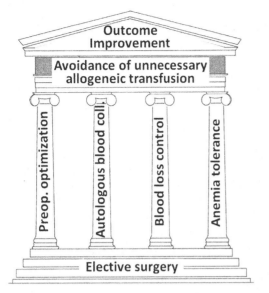

Figure 6.1 The four-column model of patient blood management (PBM) intended to avoid or minimize allogeneic transfusion in elective surgery, in order to improve the surgical patient's postoperative outcome.

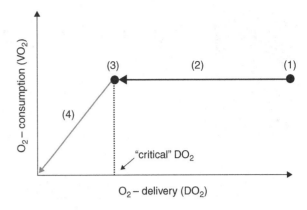

Figure 6.2 Schematic depicting the course of whole-body O_2 delivery (DO_2) and O_2 consumption (VO_2) during normovolemic hemodilution (e.g. replacement of intraoperative blood loss with red-blood-cell-free infusion solutions); modified according to [14]). The graphic has to be read from the right side (starting with normal DO_2) to the left (increasing dilutional anemia). Explanations in text.

concentrations (anemia tolerance, restrictive transfusion practice) (Figure 6.1).

Management of intraoperative blood losses

An acute surgical blood loss will not immediately be compensated by the transfusion of red blood cells (RBC) and/or plasma. More likely, the shed blood will initially be replaced by infusion of RBC-free crystalloid and/or colloid solutions. This procedure is intended to maintain a normal circulating intravascular volume (i.e. normovolemia); at the same time, the dilution of all circulating blood components (normovolemic hemodilution) is tolerated.

Tolerance of dilutional anemia

Under general anesthesia, "normovolemic hemodilution" is tolerated down to very low Hb concentrations and hct values, without any risk for tissue perfusion, tissue oxygenation, and organ function. This reflects the large natural anemia tolerance of the human body.

The physiological mechanisms enabling this anemia tolerance consist in:[7]

(1) the increase of cardiac output (CO) – initially via the increase of ventricular stroke volume and later via additional tachycardia – depending on the degree of hemodilution;

(2) the increase of total body oxygen (O_2) extraction;

(3) the physiological difference between macro- and microvascular (capillary) hct ("luxury hct"); the microvascular hct falls below its normal value only after a 30–50% reduction of the macrovascular hct;

(4) the physiological over-supply of organ tissues with O_2 ("luxury" O_2 delivery, DO_2). Under normal conditions, DO_2 exceeds tissue O_2 requirements by a factor of 3 to 4 (point (1) in Figure 6.2). Thus DO_2 can be reduced over a wide range without impairment of tissue oxygenation. Tissue O_2 demand is satisfied, and tissue O_2 consumption (VO_2) remains constant (so-called O_2 supply-independency of VO_2) (Figure 6.2, segment (2)).

The compensatory mechanisms described are decisive for the extent of anemia tolerance. Several studies show that these mechanisms likewise exist in infants,[8] children,[9,10] elderly patients,[11] patients with cardiopulmonary disease,[12] and patients under pharmacological beta-receptor blockade.[13]

Limits of the natural anemia tolerance: concept of the "critical DO$_2$" (DO$_{2crit}$)

At an extreme degree of hemodilution, O_2 demand will finally equal DO_2 (Figure 6.2, point (3)). The corresponding DO_2 is called "critical," DO_{2crit}. With

Table 6.1 The limit of anemia tolerance: overview of critical O_2 transport parameters (critical hemoglobin concentration, Hb_{crit}, and critical hematocrit, hct_{crit}) determined in different species during extreme normovolemic hemodilution

Author	Species	Anesthesia	FiO_2	Blood exchange fluid	Identification of DO_{2crit}	hct_{crit} (%)	Hb_{crit} (g/l)
Fontana et al. [10]	Man (child)	Isoflurane Sufentanil Vecuronium	1.0	Albumin	ST-segment depression		21
van Woerkens et al. [15]	Man (84 years)	Enflurane Fentanyl Pancuronium	0.4	Gelatin	Drop in VO_2	12	40
Zollinger et al. [47]	Man (58 years)	Propofol Fentanyl Pancuronium	1.0	Gelatin	ST-segment depression		~11
Cain [14]	Dog	Pentobarbital	0.21	Dextran	Drop in VO_2	98	33
Perez-de-Sá et al. [48]	Pig	Isoflurane Fentanyl Midazolam Vecuronium	0.5	Dextran	Drop in VO_2		23 ± 2
Meier et al. [16]	Pig	Propofol Fentanyl	0.21	HES	Drop in VO_2		31 ± 4
Pape et al. [49]	Pig	Propofol Fentanyl Pancuronium	0.21	HES	Drop in VO_2		24 ± 4
Kemming et al. [21]	Pig	Midazolam Morphine Pancuronium	0.21	HES	ST-segment depression	72 ± 12	26 ± 3
Meisner et al. [50]	Pig	Diazepam Morphine Pancuronium	0.21	Albumin	ST-segment depression	61 ± 18	20 ± 8
Meier et al. [51]	Pig	Propofol Fentanyl Pancuronium	0.21	HES	Drop in VO_2		24 ± 5

HES: hydroxyethylstarch.

ongoing hemodilution, DO_2 falls below DO_{2crit}, and the amount of O_2 delivered to the tissues becomes insufficient to meet their O_2 demand. As a consequence, the previously stable VO_2 starts to decline (so-called O_2 supply-dependency of VO_2) (Figure 6.2, segment (4)) [14]. This sudden decrease of VO_2 indirectly reflects the limit of anemia tolerance and the onset of tissue hypoxia. The energy needs of the body are now mainly met by anerobic glycolysis, and the serum lactate concentration therefore starts to rise. In analogy to DO_{2crit} the Hb and hct values corresponding to the inflection point of VO_2 are called Hb_{crit} and hct_{crit}, respectively. Without treatment (transfusion, hyperoxic ventilation) the persistence of the critical DO_2, Hb, or hct leads to death within a short period of time.[15,16]

The whole body's anemia tolerance may assume impressive proportions: in healthy awake volunteers, DO_{2crit} was not met even after hemodilution to Hb 48 g/l.[17] In healthy anesthetized animals and patients, the limit of dilutional anemia was reported at hct values between 12% and 3% (Hb 33 and 11 g/l) (Table 6.1). Infants (1–7 months) [8] and children (12.5 years) [10] tolerated Hb of 30 g/l and lower without falling below their DO_{2crit}. In pregnant sheep, fetal tissue oxygenation was preserved down to a maternal hct of 15% (Hb 50 g/l).[18]

Unfortunately, it is impossible to provide clinicians with universal numerical values for the aforementioned critical O_2 transport parameters. DO_{2crit}, Hb_{crit}, and hct_{crit} vary in and between individuals and depend on a variety of determining factors: adequate depth of anesthesia, hyperoxemia, muscular relaxation, and mild hypothermia increase anemia tolerance (see below); hypovolemia, restricted coronary reserve, heart failure, profound anesthesia, multiple trauma, and sepsis reduce anemia tolerance.

Moreover, it cannot be excluded that single organs will meet their DO_{2crit} at a higher Hb (hct) than the whole organism and develop tissue hypoxia prior to the drop of global VO_2. This would challenge whole-body global VO_2 as a global monitoring parameter for tissue oxygenation.

In anesthetized subjects, the anemia tolerance of the whole body and the brain,[19] the myocardium with intact coronary perfusion,[20,21] or the splanchnic system [19] have been found to be equal. Kidney and skeletal muscle seem to have a lower anemia tolerance.[22] The situation is also different for the compromised heart with restricted coronary reserve. In anesthetized dogs with an experimental 50–80% coronary artery stenosis, signs of myocardial ischemia and/or functional deterioration appeared at Hb 70–100 g/l.[23] In a retrospective cohort-analysis of cardiac risk patients undergoing non-cardiac surgery and refusing allogeneic transfusion for religious reasons (affiliation to Jehovah's Witnesses), a significantly higher 30-day mortality was found if the postoperative Hb fell below 80 g/l.[24] In otherwise healthy anesthetized rats, the limit of renal anemia tolerance was identified between Hb 4 and 70 g/l,[25] and in patients undergoing cardiac surgery at Hb between 70 and 80 g/l.[26,27]

In clinical practice it is difficult to identify the limit of the individual anemia tolerance of a single patient. Continuous measurement of VO_2 is technologically complex, costly, and therefore restricted to scientific questions. Indirect clinical signs reflecting DO_{2crit}, such as ECG changes (ST-segment deviation, arrhythmia), echocardiographic regional myocardial wall motion disturbance, lactacidosis and a decrease of mixed-venous or central-venous O_2 saturation, are uncertain.

Support in estimating the significance of perioperative dilutional anemia quoad vitam is provided with the results of large clinical studies (generally performed on Jehovah's Witnesses) investigating the relation between postoperative anemia and mortality. Until a postoperative Hb of 80 g/l no statistical relation between anemia and mortality could be detected even in older patients with pre-existing cardiopulmonary disease [24,28,29] and intensive care patients

with multiple morbidity.[1,30,31] In anemic patients (Hb < 80 g/l) whose death was causally related to anemia, the Hb was always found to be below 50 g/l.[32] At Hb 30 g/l, mortality has been shown to increase up to 50% without transfusion.[33] Nevertheless, in individual cases much lower Hb (15 g/l and lower) has been survived without transfusion.

Therapeutic increase of anemia tolerance

In cases of unexpected massive blood losses and/or logistic difficulties impeding an immediate start of transfusion, the anemia tolerance of the patient can be effectively increased by the following measures:[34]

(1) *Restoration and/or maintenance of normovolemia:* the basic prerequisite for the effective compensation of dilutional anemia is normovolemia. In "*hypo*volemic hemodilution" the whole body's O_2 demand increases, mediated by catecholamines. Under hypovolemic conditions, DO_{2crit} is met at higher values than under normovolemia, and anemia tolerance is reduced.

(2) *Myocardial function:* another basic prerequisite for optimal cardiac compensation of dilutional anemia is the increase of myocardial blood flow (MBF) realized by maximal coronary dilation as well as by the maintenance of adequate coronary perfusion pressure (CPP). Situations accompanied by an increase in myocardial O_2 demand (tachycardia, increased ventricular wall tension, increased myocardial contractility) must be avoided. The same applies for a decrease in diastolic aortic pressure due to reduction of systemic vascular resistance. Continuous application of noradrenaline increases whole-body anemia tolerance. Sympathicolysis via beta-receptor blockade or thoracic epidural anesthesia leaves anemia tolerance unaffected.[35]

(3) *Inspiratory oxygen fraction (FiO₂):* ventilation with supranormal FiO_2 (hyperoxic ventilation) increases the physically dissolved part of arterial O_2 content. Physically dissolved plasma O_2 is biologically highly available and covers up to 75% of whole-body O_2 demand in conditions of extreme dilutional anemia. Experimental and clinical studies clearly demonstrate that

hyperoxic ventilation effectively increases anemia tolerance and creates an important margin of safety for global, myocardial, gastrointestinal, and cerebral tissue oxygenation.

(4) *Muscular relaxation:* striated skeletal muscles amount to about 30% of the total body mass. Muscular relaxation significantly reduces the whole body's O_2 demand and increases anemia tolerance.

(5) *Body temperature:* hypothermia reduces the whole body's O_2 demand. In an animal experiment, anesthetized hypothermic pigs died at lower Hb than normothermic control animals. Owing to the negative impact of hypothermia on coagulation, however, the intentional induction of hypothermia in bleeding patients in order to increase anemia tolerance cannot be recommended.

(6) *Choice of anesthetic drugs and depth of anesthesia:* almost all anesthetic drugs investigated suppress the CO response to dilutional anemia. In animal experiments, a dose-related reduction in anemia tolerance could be demonstrated for halothane, enflurane, isoflurane, ketamine, propofol, etomidate, and pentobarbital. Inadequately profound anesthesia has to be avoided to the same extent as too light anesthesia (increased sympathetic tone and O_2 consumption).

(7) *Choice of the infusion solution:* the choice of the solution infused to compensate blood losses seems to influence anemia tolerance. While 3% gelatin and 6% hydroxyethyl starch (HES) 200.000/0.5 did not affect anemia tolerance in animals, an advantage could be demonstrated for 6% HES 130.000/0.4 over 3.5% gelatin, 6% HES 450.000/0.7, and Ringer's lactate. Application of infusion solutions with intrinsic O_2 transport capacity (artificial O_2 carriers based on human or bovine Hb; perfluorocarbons) increased anemia tolerance in animals and patients.[36] Unfortunately, no artificial O_2 carrier is approved in the United States or Europe.

Coagulation management

In analogy to dilutional anemia, the replacement of blood losses with crystalloid and/or colloid infusion solutions causes dilution of all components of the coagulatory and fibrinolytic system. This finally results in "dilutional coagulopathy."

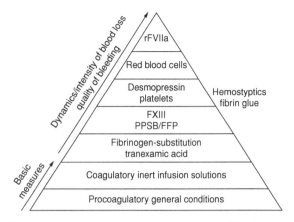

Figure 6.3 Graduated scheme ("coagulation pyramid") for the stabilization of coagulation in cases of major blood loss. The time sequence of therapeutic interventions beyond the basic measures is based on the intensity and dynamics of blood losses and on the quality of bleeding.

It has been demonstrated in animal experiments and in human patients that the first procoagulatory factor to decrease below a level requiring substitution is fibrinogen (i.e. <1.5 g/l), followed by the activity of coagulation factors of the prothrombin complex, and finally the platelet count.[37,38] Fibrinogen and fibrin are essential for clot formation at the site of the vessel damage. The lack of fibrinogen results in the formation of unstable clots that are unable to resist blood flow and to stop bleeding.[39] In addition, plasma fibrinogen concentration is reduced by infusion of HES-based colloidal infusion solutions.[40] Because of problems related to its processing, fresh frozen plasma (FFP) contains coagulation factors at a reduced concentration. This means that FFP has to be infused in large quantities to stabilize or improve coagulation, often resulting in transfusion-related cardiac overload (TACO). The infusion of small amounts of FFP to improve coagulation has to be considered meaningless.[41]

In the situation of the massively bleeding patient, it is difficult or even impossible to monitor and detect the "critical" reduction of the different components of the coagulation system. Moderate dynamics of blood losses allow differentiated coagulation management on the basis of results obtained from viscoelastic coagulation tests (thromboelastometry/-graphy),[42] but the lack of this analytic measure and/or the presence of more severe blood losses require "empirical" coagulation management based on the intensity and dynamics of the blood loss and the quality of bleeding

Table 6.2 Dosage of procoagulatory drugs in massive blood loss

Fresh frozen plasma (FFP)	>30 ml/kg BW Target: quick value (prothrombin time, PT) >40%; increased observation recommended in range 30–40%
Fibrinogen concentrate	25–50 mg/kg BW; 2–4 g; Target: plasma fibrinogen concentration >2 g/l; increased observation recommended in range 1.5–2 g/l
Prothrombin complex concentrate (PCC)	20–25 IU/kg BW Target: quick value (PT) >40% Increased observation recommended in range 30–40%
Tranexamic acid	Initial bolus 10–20 mg/kg BW Followed by 1–5 mg/kg BW per hour
Desmopressin	0.3 µg/kg BW over 30 min
Factor XIII concentrate	10–20 IU/kg BW
Recombinant human factor VIIa	90 µg/kg BW

("diffuse" bleeding tendency, rebleeding of formerly "dry" wounds).

After the establishment of procoagulatory general conditions (e.g. normothermia, normal pH) the following measures are taken, following a graduated scheme (Figure 6.3): the early and calculated administration of fibrinogen concentrate, prothrombin complex concentrate (PCC), vitamin-K-dependent coagulation factor concentrate (PPSB), FFP, and antifibrinolytic drugs (e.g. tranexamic acid).[43] The administration of desmopressin [44] mobilizes stocks of factor VIII, increases the activity of von Willebrand factor, and stimulates aggregatory platelet function. Clot stability may be additionally increased by application of factor XIII concentrate.[45] In cases of massive bleeding, the early administration of recombinant human factor VIIa ("off-label use") may be considered [46] (Table 6.2). However, the maximum effectiveness of this substance depends on stable general conditions for coagulation, in particular normothermia, normal pH, and adequate platelet count.

References

1. Vincent JL, Baron J-F, Reinhart K, *et al.* Anemia and blood transfusion in critically ill patients. *JAMA* 2002; 288: 1499–507.

2. Corwin HL, Gettinger A, Pearl RG, *et al.* The CRIT study: anemia and blood transfusion in the critically ill – current clinical practice in the United States. *Crit Care Med* 2004; 32: 39–52.

3. Hopewell S, Omar O, Hyde C, *et al.* A systematic review of the effect of red blood cell transfusion on mortality: evidence from large-scale observational studies published between 2006 and 2010. *BMJ Open* 2013; 3: e002154.

4. Marik PE, Corwin HL. Efficacy of red blood cell transfusion in the critically ill: a systematic review of the literature. *Crit Care Med* 2008; 36: 2667–74.

5. Cata JP, Wang H, Gottumukkala V, *et al.* Inflammatory response, immunosuppression, and cancer recurrence after perioperative blood transfusion. *Br J Anesth* 2013; 110: 690–701.

6. Shander A, Goodnough LT. Why an alternative to blood transfusion? *Crit Care Clin* 2009; 25: 261–77.

7. Habler O, Messmer K. The physiology of oxygen transport. *Transfus Sci* 1997; 18: 425–35.

8. Schaller RT, Schaller J, Furman EB. The advantages of hemodilution anesthesia for major liver resection in children. *J Pediatr Surg* 1984; 19: 705–10.

9. Aly Hassan A, Lochbuehler H, Frey L, Messmer K. Global tissue oxygenation during normovolemic hemodilution in young children. *Paediatr Anaesth* 1997; 7: 197–204.

10. Fontana JL, Welborn L, Mongan PD, *et al.* Oxygen consumption and cardiovascular function in children during profound intraoperative normovolemic hemodilution. *Anesth Analg* 1995; 80: 219–25.

11. Spahn DR, Zollinger A, Schlumpf RB, *et al.* Hemodilution tolerance in elderly patients without known cardiac disease. *Anesth Analg* 1996; 82: 681–6.

12. Licker M, Ellenberger C, Sierra C, *et al.* Cardiovascular response to acute normovolemic hemodilution in patients with coronary artery disease: assessment with transoesophageal echocardiography. *Crit Care Med* 2005; 33: 591–7.

13. Spahn DR, Schmid ER, Seifert B, Pasch T. Hemodilution tolerance in patients with coronary artery disease who are receiving chronic beta-adrenergic blocker therapy. *Anesth Analg* 1996; 82: 687–94.

14. Cain SM. Oxygen delivery and uptake in dogs during anemic and hypoxic hypoxia. *J Appl Physiol* 1977; 42: 228–34.

15. van Woerkens ECSM, Trouwborst A, Van Lanschot JJB. Profound hemodilution: what is the critical level of hemodilution at which oxygen delivery-dependent oxygen consumption starts in an anesthetized human? *Anesth Analg* 1992; 75: 818–21.

16. Meier J, Kemming GI, Kisch-Wedel H, *et al.* Hyperoxic ventilation reduces 6-hour mortality at the critical hemoglobin concentration. *Anesthesiology* 2004; 100: 70–6.

17. Lieberman JA, Weiskopf RB, Kelley SD, *et al*. Critical oxygen delivery in conscious humans is less than 7.3 ml $O_2 \times kg^{-1} \times min^{-1}$. *Anesthesiology* 2000; 92: 407–13.

18. Paulone ME, Edelstone DI, Shedd A. Effects of maternal anemia on uteroplacental and fetal oxidative metabolism in sheep. *Am J Obstet Gynecol* 1987; 156: 230–7.

19. van Bommel J, Trouwborst A, Schwarte L, *et al*. Intestinal and cerebral oxygenation during severe isovolemic hemodilution and subsequent hyperoxic ventilation in a pig model. *Anesthesiology* 2002; 97: 660–70.

20. Habler OP, Kleen M, Hutter J, *et al*. IV perflubron emulsion versus autologous transfusion in severe normovolemic anemia: effects on left ventricular perfusion and function. *Res Exp Med* 1998; 197: 301–18.

21. Kemming GI, Meisner FG, Kleen M, *et al*. Hyperoxic ventilation at the critical hematocrit. *Resuscitation* 2003; 56: 289–97.

22. Lauscher P, Kertscho H, Schmidt O, *et al*. Determination of organ-specific anemia tolerance. *Crit Care Med* 2013; 41: 1037–45.

23. Levy PS, Kim SJ, Eckel PK, *et al*. Limit to cardiac compensation during acute normovolemic hemodilution: influence of coronary stenosis. *Am J Physiol* 1993; 265: H340–9.

24. Carson JL, Duff A, Poses RM, *et al*. Effect of anemia and cardiovascular disease on surgical mortality and morbidity. *Lancet* 1996; 348: 1055–60.

25. Johannes T, Mik EG, Nohe B, *et al*. Acute decrease in renal microvascular pO_2 during acute normovolemic hemodilution. *Am J Physiol Renal Physiol* 2007; 292: F796–803.

26. Habib RH, Zacharias A, Schwann TA, *et al*. Role of hemodilutional anemia and transfusion during cardiopulmonary bypass in renal injury after coronary revascularization: implications on operative outcome. *Crit Care Med* 2005; 33: 1749–56.

27. Ranucci M, Romitti F, Isgro G, *et al*. Oxygen delivery during cardiopulmonary bypass and acute renal failure after coronary operations. *Ann Thorac Surg* 2005; 80: 2213–20.

28. Carson JL, Duff A, Berlin JA, *et al*. Perioperative blood transfusion and postoperative mortality. *JAMA* 1998; 279: 199–205.

29. Carson JL, Terrin ML, Noveck H, *et al*. Liberal or restrictive transfusion in high risk patients after hip surgery. *N Engl J Med* 2011; 29: 2453–62.

30. Hebert PC, Wells G, Blajchman MA, *et al*. A multicenter, randomized, controlled clinical trial of transfusion requirements in critical care. *N Engl J Med* 1999; 340: 409–17.

31. Carson JL, Noveck H, Berlin JA, Gould SA. Mortality and morbidity in patients with very low postoperative Hb levels who decline blood transfusion. *Transfusion* 2002; 42: 812–18.

32. Viele MK, Weiskopf RB. What can we learn about the need for transfusion from patients who refuse blood? The experience with Jehovah's Witnesses. *Transfusion* 1994; 34: 396–401.

33. Shander A, Javidroozi M, Naqvi S, *et al*. An update on mortality and morbidity in patients with very low postoperative hemoglobin levels who decline blood transfusion. *Transfusion* 2014; 54: 2688–95.

34. Habler O, Meier J, Pape A, *et al*. Perioperative anemia tolerance – mechanisms, influencing factors, limits. *Anaesthesist* 2006; 55: 1142–56.

35. Pape A, Weber CF, Laout M, *et al*. Thoracic epidural anesthesia with ropivacain does not compromise the tolerance of acute normovolemic anemia in pigs. *Anesthesiology* 2014; 121: 765–72.

36. Habler O, Pape A, Meier J, Zwißler B. Artificial oxygen carriers as an alternative to red blood cell transfusion. *Anaesthesist* 2005; 54: 741–54.

37. McLoughlin TM, Fontana JL, Alving B, *et al*. Profound normovolemic hemodilution: hemostatic effects in patients and in a porcine model. *Anesth Analg* 1996; 83: 459–65.

38. Hiippala ST, Myllylä GJ, Vahtera EM. Hemostatic factors and replacement of major blood loss with plasma-poor red cell concentrates. *Anesth Analg* 1995; 81: 360–5.

39. Fries D, Velik-Salchner C, Lindner K, Innerhofer P. Management of coagulation after multiple trauma. *Anaesthesist* 2005; 54: 137–44.

40. De Lorenzo C, Calatzis A, Welsch U, Heindl B. Fibrinogen concentrate reverses dilutional coagulopathy induced *in vitro* by saline but not by hydroxyethyl starch 6%. *Anesth Analg* 2006; 102: 1194–200.

41. Abdel-Wahab OI, Healy B, Dzik WH. Effect of fresh-frozen plasma transfusion on prothrombin time and bleeding in patients with mild coagulation abnormalities. *Transfusion* 2006; 46: 1279–85.

42. Grashey R, Mathonia P, Mutschler W, Heindl B. Perioperative coagulation management controlled by thrombelastography. *Unfallchirurg* 2007; 110: 259–63.

43. Kozek-Langenecker SA, Afshari A, Albaladejo P, *et al*. Management of severe perioperative bleeding. Guidelines from the European Society of Anesthesiology. *Eur J Anaesthesiol* 2013; 30: 270–82.

44. Franchini M. The use of desmopressin as a hemostatic agent: a concise review. *Am J Hematol* 2007; 82: 731–5.

45. Gödje O, Gallmeier U, Schelian M, *et al.* Coagulation factor XIII reduces postoperative bleeding after coronary surgery with extracorporeal circulation. *Thorac Cardiovasc Surg* 2006; 54: 26–33.

46. Franchini M, Franchi M, Bergamini V, *et al.* A critical review on the use of recombinant factor VIIa in life-threatening obstetric postpartum hemorrhage. *Semin Thromb Hemost* 2008; 34: 104–12.

47. Zollinger A, Hager P, Singer T, *et al.* Extreme hemodilution due to massive blood loss in tumor surgery. *Anesthesiology* 1997; 87: 985–7.

48. Perez-de-Sá V, Roscher R, Cunha-Goncalves D, *et al.* Mild hypothermia has minimal effects on the tolerance to severe progressive normovolemic anemia in swine. *Anesthesiology* 2002; 97: 1189–97.

49. Pape A, Meier J, Kertscho H, *et al.* Hyperoxic ventilation increases the tolerance of acute normovolemic anemia in anesthetized pigs. *Crit Care Med* 2006; 34: 1475–82.

50. Meisner FG, Kemming GI, Habler OP, *et al.* Diaspirin crosslinked hemoglobin enables extreme hemodilution beyond the critical hematocrit. *Crit Care Med* 2001; 29: 829–38.

51. Meier J, Pape A, Loniewska D, *et al.* Norepinephrine increases tolerance to acute anemia. *Crit Care Med* 2007; 35: 1484–92.

Chapter

7

Body volumes and fluid kinetics

Robert G. Hahn

Summary

Body fluid volumes can be measured and estimated by using different methods. A key approach is to use a tracer by which the volume of distribution of an injected substance is measured. Useful tracers occupy a specific body fluid space only. Examples are radioactive albumin (plasma volume), iohexol (extracellular fluid space), and deuterium (total body water). The transit time from the site of injection to the site of elimination must be considered when using tracers with a rapid elimination, such as the indocyanine green dye. The volume effect of an infusion fluid can be calculated by applying a tracer method before and after the administration.

Guiding estimates of the sizes of the body volumes can be obtained by bioimpedance measurements and anthropometric equations.

The blood hemoglobin (Hb) concentration is a frequently used endogenous tracer of changes in blood volume. Hb is the inverse of the blood water concentration, and changes in Hb indicate the volume of distribution of the infused fluid volume. Certain assumptions have to be made to convert the Hb dilution to a change in blood volume. Volume kinetics is based on mathematical modeling of Hb changes over time which, together with measurements of the urinary excretion, can be used to analyze and simulate the distribution and elimination of infusion fluids.

Infusion fluids exert their therapeutic effects primarily by expanding one of the three body fluid compartments (spaces), namely the *plasma volume* and the *interstitial* and *intracellular* fluid (ICF) volumes. The

sum of the plasma and interstitial fluid volumes is called the *extracellular fluid* (ECF) volume (Figure 7.1).

The sizes of these body fluid volumes have been measured under steady state conditions by the use of *tracer methods*. In an adult weighing 75 kg, they average 3 liters for the plasma, 12 liters for the interstitial fluid, and 30 liters for the ICF volume. Hence, the sum of the plasma and interstitial fluid volumes (the ECF volume) amounts to 15 liters, or 20% of the body weight.

Measures and estimates of body fluid volumes are of interest to basic research, while clinical guidance for fluid therapy is mostly guided by hemodynamic measurements, sometimes combined with fluid bolus infusions.

Tracers

Substances known to distribute solely within one body fluid compartment can be injected and the size of the compartment can be calculated by means of dilution of the substance.

The substance is then used as a tracer. The basic equation for such calculations is:

$$\text{Size of compartment} = \frac{\text{Injected dose of tracer}}{\text{Plasma concentration of tracer}}$$

Examples of such tracers include bromide and iohexol for measurements of the ECF volume. Radioiodated albumin and indocyanine green (ICG) are used for measurement of the plasma volume.

Bromide has a very slow turnover, which means that the measurement might be problematic to repeat several times. Iohexol has a shorter half-life, only 100 min, but this also implies that an estimation of the ECF volume has to be based on several plasma

Clinical Fluid Therapy in the Perioperative Setting, Second Edition, ed. Robert G. Hahn. Published by Cambridge University Press. © Cambridge University Press 2016.

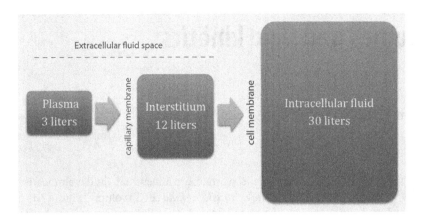

Figure 7.1 Schematic drawing of our three body fluid compartments.

samples to account for the elimination during the period of mixing. Sampling cannot start within 30–40 min because the kinetics shows a clear distribution phase.[1]

The *total body water* (sum of ECF and ICF) can be measured with water isotopes, which include tritium (radioactive) and deuterium (not radioactive). One problem is that even distribution of these molecules in the body requires about 3 hours to be completed. An alternative approach is to use ethanol, but the relatively short half-life requires frequent sampling in blood or in the expired air.[2]

The *plasma volume* has frequently been measured by radioactive iodated albumin. After 10 min of distribution of the injected substance, 3–4 samples are taken every 10 min to account for the exponential elimination. As the time window for the measurement is 30 to 40 min, the plasma volume needs to be in a reasonably steady state during that time to yield a correct result.

Plasma tracer results slightly overestimate the plasma volume. Therefore, the result should be multiplied by 0.91 (the "hematocrit factor").

Evans blue is a dye that has been used as a substitute for the albumin method because the measurement does not involve exposure to radioactivity. The dye binds to albumin, just like iodine, and the concentration is measured by light absorption.

There are several possibilities for labeling erythrocytes with radioactive tracers to calculate red cell mass. Such tracers include chromium and technetium.

Carbon monoxide binds to hemoglobin and can also be used to measure red cell mass. Drawbacks are mainly safety issues, as carbon monoxide is toxic.

The size of the interstitial fluid space and the ICF volume cannot be measured by tracers. They have to be inferred as the difference between body fluid spaces that can be measured, i.e. the plasma volume, the ECF volume, and the total body water.

These conventional tracer methods of measuring body fluid volumes have limited application in perioperative medicine. A comparison with standard values would indicate whether the patient is dehydrated or hyperhydrated before or after an operation. However, conventional tracers cannot be used to reflect what happens during surgery because the situation is too unstable. During the mixing period there must be steady state with regard to fluid shifts, a situation that is hardly ever met in the operating room. It is unlikely that the results can be accurate in the early postoperative period. The only possible exception to this rule could be the ICG tracer because steady state is then needed only for a few minutes.

If applied during steady state conditions, the tracer methods have an accuracy of between 1% (total body water) and 10% (radioiodinated albumin).

A common way to determine the volume effect of an infusion fluid in the experimental setting is to measure the plasma volume at baseline and then again after an infusion fluid has been administered. With crystalloid fluid there is no meaningful way of measuring the volume effect with a tracer until equilibration with the interstitial fluid has occurred, because the fluid shifts are so fast. There is equilibrium 30 min after ending an infusion.

Indocyanine green

Indocyanine green (ICG) is a dye that binds to plasma albumin. The half-life is only 3 min, owing to rapid uptake by the liver. The rate of elimination is directly dependent on the liver blood flow. Therefore, ICG can be used to measure both liver blood flow (elimination

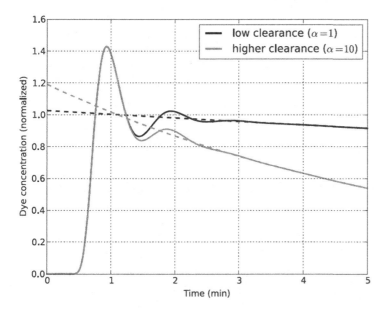

Figure 7.2 Why errors arise when back-extrapolation of the concentration–time curve of indocyanine green (ICG) overlooks the 1-min transit time for the dye to travel from the site of injection (time zero) to reach the site of elimination in the liver. α is the slope of the line. From Polidori and Rowley [6].

slope) and plasma volume. Attempts have also been made to measure cardiac output with ICG.

To measure the plasma volume, steady state with regard to the fluid balance is required for only a few minutes.[3] Therefore, the ICG method can be applied during surgery.[4] The ICG concentration can be measured both in the blood and by pulse oximetry (pulse dye densitometry).[5] The precision is claimed to be a few percent.

Drawbacks include that the circulation time (about 1 min in normal humans) becomes crucial. ICG is best injected via a central venous catheter, and backward extrapolation should be made to 1 min and not to time zero, as elimination begins only after the tracer has reached the liver. Polidori and Rowley [6] have shown that extrapolation to time zero results in an underestimation of the true plasma volume in the normal human (Figure 7.2). In a cohort of patients they found the average error to be 25%. When comparing the plasma volume before and after volume expansion, the calculations will further be dependent on a constant relationship between changes in the liver blood flow and the time required for transport of the ICG to the liver.

Double-tracer techniques

Measurement of the blood volume (BV) by a double-tracer technique means that the erythrocyte and plasma volumes are determined by separate tracer methods and that the BV is the sum of them. Various combinations of tracers can be used, of which tagging of the erythrocytes with chromium and determination of the plasma volume with radioactive albumin or ICG are the most common.

A problem with all double-tracer techniques is that the hematocrit in sampled peripheral blood is higher than the hematocrit deduced from direct measurement of the plasma and erythrocyte volumes. To account for this discrepancy, a correction factor ("hematocrit factor") of 0.91 has been introduced. This factor appears to be quite stable under various physiological circumstances [7] but has been given a number of different interpretations over the years.

In the 1950s and 1960s it was believed that the hematocrit in large vessels simply was higher than in the body as a whole. The hematocrit is lower in the capillaries, but the BV residing in them (5% of total) is too small to explain the hematocrit factor. A simplistic explanation is that that albumin but not the erythrocytes easily enters the liver sinusoids and some other perivascular spaces, which slightly exaggerates the plasma volume when measured by plasma-bound tracers.

A recent view was that only ICG but not erythrocytes and albumin penetrates the non-circulating plasma bound in the endothelial surface layer.[4] This is not a full explanation either, because the hematocrit factor is present also when measuring the plasma volume with the radioactive albumin method, where the tracer (albumin) is excluded from the endothelial surface.

Bioimpedance

In bioimpedance (BIA) measurements, a series of weak electrical currents of different frequency are passed through the body, typically running from the arm to the foot.[8] Use of the method for measuring body fluid volumes is based on the fact that currents have more difficulty passing through large amounts of water than small. An estimate of both the ICF and ECF volumes can be made as various frequencies pass through and outside cells with varying ease.

Bioimpedance is often applied while the patient is in bed before and after surgery, but rarely perioperatively owing to the risk of mechanical and electrical interference. In the author's experience, BIA can provide useful data only for groups and has a place mainly as an adjunct to more precise methods.

Anthropometry

Empirical relationships may be used to estimate the size of the body fluid compartments at baseline.

The simplest of these states that the plasma volume corresponds to 4.5% of the body weight, the BV is 7% of the body weight, and the ECF volume makes up 20% of the body weight.[1] Total body water represents 50% of the body weight in the adult female. The percentage is 60% in young adult men and 50% in older men. Children have a higher percentage. Such rules are simple but useful for the clinician to remember.

More precise information can be obtained by *regression equations*. These are typically based on tracer measurements of body fluid volumes performed in a large number of humans, and usually employ the sex, body weight, and height of the subject as predictors. Below is an example of such equations for estimation of the BV in women and men.[9]

$$\text{BV (liters, female)} = 0.03308 \text{ weight (kg)} \\ + 0.3561 \text{ height}^3\text{(m)} + 0.1833$$

$$\text{BV (liters, male)} = 0.03219 \text{ weight (kg)} \\ + 0.3669 \text{ height}^3\text{(m)} + 0.6041$$

Sodium method

The distribution of infused fluid between the ICF and ECF may be estimated based on the use of serum sodium (SNa) as the marker. Sodium is then used as an endogenous tracer.

If all infused fluid and sodium, as well as all voided amounts, are known, the change in ICF volume can be estimated based on the assumption that sodium is evenly distributed in the ECF volume, which makes up 20% of the body weight. From time 0 to time t, we get:

$$\Delta \text{ICF} = \text{ECF} + (\text{infused} - \text{voided}) \text{ volume} \\ - \frac{(\text{SNa} \times \text{ECF} - (\text{added} - \text{voided}) \text{ Na})}{\text{SNa}(t)}$$

This *mass balance equation* has mostly been used to calculate the intracellular distribution of electrolyte-free irrigating fluids,[10] but it can be used to estimate the intracellular distribution of any infusion fluid.[11] For example, the sodium method was used to demonstrate that acetated Ringer's solution does not expand the ICF volume in volunteers, despite the fact that the fluid is slightly hypo-osmolar; the reason is that the urine excreted during the first 30 min after the infusions contained much lower concentrations of sodium than the infused fluid, while there was only a marginal concomitant increase in SNa.[12]

Translocation of fluid from the ICF space when infusing hypertonic saline can also be estimated without measuring SNa. This calculation is then based on the osmolar balance between the ECF and ICF spaces, of which one space gradually becomes expanded and the other concentrated as more fluid is infused.[13]

Central blood volume

Measurement of the *intrathoracic* or *central BV* is possible with several modern hemodynamic monitoring systems, such as the PiCCO and LiDCO. These apparatuses are used mainly to measure central flow rates and blood pressures, while the central BV is provided as an adjunct output. A central venous pressure line or arterial catheterization is needed to obtain the data on body fluid volumes.

Measurement of the central BV is of interest because it is more clearly related to hypovolemia-related physiological responses than to total circulating BV. However, little has been published on intrathoracic BV in connection with infusion fluids.

Fluid "efficiency"

The *volume effect* of an infusion fluid implies how much of the infused volume is retained in the bloodstream and expands the BV. The strength and the duration of BV expansion are the properties that represent the *efficiency* of the fluid. One may also talk about *potency* when comparing the efficiency of various fluids.

For this purpose, physiological endpoints may be used. For example, a certain amount of blood can be withdrawn and the amount of fluid then required to restore baseline physiological parameters (such as cardiac output) can be taken to represent the "efficiency".[14]

Tracer methods (mostly radioiodinated albumin) have also been used to determine the efficiency of infusion fluids. This implies that the tracer method is applied twice and that the result before and after the infusion is compared. Assessment of colloid fluids is likely to work well by this approach. Studying the volume effect of crystalloids is more difficult because changes are more rapid; there is both a distribution phase, which cannot be covered by exogenous tracers, and, at least in conscious humans, a fairly rapid elimination. Most data relying on tracers refer to the period when distribution has already been completed and voiding has eliminated more than a negligible fraction of the infused crystalloid fluid volume.

Blood hemoglobin

A third and more simplistic approach to quantify the volume effect of an infusion fluid is to measure the blood hemoglobin (Hb) concentration before and after the infusion. Hemoglobin can be used as an endogenous tracer as it remains completely in the bloodstream, and it is reasonable to assume that dilution of its concentration is due to the infused fluid volume.

The use of Hb to calculate the efficiency of an infusion fluid is a frequently misunderstood method. Hemodilution is not a measure of the BV. In fact, Hb changes will be the same regardless of whether the BV is 1, 2, or 5 liters, as long as the number of Hb molecules within that volume remains unchanged. Hb changes are rather the inverse of the water concentration and indicate the volume amount of the infused water that is easily exchangeable with the water in the sampled (usually venous) blood. The water concentration of whole blood is about 80% and almost all the rest is Hb (about 1 kg); electrolytes and plasma proteins constitute only a few percent of the total. The water concentration is always increased when a plasma volume expander is infused because the main constituent

of an infused fluid is water. The dilution of Hb is a much easier way to indicate the increase in water concentration than to desiccate blood samples to determine the water concentration, but the two methods yield the same result.[15]

The potential error that can arise is when the hemodilution is interpreted in terms of a change in BV and the hemodilution is then multiplied by the BV at baseline. Radio-albumin, Evans blue, and carbon monoxide may be used to measure BV before an infusion is provided. More frequently, one assumes the BV before the infusion based on some anthropometric equation.

The Hb concentration is measured before (Hb) and after (Hb(t)) the infusion:[16]

$$\Delta BV = BV(Hb/Hb(t)) - BV$$

The amount of fluid retained in the blood is then given by:

$$Fluid\ retained\ (\%) = 100 \times \Delta BV/infused\ volume$$

The fraction of fluid retained over time is the *efficiency*.

If the urinary output is known, the difference between the infused volume and the sum of the urine and blood volumes represents the change in interstitial fluid volume.[17]

Accounting for blood loss

The Hb dilution concept can be developed to account for blood loss, if known. This is (usually) necessary when calculating fluid shifts based on Hb during surgery. One then calculates the total Hb mass and subsequently subtracts all losses (or adds transfused erythrocytes):

$$Hb\ mass = BV \times Hb$$
$$BV(t) = \frac{Hb\ mass - loss\ of\ Hb\ mass}{Hb(t)}$$
$$\Delta BV(t) = BV(t) - BV$$

These simple equations can be entered into a pocket calculator and may be helpful for the clinician when assessing whether a patient is hypervolemic or hypovolemic. The calculations can be applied repeatedly during surgery without loss of accuracy.[18]

These basic relationships shown above can, in turn, be further elaborated upon to quantify the efficiency of infusion fluids during ongoing surgery. An approach of that kind uses a multiple regression equation to separate the effects of various factors that influence the BV.

$$\Delta BV(t) = A \times (\text{infused fluid volume})$$
$$- B \times (\text{blood loss})$$

Data may be entered for an entire operation or for shorter periods of time. For example, this approach was used to show that acetated Ringer's solution expands the BV by as much as 60% of the infused amount during transurethral resection of the prostate performed under general anesthesia.[19] The deviation from the expected 20–25% can be explained by the fact that the measurements were performed every 10 min, whereas the 20–25% efficacy refers to complete distribution of the crystalloid fluid, which takes around 30 min.

The Hb method may be more difficult to apply in animals than in humans because several species (such as sheep and dogs) have reservoirs of erythrocytes in the spleen that are mobilized in stressful situations, including hemorrhage. In humans, such recruitment is very small.[20]

Volume kinetics

Drug regimens are commonly based on pharmacokinetic analysis. For this purpose, the Hb mathematics presented above has been elaborated upon to create a pharmacokinetic system for the analysis and simulation of the distribution and elimination of infusion fluids.[21] Serial analyses of the Hb concentration in whole blood are then recalculated to give the dilution of the plasma resulting from an infusion, the reason being that it is the plasma rather than whole blood that equilibrates with other body fluids.

From baseline at time 0 to time t, the dilution of the plasma can be expressed as:

$$\text{Plasma dilution}(t) = \frac{\left(\dfrac{\text{Hb} - \text{Hb}(t)}{\text{Hb}(t)} \right)}{(1 - \text{hematocrit})}$$

The plasma dilution data are then fitted to the solutions of differential equations describing the situation in a kinetic model that describes (reasonably well) what happens in the body (Figure 7.3). The distribution of fluid between a *central* and a *peripheral* compartment (V_c and V_t, respectively) is proportional to the difference in dilution between them multiplied by the intercompartment clearance, Cl_d. *Elimination* occurs from the V_c and is proportional to the plasma

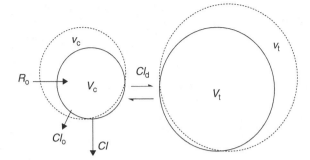

Figure 7.3 Schematic drawing of the two-compartment volume kinetic model that is applicable for analysis of the distribution and elimination of crystalloid infusion fluids during anesthesia and surgery. Note the expandable walls. Cl, elimination clearance; Cl_d, intercompartment clearance; Cl_o, baseline fluid loss; R_o, infusion rate; v_c, volume expanded state of central compartment; V_c, central compartment; v_t, volume-expanded state of peripheral compartment; V_t, peripheral compartment.

dilution multiplied by the elimination clearance, Cl. When distribution is completed, the continued elimination reverses the direction of the flow from the V_t to V_c, which is a process called *redistribution*. If urinary excretion is measured, the excreted volume divided by the area under the curve of the plasma dilution gives renal clearance. Accumulation of fluid in the body is given by the difference between Cl and renal clearance. A complete volume kinetic analysis yields five parameters: the sizes of V_c and V_t along with three clearances (the intercompartmental clearance, elimination clearance, and renal clearance).

The kinetic analysis can also use *micro-constants*, by which uneven flow to and from the interstitial fluid compartment can be studied. A micro-constant and the half-life are inversely related to each other. A benefit of this approach, which has still been used only sparingly, is that a full simulation of the distribution of fluid in the body can be performed using only three micro-constants. The sizes of the body fluid spaces between which the fluid distributes do not have to be assumed or measured.

The parameters in the models are estimated by a mathematical procedure called nonlinear-least squares regression. This minimizes the difference between the experimental concentration–time data and theoretical values generated by a computer. When the parameters in the kinetic model have been estimated, the effect of various infusion regimens on the body fluid compartments can be predicted and compared by computer simulation.

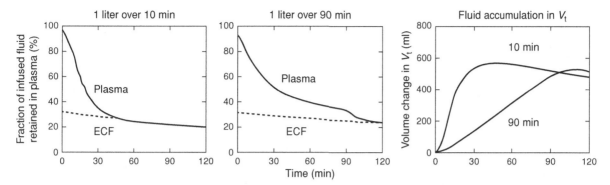

Figure 7.4 The effectiveness of Ringer's solution as a plasma volume expander is greater when given slowly. Computer simulation based on volume kinetic data from thyroid surgery,[11] showing how much of the infusion that resides in the plasma when 1 liter of Ringer's acetate is infused over 10 min (left) and 90 min (middle). The hatched lower line shows the theoretical percentage of the infused fluid that would remain in the plasma if all fluid had immediately been distributed over the ECF space. Right panel: the expansion of the interstitial fluid space. Note the slow elimination of infused Ringer's during surgery.

The working process is very similar to drug pharmacokinetics, albeit there are certain differences with regard to underlying assumptions. One difference is that drugs do not expand their volume of distribution, while infusion fluids exert their most important therapeutic effect by doing just that.

The body fluid spaces expanded by infused fluid are called "functional" as they may not correspond exactly to the physiological plasma volume and interstitial fluid volumes. Studies performed in volunteers provide data in which crystalloid fluid infused at a rate of about 30 ml/min expands a V_c that correlates closely with the expected size of the plasma volume. The size of the central space is 4–5 liters when the rate of infusion is higher, which suggests that the infused water volume easily equilibrates with body water that resides outside the plasma volume (presumably perivascular spaces). As stated previously, exchange with the V_t (presumably the interstitial fluid space) requires 25–30 min to be completed. The size of V_t space is usually only twice as large as V_c, and consequently smaller than the interstitial fluid space as measured with tracers. This difference might be explained by the fact that volume kinetics only measures the size of spaces that can be expanded, which is not the case for all parts of the ECF.

Volunteer studies

More than 50 studies of volume kinetics have been performed.[21]

Key findings show that distribution of *crystalloid fluids*, such as the Ringer's solutions, results in a 50–75% larger plasma dilution during an infusion of crystalloid fluid than would be expected if distribution had been immediate. It is often claimed that only 20–25% of the fluids expand the plasma volume, but these figures are valid only some 25–30 min after the infusion has been turned off.

The distribution effect of crystalloid fluid means that its efficiency is much better during an actual infusion than after it is completed. The efficiency of the fluid is also much better, and the peripheral edema less pronounced, if Ringer's solution is infused slowly (Figure 7.4).

Comparisons between infusion fluids in volunteers have been made to quantify their relative efficiency to expand the plasma volume over time. This can be made both by an area method and by computer simulation to a target dilution.[15] This conclusion is not specific for infusion fluids but applies to all drugs with exponential elimination (which is almost all drugs).

Acetated and lactated Ringer's have a potency of 0.9 compared with the reference, which was normal saline. This difference is due to the slower elimination of normal saline as compared with Ringer's. Hypertonic (7.5%) saline is four times more potent, and hypertonic saline in 6% dextran 70 is seven times more potent, than normal saline.[13]

Repeated infusions of crystalloid fluid are followed by a slightly higher Cl. In contrast, hemorrhage of up to

Table 7.1 The half-life ($T_{1/2}$) of the buffered Ringer's solutions after infusing the fluid (usually 25 ml/kg) over 30 min in the conscious and anesthetized state

Fluid	Subjects	Subjects	Median $T_{1/2}$ (min)	Ref.
Ringer's acetate				
	Volunteers	20	23	31
	Volunteers	10	27	32
	Volunteers	8	40	15
	Volunteers	10	46	22
	Dehydrated volunteers	20	76	31
	Thyroid surgery; isoflurane	15	327	11
	Thyroid surgery; TIVA	14	345	11
	Laparoscopic cholecystectomy	12	268	24
Ringer's lactate				
	4 hours after laparoscopy	20	17	33
	Gynecological laparoscopy	20	346	34

TIVA, total intravenous anesthesia.

900 ml reduces *Cl* by 50% although the blood pressure is unchanged.[22]

Colloid fluids differ from crystalloids in that they lack a marked distribution phase. The kinetics then becomes quite simple. The infused fluid only occupies one body fluid space, which has a size fairly similar to the expected plasma volume, from which elimination occurs according to a mono-exponential function.

Anesthesia and surgery

Anesthesia and surgery exert several effects on the distribution and elimination of crystalloid fluids. The anesthesia-induced reduction of the arterial pressure makes the distribution clearance (Cl_d) drop by approximately 50% during the onset of spinal, epidural, and general anesthesia,[23] which increases the plasma volume expansion resulting from an ongoing infusion. Cl_d is even expected to become zero in response to a constant reduction of the mean arterial pressure to 80% of baseline, which means that all infused fluid remains in the bloodstream.[21] The distribution clearance normalizes later, when a new Starling equilibrium has been reached, and this occurs after perhaps 30 min (depending on the rate of infusion). However, the anesthesia-related reduction in arterial pressure still promotes additional fluid accumulation in the plasma volume, owing to a persistent reduction of *Cl*.

The most significant finding during surgery is that the renal clearance is very low, which has been found during several types of surgery (Table 7.1).[11,24]

One can expect that only 10–20% of a volume load would be excreted within 2 hours during surgery, while this fraction is 50–80% in conscious subjects. Hormonal changes, such as aldosterone release, are probably responsible for much of this reduction, half of which can be seen also during experimental anesthesia.[25] Vasodilatation caused by the anesthetic drugs may also play a role by lowering the baseline for the Hb concentration.

Low renal clearance increases the plasma volume expansion in response to crystalloid fluid, and acts to retain infused fluid during surgery (Figure 7.5). Hence, it is a delicate balance to provide the patient with an optimal dose of crystalloid fluid, as the normal mechanisms for elimination of excess fluid operate poorly. Low renal clearance also implies that monitoring of the urine flow can only indicate hypovolemia but not hypervolemia.

It is unknown whether colloid fluid is excreted more slowly during anesthesia and surgery as compared with the unstressed conscious state. However, the intravascular persistence of colloid fluid is clearly decreased in the postoperative phase of major surgery, owing to the trauma-related inflammatory response.

"Non-functional" fluid spaces

Volume kinetic studies performed in the perioperative setting indicate that a single clearance parameter is not always sufficient to describe the distribution of fluid between the central and the peripheral fluid space. One constant would suffice if there is free flow of

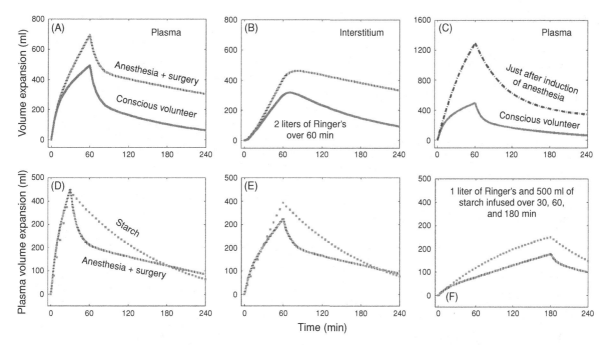

Figure 7.5 Volume kinetic simulations. A, B: Expansion of the plasma and interstitial fluid volumes when 2 liters of Ringer's acetate is infused over 60 min in an adult patient weighing 80 kg, depending on the presence of anesthesia and surgery. **C**: As for A, but using the kinetics seen just after induction of anesthesia when associated with a decrease in mean arterial pressure to 85% of baseline. **D, E, F**: Plasma volume expansion when infusing 1 liter of Ringer's acetate or 500 ml of hydroxyethyl starch 130/0.4 (Voluven) over 30 min, 60 min, and 180 min. The starch generally expands the plasma volume by twice as much as Ringer's does during anesthesia and surgery, but the difference is greater in conscious subjects.

fluid between compartments, but fluid seems to accumulate in the periphery when the rate of infusion is high.

Fluid accumulation may be interpreted as allocation of fluid to non-functional spaces, a finding with similarities to the *third space* that was described in the 1960s.[26] In kinetic terms, accumulation implies that a fraction of the infused fluid is not available for excretion, at least not within the period of study. In patients undergoing thyroid surgery, such allocation to non-functional spaces amounted to 2 ml/min or approximately 20% of the infused fluid volume, regardless of whether anesthesia was performed with propofol or isoflurane.[11]

The likely explanation for the poor return of infused fluid from the interstitium to the plasma is a qualitative change of the elastic fibers in the interstitial fluid gel. The matrix has initially a low compliance or volume expansion, but this is lost when the hydrostatic pressure increases. Eventually, free fluid appears in lacunae in the tissues, which slows down the redistribution process.[27] Current evidence suggests

that the problem increases when the rate of infusion of crystalloid fluid is high. A contributing mechanism could be that exclusion of albumin from the matrix is reduced upon plasma volume expansion, which binds fluid in the meshwork by oncotic forces.[28]

Glucose solutions and hypertonic saline

Glucose and hypertonic saline contain molecules that govern the distribution of the accompanying fluid volume by virtue of osmosis. These fluid shifts may be included in volume kinetic analysis, and the forces due to osmosis and those due to the fluid volume alone can be separated.[29]

The duration of plasma volume expansion by glucose solution is only partly governed by the half-life of infused glucose – renal elimination also operates alongside the osmotic-driven translocation of water to the ICF.[29] In contrast, renal capacity to excrete sodium strongly governs the rate of restoration of baseline plasma volume after infusion of 7.5% saline.[30]

References

1. Zdolsek J, Lisander B, Hahn RG. Measuring the size of the extracellular space using bromide, iohexol and sodium dilution. *Anesth Analg* 2005; 101: 1770–7.

2. Norberg Å, Sandhagen B, Bratteby L-E, *et al.* Do ethanol and deuterium oxide distribute into the same water space in healthy volunteers? *Alcohol Clin Exp Res* 2001; 25: 1423–30.

3. Menschen S, Busse MW, Zisowsky S, Panning B. Determination of plasma volume and total blood volume using indocyanine green: a short review. *J Med* 1993; 24: 10–27.

4. Rehm M, Haller M, Orth V, *et al.* Changes in blood volume and hematocrit during acute perioperative volume loading with 5% albumin or 6% hetastarch solutions in patients before radical hysterectomy. *Anesthesiology* 2001; 95: 849–56.

5. Reekers M, Simon MJG, Boer F, *et al.* Pulse dye densitometry and indocyanine green plasma disappearance in ASA physical status I-II-patients. *Anesth Analg* 2010; 110: 466–72.

6. Polidori D, Rowley C. Optimal back-extrapolation method for estimating plasma volume in humans using the indocyanine green dilution method. *Theor Biol Med Model* 2014; 11: 33.

7. Chaplin H Jr, Mollison PL, Vetter H. The body/venous hematocrit ratio: its constancy over a wide hematocrit range. *J Clin Invest* 1953; 32: 1309–16.

8. De Lorenzo A, Andreoli A, Matthie J, Withers P. Predicting body cell mass with bioimpedance by using theoretical methods. *J Appl Physiol* 1997; 82: 1542–58.

9. Nadler SB, Hidalgo JU, Bloch T. Prediction of blood volume in normal human adults. *Surgery* 1962; 51: 224–32.

10. Sandfeldt L, Riddez L, Rajs J, *et al.* High-dose intravenous infusion of irrigating fluids containing glycine and mannitol in the pig. *J Surg Res* 2001; 95: 114–25.

11. Ewaldsson C-A, Hahn RG. Kinetics and extravascular retention of acetated Ringer's solution during isoflurane and propofol anesthesia for thyroid surgery. *Anesthesiology* 2005; 103: 460–9.

12. Hahn RG, Drobin D. Rapid water and slow sodium excretion of Ringer's solution dehydrates cells. *Anesth Analg* 2003; 97: 1590–4.

13. Drobin D, Hahn RG. Kinetics of isotonic and hypertonic plasma volume expanders. *Anesthesiology* 2002; 96: 1371–80.

14. Riddez L, Hahn RG, Brismar B, *et al.* Central and regional hemodynamics during acute hypovolemia and volume substitution in volunteers. *Crit Care Med* 1997; 25: 635–40.

15. Svensén C, Hahn RG. Volume kinetics of Ringer solution, dextran 70 and hypertonic saline in male volunteers. *Anesthesiology* 1997; 87: 204–12.

16. Hahn RG. Haemoglobin dilution from epidural-induced hypotension with and without fluid loading. *Acta Anaesthesiol Scand* 1992; 36: 241–4.

17. Tollofsrud S, Elgo GI, Prough DS, *et al.* The dynamics of vascular volume and fluid shifts of lactated Ringer's solution and hypertonic-saline-dextran solutions infused in normovolemic sheep. *Anesth Analg* 2001; 93: 823–31.

18. Hahn RG. Blood volume at the onset of hypotension in TURP performed during epidural anaesthesia. *Eur J Anaesth* 1993; 10: 219–25.

19. Hahn RG. Volume effect of Ringer solution in the blood during general anaesthesia. *Eur J Anaesth* 1998; 15: 427–32.

20. Ebert RV, Stead EA. Demonstration that in normal man no reserves of blood are mobilized by exercise, epinephrine, and hemorrhage. *Am J Med Sci* 1941; 201: 655–64.

21. Hahn RG. Volume kinetics of infusion fluids (review). *Anesthesiology* 2010; 113: 470–81.

22. Drobin D, Hahn RG. Volume kinetics of Ringer's solution in hypovolemic volunteers. *Anesthesiology* 1999; 90: 81–91.

23. Li Y, Zhu S, Hahn RG. The kinetics of Ringer's solution in young and elderly patients during induction of general and epidural anesthesia. *Acta Anaesthesiol Scand* 2007; 51: 880–7.

24. Olsson J, Svensén CH, Hahn RG. The volume kinetics of acetated Ringer's solution during laparoscopic cholecystectomy. *Anesth Analg* 2004; 99: 1854–60.

25. Norberg Å, Hahn RG, Li H, *et al.* Population volume kinetics predicts retention of 0.9% saline infused in awake and isoflurane-anesthetized volunteers. *Anesthesiology* 2007; 107: 24–32.

26. Shires GT, Williams J, Brown F. Acute changes in extracellular fluids associated with major surgical procedures. *Ann Surg* 1961; 154: 803–10.

27. Guyton AC, Hall JE. *Textbook of Medical Physiology.* 9th edn. Philadelphia: W.B. Saunders Company, 1996: 310–13.

28. Parker JC, Falgout HJ, Oarker RE, Granger N, Taylor AE. The effect of fluid volume loading on exclusion of interstitial albumin and lymph flow in the dog lung. *Circ Res* 1979; 45: 440–50.

29. Sjöstrand F, Edsberg L, Hahn RG. Volume kinetics of glucose solutions given by intravenous infusion. *Br J Anaesth* 2001; 87: 834–43.

30. Svensén CH, Waldrop KS, Edsberg L, Hahn RG. Natriuresis and the extracellular volume expansion

by hypertonic saline. *J Surg Res* 2003; 113: 6–12.

31. Zdolsek J, Li Y, Hahn RG. Detection of dehydration by using volume kinetics. *Anesth Analg* 2012; 115: 814–22.

32. Hahn RG, Lindahl C, Drobin D. Volume kinetics of acetated Ringer's solution during experimental spinal anesthesia. *Acta Anaesthesiol Scand* 2011; 55: 987–94.

33. Holte K, Hahn RG, Ravn L, *et al.* Influence of liberal vs. restrictive fluid management on the elimination of a postoperative intravenous fluid load. *Anesthesiology* 2007; 106: 75–9.

34. Li Y, Zhu HB, Zheng X, *et al.* Low doses of esmolol and phenylephrine act as diuretics during intravenous anesthesia. *Crit Care* 2012; 16: R18.

Chapter

8

Acid–base issues in fluid therapy

Niels Van Regenmortel and Paul W. G. Elbers

Summary

Solutions such as NaCl 0.9% are an established cause of metabolic acidosis. The underlying mechanism, a reduction in plasma strong ion difference, [SID], is comprehensibly explained by the principles of the Stewart approach. Fluid-induced metabolic acidosis can be avoided by the use of so-called balanced solutions that do not cause alterations in plasma [SID]. Many balanced solutions are commercially available, their only drawback being their higher cost. Since NaCl 0.9% remains the first choice of resuscitation fluid in large parts of the world, there remains an important question over whether a large-scale upgrade to balanced solutions should be at hand. There is a lack of high-quality data at the time of writing, but there is increasing evidence that hyperchloremia has a detrimental effect on renal function and has an economic impact of its own. Therefore, until we have more definitive data, the use of balanced solutions in patients who need a relevant amount of fluid therapy seems to be a pragmatic choice.

It is widely appreciated that the administration of intravenous fluids can affect the human acid–base status. In this chapter we will try to elucidate the mechanisms behind this phenomenon and whether it can be avoided by so-called balanced solutions. Finally we will discuss whether there is a clinical impact of adopting an acid–base neutral fluid strategy.

An introduction to the Stewart approach

While the following introduction should be sufficient to provide the reader with the necessary basics to understand the effect of fluid infusion on a patient's acid–base state, a more elaborate explanation can be found in dedicated scientific literature.[1]

There are three popular methods of assessing disturbances in acid–base physiology. These are the bicarbonate centered approach, the base excess method, and the Stewart approach. Essentially, these are all mathematically compatible. However, for patients with many co-existing acid–base disorders, the Stewart approach arguably provides the best overview. A potential drawback lies in its perceived complexity. But, as discussed below, it demystifies the interaction between acid–base balance and electrolyte physiology, and hence demystifies the acid–base effects of fluids. The Stewart approach argues that bicarbonate does not play a causal role in acid–base disturbances. Instead, acid–base and electrolyte balance are governed by a number of physicochemical equations, derived from basic principles of physics and chemistry (Table 8.1). These must be satisfied simultaneously.

Table 8.1 The Stewart equations

Water dissociation equilibrium	$[H^+] \times [OH^-] = K'_W$
Weak acid dissociation equilibrium	$K_A \times [HA] = [H^+] \times [A^-]$
Conservation of mass for A	$A_{TOT} = [A^-] + [HA]$
Bicarbonate ion formation equilibrium	$pCO_2 \times K_C = [H^+] \times [HCO_3^-]$
Carbonate ion formation equilibrium	$K_3 \times [HCO_3^-] = [H^+] \times [CO_3^{2-}]$
Electrical neutrality equation	$[SID] + [H^+] - [HCO_3^-] - [A^-] - [CO_3^{2-}] - [OH^-] = 0$

All equations reflect chemical equilibria that need to be satisfied simultaneously. Constants are represented by K. Units are mEq/l for ions, mM for HA and A_{TOT}, and kPa or mmHg for PCO_2. [SID], strong ion difference.

Clinical Fluid Therapy in the Perioperative Setting, Second Edition, ed. Robert G. Hahn. Published by Cambridge University Press. © Cambridge University Press 2016.

Two important concepts thus emerge. Firstly, water is abundantly present in the body and is a virtually inexhaustible source of $[H^+]$ formation or reuptake. This is described by the water equilibrium equation. Secondly, as all equations must be simultaneously satisfied, it follows that only three independent parameters will ultimately determine the final equilibrium of water dissociation, and therefore also $[H^+]$ or pH. This can be mathematically expressed as:

$$[H^+]^4 + [H^+]^3 \times ([K_A] + [SID]) + [H^+]^2$$
$$\times ([K_A] \times ([SID] - [A_{TOT}]) + (K_C \times pCO_2$$
$$+ K'_W)) + [H^+] \times (K_A \times (K_C \times pCO_2$$
$$+ K'_W) + K_3 \times K_C \times pCO_2) - K_A \times K_3 \times K_C$$
$$\times pCO_2 = 0$$

For bedside purposes, it is sufficient to remember that this daunting equation may be functionally represented as $[H^+] = f(pCO_2, [SID], A_{TOT})$. This implies that $[H^+]$ (and also $[HCO_3^-]$) are dependent parameters, which can only be modified by changes in the three following independent parameters:

pCO$_2$, the partial pressure of CO$_2$. It follows from the Stewart equations that if pCO_2 increases, $[H^+]$ must increase as well. This is not different from other approaches to acid base–physiology.

[SID], the strong ion difference. Strong ions are essentially completely dissociated and thus exist in charged form only. Important examples include Na^+, K^+, Ca^{2+}, Mg^{2+}, Cl^-, lactate, and ketoacids. In contrast, weak ions can exist both in charged and uncharged forms. Examples include HCO_3^-, albumin, and inorganic phosphate. [SID] is the sum of strong cations minus the sum of strong anions. In plasma, it is mainly determined by $[Na^+]$ and $[Cl^-]$ and its normal value is about 40 mEq/l. It follows from the Stewart equations, that if [SID] decreases, $[H^+]$ must increase and vice versa. Any pathological process that disturbs the balance between strong cations and strong anions will thus directly affect pH. This includes lactic acidosis, ketoacidosis, renal acidosis, vomiting-induced alkalosis, contraction alkalosis, and most importantly iatrogenic fluid administration.

[A$_{TOT}$], the total amount of weak acids. Weak acids are molecules that exist in incompletely

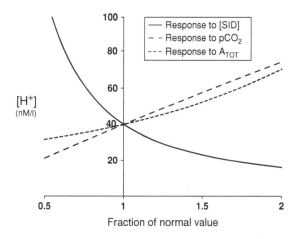

Figure 8.1 Spider plot showing the dependence of plasma pH on changes in the three independent variables: strong ion difference [SID] (normal value = 40 mEq/l), pCO$_2$ (normal value = 40 mmHg), and total concentration of non-volatile weak acids (A$_{TOT}$) (normal value = 17.2 mmol/l).

ionized forms. They are grouped as A_{TOT}, the total amount of weak acids, and consist mainly of plasma proteins. From an acid–base perspective, albumin and to a lesser extent phosphate are the most important contributors. It follows from the Stewart equations that if A_{TOT} increases, $[H^+]$ must also increase. This implies that hypoalbuminemia of any cause contributes to alkalosis. Similarly, hyperphosphatemia, as seen in renal failure, causes acidosis.

The effect of the different parameters on acidity is summarized in Figure 8.1. It is easily appreciated that a decrease in [SID] exerts the strongest effect.

Impact of fluids on acid–base status

The pivotal role of crystalloid [SID]

If a patient is being resuscitated with large amounts of fluids, plasma [SID] will be forced in the direction of the [SID] of the fluid. For example, NaCl 0.9% has a [SID] of 0 mEq/l. Thus, giving large amounts of NaCl 0.9% will lower the normal plasma [SID]. This directly causes $[H^+]$ to rise (acidosis). Therefore, it is important to consider [SID] when choosing fluids for resuscitation.

Importantly, it is the [SID] rather than the chloride content *per se* that causes this effect. Hyperchloremic acidosis is, as such, a poor descriptor. Theoretically it would be perfectly possible to produce a solution that is hyperchloremic as opposed to plasma and yet would (seemingly paradoxically) lead to metabolic alkalosis, provided it contained enough cations to enlarge its [SID]. A fluid containing 120 mEq/l of chloride and 160 mEq/l of sodium in the absence of other strong ions is an example of such a solution. On the other hand, the use of a chloride-free solution will not in itself avoid acidosis. For example, glucose and dextrose 5% do not contain any chloride, but owing to the concomitant absence of strong cations, the [SID] amounts to 0 mEq/l. The acid–base effect of such a solution will be the same as NaCl 0.9%, maybe slightly less important at most owing to an increased distribution of the fluid towards the intracellular compartment.

The only way to avoid fluid-based manipulations of the acid–base equilibrium is by using fluids that respect the human [SID] after being administered. We call these solutions "balanced." Their common characteristic lies in the fact that they contain more strong cations (mostly sodium) than strong anions (mostly chloride), and the electrical "gap" hereby created is filled by alkalizing agents, such as lactate, acetate, and gluconate, among others. These agents, sometimes called "buffers" (which is not the completely correct term from a chemical point of view) are metabolized after administration, exposing the solution's *in vivo* [SID] (versus the [SID] "in the bag," which is often 0 since lactate acts as strong anion). Classic examples of balanced solutions are Ringer's acetate and Hartmann's solution. More recent formulations are Plasma-Lyte® (Baxter, Deerfield Illinois, USA) or Sterofundin ISO® (B. Braun, Melsungen, Germany). An overview of the most common fluids with their respective [SID] is given in Table 8.2. The use of acetate as a buffer solution was treated with some skepticism, especially after it was abandoned in the field of hemodialysis, but nowadays is generally regarded as safe.[2] There is almost no research on the more recently used agents such as gluconate (an ubiquitous food additive) and malate, but they too seem to be without important safety issues. It would seem more straightforward to avoid the need for this extra metabolization step and use bicarbonate as the buffer of choice in balanced solutions. This is not commonly done, since it would be obligatory to use glass bottles in place of the much more flexible plastic bags.

A relevant question is at which *in vivo* [SID] a solution would be completely acid–base neutral. An intuitive answer would be a [SID] comparable to that of human plasma, around 40 mEq/l. This is not correct, however, as fluid administration not only manipulates the patient's [SID] but also another independent variable, A_{TOT}, while pCO_2 is kept constant due to respiration. Morgan *et al.* experimentally deduced that a solution that does not alter acid–base profile needs to have a [SID] of 24 mEq/l.[3,4] Gattinoni and Carlesso *et al.* confirmed this finding mathematically and argued that to avoid a change in pH by diluting plasma with fluids, the [SID] of the solution has to equal the patient's bicarbonate concentration.[5,6] Plasma-Lyte® has a higher *in vivo* SID of 50 mEq/l and could thus give rise to metabolic alkalosis. On the other hand, its high [SID] can be useful in situations where hyperchloremic or other forms of metabolic acidosis are already present or in cases of concomitant use of unbalanced solutions such as NaCl 0.9%, e.g. as diluents for medication.

Acid–base effects of colloid solutions

An important fact to acknowledge is that the acid–base effect of some colloid solutions is not only determined by their [SID], but that the colloid itself can be a source of A_{TOT}. For example, gelatins are proteins that exert weak acid activity. In the bag their net negative charge leads to a positive [SID] of the carrier crystalloid solution. For example, Gelofusine® (B. Braun, Melsungen, Germany), a succinylated gelatin, contains 154 mEq/l sodium and 120 mEq/l chloride, while the gelatin itself accounts for the remainder of the negative charge to ensure electroneutrality. Technically this makes the gelatins "spontaneously" balanced solutions, although sometimes their core solutions are balanced as well. Their effect on acid–base status is difficult to predict: at least until the gelatin molecules are metabolized, they exert an acidifying effect through an increase in A_{TOT}. Human albumin, whether in a concentration of 4% or 20%, follows the same principle. Hydroxyethyl starches have no weak acid activity, which makes their [SID] solely dependent on that of their carrier fluids. In an attempt to optimize these products, the latest-generation starches were improved by balancing their vehicle solution, e.g. Volulyte® is Voluven® (both from Fresenius Kabi, Bad Homburg, Germany) in a balanced core solution. An overview of the most frequently used colloids can be found in Table 8.2, bottom.

Table 8.2 Composition and [SID] of fluids that are frequently used across Europe. Not all solutions are available in every country

			Nutrients	Cations (mEq/l)				Anions (mEq/l)									
			Glucose (g)	Na+	K+	Ca^{2+}	Mg^{2+}	Cl$^-$	HPO$_4^{2-}$	HCO$_3^-$	Lactate	Acetate	Gluconate	Malate	SID (mEq/l)	pH	Osmolarity (mosmol/l)
Unbalanced	Hypotonic	Glucose 5%	50	0	0	0	0	0	0	0	0	0	0	0	0	4.20	278
		NaCl 0.45% in glucose 5%	50	77	0	0	0	77	0	0	0	0	0	0	0	4.30	432
		GNak[1]	50	51	40	0	0	91	0	0	0	0	0	0	0	4.50	460
		Glucidion[2]/Bionolyte[3] 5%	50	68.4	26.8	0	0	95.2	0	0	0	0	0	0	0	4.80	467
	Isotonic	NaCl 0.9%	0	154	0	0	0	154	0	0	0	0	0	0	0	5.50	308
		NaCl 0.9% in glucose 5%	50	154	0	0	0	154	0	0	0	0	0	0	0	3.5–6.5	585
		Tutofusin[1]	0	140	5	5	3	153	0	0	0	0	0	0	0	4.3–6.5	300
	Hypertonic	NaCl 3%	0	513	0	0	0	513	0	0	0	0	0	0	0	5.50	1,026
		Mannitol 15%	0	0	0	0	0	0	0	0	0	0	0	0	0	4.5–7	823
	Colloid	Voluven[3]	0	154	0	0	0	154	0	0	0	0	0	0	0	4–5.5	308
Balanced	Hypotonic	Glucion 5%[1]	50	54	26	0	5.2	55	12.4	0	25	0	0	0	30	4.90	447
		Rehydrex[3] 5%	50	70	0	0	0	45	0	0	0	25	0	0	25	6	440
	Isotonic	Hartmann's/Ringer's lactate[a]	0	131	5	4	0	111	0	0	29	0	0	0	29	5–7	278
		Ringer's acetate	0	130	5.4	1.8	2	112	0	0	0	27	0	0	27	6–8	276
		Sterofundin ISO/Ringerfundin[2]	0	145	4	5	2	127	0	0	0	24	0	5	29	5.1–5.9	309
		Plasma-Lyte[1]	0	140	5	0	3	98	0	0	0	27	23	0	50	7.40	295
		Ionolyte[3]	0	137	4	0	3	110	0	0	0	34	0	0	34	6.9–7.9	286
		Sodium bicarbonate 1.3%	0	154	0	0	0	0	0	154	0	0	0	0	154	7–8.5	308
	Hypertonic	Sodium bicarbonate 8.4%	0	1,000	0	0	0	0	0	1,000	0	0	0	0	1,000	7.0–8.5	2,000
	Colloid	Gelofusine[2]	0	154	0	0	0	120	0	0	0	0	0	0	34[b]	7.1–7.7	274
		Geloplasma[3]	0	152	5	0	3	100	0	0	30	0	0	0	64[b]	7.1–7.7	287
		Gelaspan/Isogelo[2]	0	151	4	2	2	103	0	0	0	24	0	0	56[b]	7.1–7.7	284
		Volulyte[3]	0	137	4	0	3	110	0	0	0	34	0	0	34	5.7–6.5	287
		Tetraspan[2]	0	140	4	5	2	118	0	0	0	24	0	5	33[c]	5.6–6.4	296

[1] ® Baxter, Deerfield, Illinois, USA.
[2] ® B. Braun, Melsungen, Germany.
[3] ® Fresenius Kabi, Bad Homburg, Germany.
[a] Slightly different formulations exist.
[b] Also contains weak acids and thus has an impact on A_{TOT}.
[c] Information according to product information leaflet. Electrolyte charge does not match acetate charge.

The treatment of metabolic alkalosis

A high plasma [SID], as seen for example after the loss of chloride-rich gastric juice due to vomiting or naso-gastric drainage, leads to metabolic alkalosis. NaCl 0.9% would be a fair treatment choice in an attempt to reduce [SID]. The use of fluids with a negative [SID] could be an even more effective strategy. In this case strong anions should not be accompanied by strong cations. Solutions containing ammonium chloride are good examples. In some parts of the world, dedicated preparations such as Multion Gastrique® (Baxter, Deerfield Illinois, USA) are available.

The relevance of fluid pH and bicarbonate content

Two common misconceptions can easily be dispelled in the light of the Stewart approach. The first is presumed effect of the pH of a solution, and thus its H^+ concentration, on acid–base status. The law of mass – on which the Stewart approach is based upon – dictates that protons cannot be added to or removed from aqueous media, but that they appear from the dissociation of water when forced to by the concentration of (the independent variables) [SID], A_{TOT}, and pCO_2. The pH of a solution is a characteristic relevant for the tolerability of intravenous administration, but has no predictable effect on acid–base equilibrium. Another inaccurate concept is that of the dilution of bicarbonate as the cause of metabolic acidosis due to fluid loading. Bicarbonate is a weak anion, and its concentration is again a dependent variable according to Stewart's theory. It will be generated from its main source, CO_2 (as the endpoint of aerobic metabolism), in an amount based upon the "gap" created by [SID]. Simplifying this process by calling it bicarbonate dilution is more than a terminological flaw, it goes against basic physical chemistry. Moreover, when administering sodium bicarbonate as an alkalizing agent, it is the strong cation sodium, administered without any strong anion, that increases plasma [SID] and leads to the correction of metabolic acidosis. Bicarbonate should merely be seen as a fellow companion, its only role lying in ensuring electrical neutrality of the solution. Proof of this concept can be experienced in the often encountered phenomenon that sodium bicarbonate is less effective in correcting metabolic acidosis in a patient with hypernatremia than in other patients.

The clinical relevance of balanced solutions

Numerous reports, most of them dating back to the 1990s, show a clear relationship between fluid therapy and the occurrence of metabolic acidosis.[7–9] The role of balanced solutions in avoiding this fall in base excess and resulting in a more stable acid–base profile was also established in different patient populations many years ago.[10] The clinical relevance of these findings, on the other hand, was debated and openly doubted, especially in the light of a lack of high-quality evidence.[11,12] It was the presumed negative effect of hyperchloremia on kidney function, induced by vasoconstriction of the afferent arteriole of the renal glomerulus, that led to persistent research.[13] At first, the only available data that showed an impact on clinically relevant endpoints came from animal studies and experiments in normal volunteers.[14–17] Nephrological literature provided further, although circumstantial, evidence for the deterioration of kidney function when long-term hyperchloremic metabolic acidosis was left untreated.[18] In an experimental setting, the effects of fluid type on renal parameters could be reproduced in humans.[19]

In 2012, a large-scale propensity-matched observational analysis of US insurance data showed that the use of Plasma-Lyte® versus normal saline on the first day of major abdominal surgery led to significantly fewer postoperative infections and incidences of renal failure requiring dialysis.[20] The authors also argued that the economic impact of "upgrading" of NaCl 0.9% to balanced solutions could be counterbalanced by reducing acidosis-related investigations and interventions such as blood gas analyses, lactate measurements, blood transfusions, and bicarbonate administration. Although the nature of the data and the design of the study made it difficult to exclude potential unmeasured confounders, this paper is regarded as extending concern about the safety of NaCl 0.9% to a clinical situation. Further evidence came from a prospective open-label sequential experiment in which patients, admitted to a tertiary intensive care unit, were treated during two distinct 6-month periods, first with the standard chloride-rich fluid regimen, and then with this regimen switched to a set of chloride-poor solutions.[21] After this second period a significant risk reduction of acute kidney injury (AKI) based on RIFLE criteria and a significant decrease in the need for renal replacement therapy was shown. Although some limitations, such as the unblinded design and a shift in fluid management that went beyond the chloride level alone (iso-oncotic albumin was replaced by hyperoncotic albumin during the intervention period, which could have a prognostic effect especially in sepsis), hindered a definitive conclusion, the trial provided clinicians with the first prospective evidence against the careless use of chloride-rich solutions.

Indirect proof against the use of unbalanced solutions can be sought by looking at the effects of hyperchloremia. This was accomplished, among others, in a large retrospective cohort trial in a surgical population.[22] Using an elegant statistical design, it was shown that postoperative hyperchloremia was associated with an increased risk of mortality at 30 days and a prolonged hospital stay. The most important issue with this kind of approach is that it does not take the amount of administered fluids into account. Being a marker of both hyperchloremia and severity of illness (or complex or complicated surgery), this is a potentially relevant confounder of outcome. As such, it is again difficult to draw a definitive conclusion.

In short, definitive proof of the added value of the use of balanced solutions has not been delivered. On the other hand, most of them have been in use for a very long time (in fact Ringer's and Hartmann's solutions were available long before the advent of NaCl 0.9%[23]) without safety issues being reported in an already extensive amount of research. Even the fact that most isotonic balanced solutions contain a small amount of potassium seems not to be an issue, even in patients with renal failure.[24–26] This makes the only reason to opt for an unbalanced fluid regimen an economic one, an incentive that clinicians should regard as short-sighted in the light of the above-mentioned findings. Until we have stronger evidence, abandoning the use of normal saline in favor of balanced isotonic crystalloids seems a pragmatic choice, especially in sicker patients or when large amounts are necessary. At the time of writing, a randomized controlled trial comparing Plasma-Lyte® with NaCl 0.9% in an intensive care population (the so-called SPLIT trial) is nearing completion and will undoubtedly contribute invaluable information. It is not clear at the moment whether the detrimental effect of unbalanced solutions such as NaCl 0.9% lies in the chloride load leading to hyperchloremia or in the acidosis induced by the reduction in plasma [SID]. There is also a lack of data on the critical dose beyond which the acid effect would become clinically relevant. The reason for the fluid to

be administered and the patient's comorbidities probably play important roles.

Conclusion

Solutions such as NaCl 0.9% are an established cause of metabolic acidosis. The underlying mechanism, a reduction in plasma [SID], is comprehensibly explained by the principles of the Stewart approach. Fluid-induced metabolic acidosis can be avoided by the use of so-called balanced solutions that do not cause major alterations in plasma [SID]. Many balanced solutions are commercially available, their only drawback being their higher cost. Since NaCl 0.9% remains the first choice of resuscitation fluid in large parts of the world, an important question remains as to whether a large- scale upgrade should be at hand. There is a lack of high-quality data at the time of writing, but there is increasing evidence that hyperchloremia has a detrimental effect on renal function and has an economic impact of its own. Therefore, as we await more definitive data, the use of balanced solutions in patients who need a relevant amount of fluid therapy seems to be a pragmatic choice.

References

1. *Stewart's Textbook of Acid–Base.* 2nd edn. Kellum J, Elbers P, eds. 2009; Amsterdam: Paul WG Elbers; AcidBase.org.

2. Hofmann-Kiefer KF, Chappell D, Kammerer T, *et al.* Influence of an acetate- and a lactate-based balanced infusion solution on acid base physiology and hemodynamics: an observational pilot study. *Eur J Med Res* 2012; 17: 21.

3. Morgan TJ, Power G, Venkatesh B, *et al.* Acid–base effects of a bicarbonate-balanced priming fluid during cardiopulmonary bypass: comparison with Plasma-Lyte 148. A randomised single-blinded study. *Anaesth Intensive Care* 2008; 36: 822–9.

4. Morgan TJ, Venkatesh B, Hall J. Crystalloid strong ion difference determines metabolic acid–base change during acute normovolaemic haemodilution. *Intensive Care Med* 2004; 30: 1432–7.

5. Carlesso E, Maiocchi G, Tallarini F, *et al.* The rule regulating pH changes during crystalloid infusion. *Intensive Care Med* 2011; 37: 461–8.

6. Gattinoni L, Carlesso E, Maiocchi G, *et al.* Dilutional acidosis: where do the protons come from? *Intensive Care Med* 2009; 35: 2033–43.

7. Liskaser FJ, Bellomo R, Hayhoe M, *et al.* Role of pump prime in the etiology and pathogenesis of

cardiopulmonary bypass-associated acidosis. *Anesthesiology* 2000; 93: 1170–3.

8. O'Dell E, Tibby SM, Durward A, *et al.* Hyperchloremia is the dominant cause of metabolic acidosis in the postresuscitation phase of pediatric meningococcal sepsis. *Crit Care Med* 2007; 35: 2390–4.

9. Scheingraber S, Rehm M, Sehmisch C, *et al.* Rapid saline infusion produces hyperchloremic acidosis in patients undergoing gynecologic surgery. *Anesthesiology* 1999; 90: 1265–70.

10. Waters JH, Gottlieb A, Schoenwald P, *et al.* Normal saline versus lactated Ringer's solution for intraoperative fluid management in patients undergoing abdominal aortic aneurysm repair: an outcome study. *Anesth Analg* 2001; 93: 817–22.

11. Handy JM, Soni N. Physiological effects of hyperchloraemia and acidosis. *Br J Anaesth* 2008; 101: 141–50.

12. Roth JV. What is the clinical relevance of dilutional acidosis? *Anesthesiology* 2001; 95: 810–12.

13. Hansen PB, Jensen BL, Skott O. Chloride regulates afferent arteriolar contraction in response to depolarization. *Hypertension* 1998; 32: 1066–70.

14. Aksu U, Bezemer R, Yavuz B, *et al.* Balanced vs. unbalanced crystalloid resuscitation in a near-fatal model of hemorrhagic shock and the effects on renal oxygenation, oxidative stress, and inflammation. *Resuscitation* 2012; 83: 767–73.

15. Kellum JA, Song M, Almasri E. Hyperchloremic acidosis increases circulating inflammatory molecules in experimental sepsis. *Chest* 2006; 130: 962–7.

16. Wilcox CS. Regulation of renal blood flow by plasma chloride. *J Clin Invest* 1983; 71: 726–35.

17. Williams EL, Hildebrand KL, McCormick SA, *et al.* The effect of intravenous lactated Ringer's solution versus 0.9% sodium chloride solution on serum osmolality in human volunteers. *Anesth Analg* 1999; 88: 999–1003.

18. de Brito-Ashurst I, Varagunam M, Raftery MJ, *et al.* Bicarbonate supplementation slows progression of CKD and improves nutritional status. *J Am Soc Nephrol* 2009; 20: 2075–84.

19. Chowdhury AH, Cox EF, Francis ST, *et al.* A randomized, controlled, double-blind crossover study on the effects of 2-L infusions of 0.9% saline and plasma-lyte(R) 148 on renal blood flow velocity and renal cortical tissue perfusion in healthy volunteers. *Ann Surg* 2012; 256: 18–24.

20. Shaw AD, Bagshaw SM, Goldstein SL, *et al.* Major complications, mortality, and resource utilization after open abdominal surgery: 0.9% saline compared to Plasma-Lyte. *Ann Surg* 2012; 255: 821–9.

21. Yunos NM, Bellomo R, Hegarty C, *et al.* Association between a chloride-liberal vs. chloride-restrictive intravenous fluid administration strategy and kidney injury in critically ill adults. *JAMA* 2012; 308: 1566–72.

22. McCluskey SA, Karkouti K, Wijeysundera D, *et al.* Hyperchloremia after noncardiac surgery is independently associated with increased morbidity and mortality: a propensity-matched cohort study. *Anesth Analg* 2013; 117: 412–21.

23. Awad S, Allison SP, Lobo DN. The history of 0.9% saline. *Clin Nutr* 2008; 27: 179–88.

24. Hadimioglu N, Saadawy I, Saglam T, *et al.* The effect of different crystalloid solutions on acid–base balance and early kidney function after kidney transplantation. *Anesth Analg* 2008; 107: 264–9.

25. Khajavi MR, Etezadi F, Moharari RS, *et al.* Effects of normal saline vs. lactated ringer's during renal transplantation. *Ren Fail* 2008; 30: 535–9.

26. O'Malley CM, Frumento RJ, Hardy MA, *et al.* A randomized, double-blind comparison of lactated Ringer's solution and 0.9% NaCl during renal transplantation. *Anesth Analg* 2005; 100: 1518–24.

Chapter

9

Fluids and coagulation

Sibylle A. Kozek-Langenecker

Summary

Infusion therapy is essential in intravascular hypovolemia and extravascular fluid deficits. Crystalloid fluids and colloidal volume replacement affect blood coagulation when infused intravenously. Questions remain over whether unspecific dilution and specific side effects of infusion therapy are clinically relevant in patients with and without bleeding manifestations, and whether fluid-induced coagulopathy is a risk factor for anemia, blood transfusion, mortality, and a driver for resource use and costs. In this chapter, pathomechanisms of dilutional coagulopathy and evidence for its clinical relevance in perioperative and critically ill patients are reviewed. Furthermore, medico-legal aspects are discussed. The dose-dependent risk of dilutional coagulopathy differs between colloids (dextran > hetastarch > pentastarch > tetrastarch, gelatins > albumin). Risk awareness includes monitoring for early signs of side effects. With rotational thromboelastometry/thromboelastography not only the deterioration in clot strength can be assessed but also in clot formation and platelet interaction. Fibrinogen concentrate administration may be considered in severe bleeding as well as relevant dilutional coagulopathy. Targeted doses of gelatins and tetrastarches seem to have no proven adverse effect on anemia and allogeneic blood transfusions. Further studies implementing goal-directed volume management and careful definition of triggers for transfusions and alternative therapies are needed.

Introduction

Perioperative bleeding in trauma and surgery may be due to ruptured or cut vessels – often referred to as surgical bleeding – and/or may be induced by deteriorations in hemostatic competence – often referred to as coagulopathic bleeding. Perioperative acquired coagulopathy is complex and has been reviewed recently.[1] Changes in hemostasis in the perioperative period include, for example, hyperfibrinolysis, coagulopathy due to blood loss, consumption, dilution, hypothermia, acidosis, hypocalcemia, and anticoagulation. These coagulopathic changes in massive bleeding may result in (1) a defect in clot firmness due to deficiency in the substrate fibrinogen (an early phenomenon) and thrombocytopenia, (2) impaired clot stability due to hyperfibrinolysis and factor XIII deficiency (a late phenomenon), and (3) prolonged clot generation due to various deficiencies in coagulation factor enzymes.

Obviously, patients with surgical and coagulopathic bleeding are susceptible to additional impacts on the clotting system. For example, coagulopathic bleeding may be aggravated by inherited bleeding diasthesis or pre-existing antithrombotic (anticoagulant, anti-platelet) medication.[2,3] Intravenous infusions of clear fluids, not containing coagulation factors or cellular pro-coagulant surfaces, may also impair coagulation (1) by non-specific dilution of the coagulation potential (enzymes, substrates, cell surfaces, calcium ions), and (2) by specific antithrombotic side effects. The current review will focus on the resulting dilutional coagulopathy – the unwanted side effect of colloids. In contrast to colloids, crystalloids have no specific side effects beyond pure dilution.

Hemostatic strategies to stop severe bleeding in elective surgery and in peri-partum hemorrhage have been summarized in the respective evidence-based guidelines from the European Society of Anaesthesiology (ESA).[2] The European Trauma guidelines describe the management of trauma-induced coagulopathy.[3] A prerequisite for targeted bleeding control is a sensitive and rapid identification of the actual cause(s) of bleeding. Viscoelastic point-of-care testing such as rotational thromboelastometry (ROTEM) or thromboelastography (TEG) may guide a timely, rational, and individualized therapy including, for example, administration of antifibrinolytic drugs and/or potent coagulation factor concentrates.[1–3] Practicability and cost-effectiveness support this monitoring-guided concept.[4] There is also a medico-legal perspective: after the statement of the European Medicines Agency (EMA),[5] hydroxyethyl starch (HES) solutions are less prescribed Europe-wide because of legal considerations.

The EMA encouraged us to think twice before infusing any fluids intravenously and to acknowledge that fluids are drugs. Interestingly, other colloids are also increasingly being avoided, although the evidence for safety problems for albumin or gelatin is scarce. In the statement of the Co-ordination group for Mutual recognition and Decentralized Procedures – Human (CMDh), healthcare professionals are told: "*HES solutions should only be used for the treatment of hypovolemia due to blood loss when crystalloids alone are not considered sufficient*" (Article 2 of the statement). With this article, the authorities reinforce applying individualized medicine and using methods such as preload monitoring to assess hypovolemia. This represents a step forward from conventional pressure-based management strategies, as still recommended, for example, by the Surviving Sepsis Campaign. According to the CMDh information, blood loss is a prerequisite for colloidal HES infusion; replacement of extracellular water losses is clearly not listed as an indication for a colloidal infusion. The wording in this article leaves room for individual decision making because the lack of efficacy of crystalloids does not need to be proven in the individual patient before choosing a more potent colloid but only anticipated by the attending clinician.

Another aspect of the CMDh statement (Article 6) proposes a link between use of HES and blood coagulation, the topic of this book chapter, and will be discussed below. The article states: "HES solutions are contraindicated in severe coagulopathy. HES solutions should be discontinued at the first signs of coagulopathy. Blood coagulation parameters should be monitored carefully in case of repeated administration."

Dilutional coagulopathy

Crystalloids and colloids exert different anticoagulant side effects:

(1) Unspecific dilution and reduction of the coagulation potential is determined by the fluid's volume efficacy, with colloids having a higher efficacy than crystalloids. Although still controversial, recent landmark studies (e.g. CRYSTMAS, FIRST, CRYSTAL, CHEST) report reduced volume requirements in the colloid groups, indicating superior volume efficacy over the comparator, even though the studies were not well controlled (rational preload-based goal-directed management was not employed in these trials). Importantly, transfusion of packed red blood cell concentrates (pRBC) with or without mixing it with fresh frozen plasma (FFP) also results in hemodilution and may induce dilution.[6]

(2) Specific antithrombotic side effects have been reviewed previously, with dose-dependent differences in the risk of dilutional coagulopathy among the colloids (dextran > hetastarch > pentastarch > tetrastarch ~ gelatin > albumin).[7]

Transient decrease in factor VIII and acquired von Willebrand syndrome

In contrast to slowly degradable HES (heta-, hexa- and pentastarch), rapidly degradable HES solutions (tetrastarch) have no effect on factor VIII and von Willebrand factor (vWF) levels even at high doses of up to 50–70 ml/kg.[8] There is a physiologic increase in these acute phase parameters in the postoperative period which has been found to be diminished after slowly degradable HES but not after rapidly degradable HES. The pathogenetic mechanism responsible for the adverse effects on plasmatic coagulation is not yet understood. Association with larger HES molecules may accelerate elimination of the factor VIII/vWF-complex.[7] Pathophysiological consequences of the transient decrease in factor VIII and acquired von

Willebrand syndrome are, for example, decreased ristocetin co-factor activity and increased activated partial thromboplastin time (aPTT).

Anti-platelet effects: extracellular coating

Physicochemical differences among colloids and HES generations were found to be important for the platelet-inhibiting properties, with slowly degradable HES solutions exerting more pronounced effects than rapidly degradable HES.[7] The pathogenetic mechanism behind this has been found to be extracellular coating of the platelet surface with colloidal macromolecules.[9] Coating induces inhibition in the conformational changes and/or interaction of glycoprotein (GP) IIb-IIIa and GP Ib with their ligands, such as fibrinogen. It remains to be determined whether extracellular coating impairs not only platelet aggregation but also platelet procoagulant activity by modifying the binding of constituents of the prothrombinase and tenase complex to the negatively charged phospholipids exposed at activated platelets. Pathophysiological consequences of the mild colloidal anti-platelet effect are a prolongation in PFA-100 closure times, decrease in platelet aggregation and adhesion, as well as deterioration in clot formation time (CFT) in the ROTEM or angle alpha in the TEG.

No major effects on fibrinolysis

Clots get more susceptible to fibrinolytic breakdown in the presence of HES and albumin in *in vitro* experiments.[7] The clinical importance of a pro-fibrinolytic side effect of colloids remains unclear, especially when considering the fact that induction of lysis after *in vivo* colloid infusions has not yet been reported.

No major effect on the acceleration of clotting

Mild to moderate hemodilution has been reported to accelerate the onset of clotting. This phenomenon may either be an *in vitro* artifact, or HES may indeed serve as an additional surface able to activate coagulation factors, thus accelerating the conversion of fibrinogen to fibrin. In contrast to crystalloid-induced hypercoagulability, an imbalance between thrombin generation and antithrombin concentration is not suggested to be involved in HES-induced hypercoagulability.[10]

No major effects of hyperchloremic metabolic acidosis on coagulation

Profound acidosis may affect coagulation by pH-dependent structural changes of coagulation factor IX, impaired coagulation factor Xa and thrombin generation, impaired fibrinogen breakdown, and protein C consumption.[11] Buffered plasma-adapted composition of the crystalloid carrier solution of colloids up to 20 ml/kg increases chloride levels but appears to have only minor impact on platelet aggregation and ROTEM kinetics.[12]

Impaired fibrin polymerization and decrease in fibrinogen levels

Historically, the effects of colloids on coagulation factors VIII and vWF were identified early after the licensing of slowly degradable HES solutions, while the effects on platelets and fibrin were not detected before point-of-care coagulation tests became available. Currently, impairment in fibrin polymerization is suggested to be the most outcome-relevant side effect of colloids on coagulation. Sensitive parameter for monitoring decreased polymerization of fibrin monomers is the maximum clot firmness (MCF) or amplitude after 5 or 10 min (A5 or A10) in the ROTEM, especially in the FIBTEM test. Similar decreases in the maximum amplitude in the functional fibrinogen assay in the TEG are expected but have not been published so far. *In vitro* experiments have major limitations in assessing the effects of colloids on coagulation. However, *in vitro* trials repeatedly confirmed a decrease in MCF (in INTEM and EXTEM tests) at 10–30% dilution with HES.[13] The carrier solution of HES (electrolyte-balanced vs. non-balanced) had no effect on ROTEM parameters.[12,14]

In vivo infusion series showed a decrease in clot kinetics and clot strength after HES infusion vs. Ringer's acetate after stroke volume-directed administration in neurosurgical patients.[15,16] This decrease was found to be only transient in major abdominal surgery at doses up to 15 ml/kg HES; 24 hours after infusion, no significant differences could be detected any more.[17] Confirming the transient nature of fibrin polymerization impairment, ROTEM data in complex cardiac surgery were also comparable at the first postoperative day in the groups receiving HES vs. lactated Ringer's solution (RL) [18] or HES vs. albumin [19] for the pump prime. HES and albumin up to 50 ml/kg similarly affected clot formation and clot strength in cardiac surgery.[20] Tetrastarch and gelatin similarly affected ROTEM parameters at pump prime-doses.[21] Preloading with tetrastarch or gelatin was associated with a mild hypocoagulable effect in healthy parturients presenting for elective Cesarean section; however, all TEG parameters in both groups remained within or very close to the normal range after preloading.[22]

But albumin is also not free from side effects on fibrin polymerization: at large degrees of hemodilution, the adverse effects on fibrinogen activity are in excess of what can be explained by hemodilution alone and more impaired after albumin than after saline.[23] In small infants, clot firmness decreased significantly but remained within the normal range after both albumin and gelatin.[24] The authors concluded that from a hemostatic point of view it might be preferable to use gelatin solution as an alternative to albumin. Fibrinogen levels decrease less after HES exposure compared with indicative ROTEM parameters.[25] An explanation may be that HES macromolecules interfere more with the functional parameter of fibrinogen polymerization in whole blood samples than indicated by the fibrinogen concentration in plasma.

First signs and severe coagulopathy: FIBTEM decrease

In the CMDh statement, Article 6, the terms "first signs of coagulopathy" and "severe coagulopathy" are used:[5] *"HES solutions are contraindicated in severe coagulopathy. HES solutions should be discontinued at the first signs of coagulopathy. Blood coagulation parameters should be monitored carefully in case of repeated administration."*

Obviously, the authorities require clinicians to monitor the actual coagulation potential repeatedly, without defining the appropriate methodology for laboratory testing, grades, and pathomechanisms.

From a practical viewpoint, "severe coagulopathy" will most likely prolong global laboratory tests such as the aPTT and prothombin time above 1.5 times normal. Global coagulation tests, however, are inappropriate for assessing pathomechanisms of perioperative bleeding [2] and for identifying "first signs" of dilutional coagulopathy. The CMDh statement may suggest stopping HES infusion, at the latest, if clot strength in the FIBTEM decreases towards hospital-internal trigger values for fibrinogen substitution. Even though

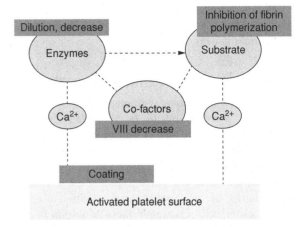

Figure 9.1 Effects of colloidal fluids on components of the cell-based model of hemostasis. The cell-based model of hemostasis describes physiology of blood coagulation. On the surface of activated platelets, coagulation enzymes – together with co-factors and calcium ions – utilize substrates in order to form a stable clot. Colloidal solutions may interfere with all these components via non-specific and/or specific effects (dark gray boxes). The net adverse effect of dextran > hetastarch > pentastarch > tetrastarch ~ gelatin > albumin may be hypocoagulability, hypoactivation, and impaired primary hemostatic capacity.

this sensitive viscoelastic parameter may deteriorate owing to many other pathomechanisms during perioperative bleeding irrespective of HES, avoidance of an additional hit on the coagulation system is rational. Once clot strength has been corrected, HES infusion may be continued if bleeding is overt, and in the presence of hypovolemia and hemodynamic instability.

Net result of specific antithrombotic effects of colloids

Unspecific dilution and specific coagulopathic changes induced by colloids are summarized in Figure 9.1. These antithrombotic changes may result in (1) a defect in clot firmness due to impaired fibrin polymerization (hypocoagulability), (2) impaired clot stability and susceptibility for fibrinolytic breakdown due to weakening of clot strength, (3) prolonged clot formation due to various deficiencies in coagulation factor enzymes and co-factors including coagulation factor VIII (hypoactivation), and (4) impaired primary hemostatic capacity due to platelet surface coating and decrease in vWF. In *in vitro* experiments, another factor may contribute to the net result: the crystalloidal carrier solution of the colloidal macromolecules may affect the homeostatic milieu, e.g. the calcium concentration in the test cuvette, thus affecting all components of the cell-based model of hemostasis.

Reversal of colloid-induced coagulopathy

Unfortunately, there is no drug in our critical care repertoire that has no potential risks or side effects. Risk awareness, co-administering prophylaxis, and targeted symptomatic treatment of side effects are routine strategies. Some medications are combined in one pill, e.g. the active painkiller with an adjuvant substance against the common side effect of obstipation. Such a pharmacological approach appears to be acceptable if efficacy, safety, and galenic compatibility of the active compound and the adjuvant are proven, and if no alternatives without such side effects exist.

If colloids are infused restrictively and according to individualized preload and/or microcirculatory targets (and if colloids are not abused for general fluid substitution), dose-dependent side effects on clot strength are suggested to be minimal and – most likely – not requiring reversal. Nevertheless, it is intriguing to consider prescribing colloids – in order to use their superiority in volume efficacy over crystalloids – together with fibrinogen concentrate in order to reverse eventual colloid-induced reductions in clot strength. Feasibility studies in *in vivo* animal experiments indicate that fibrinogen concentrate can rapidly reverse MCF to baseline values. *In vitro*, however, HES-induced FIBTEM reductions could be reversed completely by fibrinogen concentrate or cryoprecipitate in some experiments but not in others.[25,26] HES-induced MCF reductions responded less to fibrinogen concentrate compared with gelatins or albumin (also at hypothermia), and the combination with factor XIII concentrate improved reversal. These experimental findings suggest the use of fibrinogen concentrate after resuscitation with albumin and gelatins.[27] ROTEM parameters cannot be improved *in vitro* with factor XIII concentrate alone in any tested diluent.[27]

No clinical and histopathological signs for thromboembolic events could be detected, suggesting safety of factor concentrates for reversal.[26] Similarly, thrombin generation potential was not increased by fibrinogen concentrate addition, whereas it was increased for cryoprecipitate and plasma, suggesting

thrombogenic risks of a reversal approach based on allogeneic blood products.

Clinical relevance of colloid-induced coagulopathy

The question arises whether disturbances in laboratory parameters translate into clinically relevant bleeding manifestations, burdens, and harm, and whether fluid-induced coagulopathy is an independent risk factor for anemia, blood transfusion, and mortality, as well as a driver for resource use and costs. These aspects of patient safety and healthcare economics have received more attention since the World Health Organization (WHO) started supporting the multimodal therapeutic concept of patient blood management (PBM). Inherent side effects of fluids on dilution-dependent anemia and dilutional coagulopathy may counterbalance the role of fluids in PBM (to increase the tolerance to anemia) and, therefore, need careful consideration. PBM requires clinicians worldwide to apply a restrictive transfusion practise and to use physiological triggers for transfusion of pRBC instead of hemoglobin triggers.

Outcome studies report controversial results. A meta-analysis published in 2013 detected no adverse effects of tetrastarch in the surgical population: in 38 trials (3,280 patients) no increase in blood loss was found, in 20 trials (2,151 patients) no increase in allogeneic blood transfusions was found, and there was no signal for increased mortality.[28] This finding was confirmed by a recent meta-analysis.[29] More recent evidence confirms no increase in blood loss and transfusion requirements after HES exposure in major abdominal surgery [17] and cardiac surgery.[19,21,30] In neurosurgery, blood loss was not increased in patients receiving HES.[15,16] The intraoperative infusion of HES was not associated with the higher incidence of post-craniotomy intracranial hematoma formation requiring surgery, while perioperative arterial hypertension and the use of non-steroidal anti-inflammatory drugs were risk factors.[31]

Some studies, however, demonstrate increased transfusion requirements despite similar blood loss or intact coagulation in cardiac surgery.[18,20] The explanation may be the use of hemoglobin levels as transfusion triggers instead of physiological transfusion triggers; because of the higher volume efficacy, hemoglobin drops more after colloids than after crystalloids. Transfusion requirements, mortality, length of stay, and infections were all observed to be reduced in orthopedic patients resuscitated with HES.[32] However, some authors reported increased blood loss on implementing fixed-dose rather than goal-directed protocols.[33,34] Retrospective analysis suspected increased volume efficacy-related hemodilution as a contributor to increased blood loss and transfusion requirements in patients receiving HES versus crystalloids.[35]

In the critically ill and septic population, studies again reported controversial results. Mean increases of 18 ml FFP in HES-treated patients appear not clinically meaningful, despite being statistically significant.[36] In septic patients receiving tetrastarch, absence of an increase towards hypercoagulability in the TEG was hypothesized to be predictive for death and bleeding.[37] Some trials showed no effects of HES on blood loss,[38] while others found an increase in major bleeding events and transfusion rates.[37,39] However, in the latter studies, indication and dosing of the tetrastarch has been criticized; it was not the drug *per se* that was considered harmful, but rather the way it had been used.[40] Post-hoc analyses and meta-analyses aggravate methodological concerns and hide them behind the claim of high-quality evidence-based medicine. While waiting for refined trials considering denominators of quality of critical care, we have to acknowledge the alarming signs in the existing trials indicating deleterious effects of HES: patient safety management warrants the avoidance of HES in critical illness.

Increased mortality has been reported in those patients developing HES-induced clot strength reductions:[41] reduction in thromboelastographic maximum amplitude was an independent predictor for mortality. This is surprising, because, in general, viscoelastic tests have a poor predictive value and are therefore used and recommended for detecting actual pathomechanisms of bleeding manifestations rather than for prediction purposes.[2] Even more surprising is the finding that minimal changes in absolute values of thromboelastographic clot strength within the reference range have been suggested to be predictive for survival.[39] Future prospective trials will have to confirm this observation or identify potential statistical random failure. A recent meta-analysis found no increase in mortality, incidence of the need for renal replacement therapy, bleeding volumes, or in transfusion requirements in non-septic patients at the intensive care unit [42].

References

1. Kozek-Langenecker S. Coagulation and transfusion in the postoperative bleeding patient. *Curr Opin Crit Care* 2014; 20: 460–6.

2. Kozek-Langenecker S, Afshari A, Albaladejo P, *et al.* Management of severe perioperative bleeding. Guidelines from the European Society of Anaesthesiology. *Eur J Anaesthesiol* 2013; 30: 270–382.

3. Spahn D, Bouillon B, Cerny V, *et al.* Management of bleeding and coagulopathy following major trauma: an updated European guideline. *Crit Care* 2013; 17: R76.

4. Görlinger K, Kozek-Langenecker S. Economic aspects and organisation. In: Marcucci C, Schroecker P, eds. *Perioperative Hemostasis*. Berlin Heidelberg: Springer. 2015: 421–45.

5. http://www.ema.europa.eu/ema/index.jsp?curl=pages/medicines/human/referrals/Hydroxyethyl_starch-containing_solutions/human_referral_prac_000012.jsp&mid=WC0b01ac05805c516f (last accessed: 27 June 2015).

6. Ponschab M, Schöchl H, Gabriel C, *et al.* Haemostatic profile of reconstituted blood in a proposed 1:1:1 ratio of packed red blood cells, platelet concentrate and four different plasma preparations. *Anaesthesia* 2015; 70: 528–36.

7. Kozek-Langenecker SA. Effects of hydroxyethyl starch solutions on haemostasis. *Anesthesiology* 2005; 103: 654–60.

8. Neff TA, Doelberg M, Jungheinrich C, *et al.* Repetitive large-dose infusion of the novel hydroxyethyl starch 130/0.4 in patients with severe head injury. *Anesth Analg* 2013; 96: 1453–9.

9. Deusch E, Gamsjäger T, Kress HG, Kozek-Langenecker S. Binding of hydroxyethyl starch molecules to the platelet surface. *Anesth Analg* 2003; 97: 680–3.

10. Innerhofer P, Fries D, Margreiter J, *et al.* The effects of perioperatively administered colloids and crystalloids on primary platelet-mediated hemostasis and clot formation. *Anesth Analg* 2002; 95: 858–65.

11. De Robertis E, Kozek-Langenecker SA, Tufano R, *et al.* Coagulopathy induced by acidosis, hypothermia and hypocalcaemia in severe bleeding. *Minerva Anestesiol* 2015; 81: 65–75.

12. Schaden E, Wetzel L, Kozek-Langenecker S, *et al.* Effect of the carrier solution of tetrastarch on platelet

aggregation and clot formation. *Br J Anaesth* 2012; 109: 572–7.

13. Tynngard N, Berlin G, Samuelsson A, Berg S. Low dose of hydroxyethyl starch impairs clot formation as assessed by viscoelastic devices. *Scand J Clin Lab Invest* 2014; 74: 344–50.

14. Rau J, Rosenthal C, Langer E, *et al.* A calcium-containing electrolyte-balanced hydroxyethyl starch (HES) solution is associated with higher factor VIII activity than is a non-balanced HES solution, but does not affect von Willebrand factor function or thromboelastometric measurements – results of a model of *in vitro* haemodilution. *Blood Transfus* 2014; 12: 260–8.

15. Linderoos AC, Niiya T, Randell T, Niemi TT. Stroke volume-directed administration of hydroxyethyl starch (HES 130/0.4) and Ringer's acetate in prone position during neurosurgery: a randomized controlled trial. *J Anesth* 2014; 28: 189–97.

16. Linderoos AC, Niiya T, Silvasti-Lundell M, *et al.* Stroke volume-directed administration of hydroxyethyl starch (HES 130/0.4) and Ringer's acetate in sitting position during craniotomy. *Acta Anaesthesiol Scand* 2013; 57: 729–36.

17. Hung MH, Zou C, Lin FS, *et al.* New 6% hydroxyethyl starch 130/0.4 does not increase blood loss during major abdominal surgery – a randomized controlled trial. *J Formos Med Assoc* 2014; 113: 429–35.

18. Schramko A, Suojaranta-Ylinen R, Niemi T, *et al.* The use of balanced HES 130/0.4 during complex cardiac surgery: effect on blood coagulation and fluid balance: a randomized controlled trial. *Perfusion* 2014; 30: 224–32.

19. Cho JE, Shim JK, Song JVV, *et al.* Effect of 6% hydroxyethyl starch 130/0.4 as a priming solution on coagulation and inflammation following complex heart surgery. *Yonsei Med* 2014; 55: 625–34.

20. Skhirtladze K, Base E, Lassnigg A, *et al.* Comparison of the effects of albumin 5%, hydroxyethyl starch 130/0.4 6%, and Ringer's lactate on blood loss and coagulation after cardiac surgery. *Br J Anaesth* 2014; 112: 255–64.

21. Kimenai DM, Bastianen GW, Daane CR, *et al.* Effect of the colloid gelatin and HES 130/0.4 on blood coagulation in cardiac surgery patients: a randomized controlled trial. *Perfusion* 2013; 28: 512–19.

22. Turker G, Yilmazlar T, Mogol EB, *et al.* The effects of colloid pre-loading on thromboelastography prior to caesarean delivery: hydroxyethyl starch 130/0.4 versus succinylated gelatine. *J Int Med Res* 2011; 39: 143–9.

23. Pathirana S, Wong G, Williams P, *et al.* The effects of haemodilution with albumin on coagulation *in vitro* as assessed by rotational thromboelastometry. *Anaesth Intensive Care* 2015; 43: 187–92.

24. Haas T, Preinreich A, Oswald E, *et al.* Effects of albumin 5% and artificial colloids on clot formation in small infants. *Anaesthesia* 2007; 62: 1000–7.

25. Winstedt D, Thomas OD, Nilsson F, *et al.* Correction of hypothermic and dilutional coagulopathy with concentrates of fibrinogen and factor XIII: an *in vitro* study with ROTEM. *Scand J Trauma Resusc Emerg Med* 2014; 22: 73.

26. Martini J, Maisch S, Pilshofer L, *et al.* Fibrinogen concentrate in dilutional coagulopathy: a dose study in pigs. *Perfusion* 2014; 54: 149–57.

27. Schlimp CJ, Cadamuro J, Solomon C, Redl H, Schöchl H. The effect of fibrinogen concentrate and factor XIII on thromboelastometry in 33% diluted blood with albumin, gelatine, hydroxyethyl starch or saline *in vitro*. *Blood Transfus* 2013; 11: 510–17. doi: 10.2450/2012.0171-12. Epub 2012 Dec 13.

28. Van der Linden P, James M, Mythen M, Weißkops RB. Safety of modern starches used during surgery. *Anesth Analg* 2013; 116: 35–48.

29. Heler M, Arnemann PH, Ertmer C. To use or not to use hydroxyethyl starch in intraoperative care: are we ready to answer the "Gretchen question"? *Curr Opin Anaesthesiol* 2015; 28: 370–7.

30. Jacob M, Fellahi JL, Chappell D, Kurz A. The impact of hydroxyethyl starches in cardiac surgery: a meta-analysis. *Crit Care* 2014; 18: 656.

31. Jian M, Li X, Wang A, *et al.* Flurbiprofen and hypertension but not hydroxyethyl starch are associated with post-craniotomy intracranial haemoatoma requiring surgery. *Br J Anaesth* 2014; 113: 832–9.

32. Hamaji A, Hajar L, Caiero M, *et al.* Volume replacement therapy during hip arthroplasty using hydroxyethyl starch (130/0.4) compared to lactated Ringer decreased allogeneic blood transfusions and postoperative infection. *Braz J Anesthesiol* 2013; 63: 27–35.

33. Rasmussen KC, Johansson PI, Hojskov M, *et al.* Hydroxyethyl starch reduces coagulation competence and increases blood loss during major surgery: results from a randomized controlled trial. *Ann Surg* 2014; 259: 249–54.

34. Kancir AS, Johansen JK, Ekeloef NP, Pedersen EB. The effect of 6% hydroxyethyl starch 130/0.4 on renal function, arterial blood pressure and vasoactive hormones during radical prostatectomy: a randomized controlled trial. *Anesth Analg* 2015; 120: 608–18.

35. Hans GA, Ledoux D, Roediger L, *et al.* The effect of intraoperative 6% balanced hydroxyethyl starch (130/0.4) during cardiac surgery on transfusion

requirements. *J Cardiothorac Vasc Anesth* 2015; 29: 328–32.

36. Myburgh JA, Finfer S, Billot L, *et al.* Hydroxyethyl starch or saline for fluid resuscitation in intensive care. *N Engl J Med* 2012; 367: 1901–11.

37. Perner, A., Haase N, Winkel P, *et al.* Hydroxyethyl starch 130/0.42 versus Ringer's acetate in severe sepsis. *N Engl J Med* 2012; 367: 124–34.

38. Guidet B, Martinet O, Boulain T, *et al.* Assessment of hemodynamic efficacy and safety of 6% hydroxyethylstarch 130/0.4 vs. 0.9% NaCl fluid replacement in patients with severe sepsis: The CRYSTMAS study. *Crit Care* 2012; 16: R94.

39. Müller MC, Meijers JC, Vroom MB, Juffermans NP. Utility of thromboelastography and/or thromboelastometry in adults with sepsis: a systematic review. *Crit Care* 2014; 18: R30. doi:10.1186/cc13721.

40. Meybohm P, Van Aken H, De Gasperi A, *et al.* Re-evaluating currently available data and suggestions for planning controlled studies regarding the use of hydroxyethyl starch in critically ill patients – a multidisciplinary statement. *Crit Care* 2013; 17: R166.

41. Haase N, Ostrowski SR, Wetterslev J, *et al.* Thrombelastography in patients with severe sepsis: a prospective cohort study. *Intensive Care Med* 2015; 41: 77–85.

42. He B, Xu B, Xu X, *et al.* Hydroxyethyl starch versus other fluids for non-septic patients in the intensive care unit: a meta-analysis of randomized controlled trials. *Crit Care* 2015; 19: 92. doi: 10.1186/s13054–015–0833–9.

Microvascular fluid exchange

Per-Olof Grände and Johan Persson

Summary

There is always a continuous leakage of plasma fluid and proteins to the interstitium, called the transcapillary escape rate (TER). The transcapillary escape rate of albumin (TERalb) corresponds to 5–6% of total plasma albumin per hour. Plasma volume is preserved mainly because of recirculation via the lymphatic system and transcapillary absorption. During inflammation and after trauma, TER may increase up to 2–3 times and exceed the recirculation capacity, resulting in hypovolemia, low plasma concentration of proteins, and tissue edema. The present chapter discusses mechanisms controlling microvascular fluid exchange under physiological and pathophysiological conditions, including possible passive and active mechanisms controlling transcapillary fluid exchange. Options to reduce the need for plasma volume expanders while still maintaining an adequate plasma volume are presented. Consequently, this may simultaneously reduce accumulation of fluid and proteins in the interstitium. The effectiveness of available plasma volume expanders is also discussed.

Fluid and protein exchange from the intravascular to the extravascular space is a continuous process with a net fluid flow across the capillary membranes and the venules, the rate of which is called the transcapillary escape rate (TER).[1]

Under normal circumstances, accumulation of fluid and proteins in the interstitium is prevented by recirculation back to the intravascular space mainly via the lymphatic system, but also via fluid absorption across the capillary wall. Under normal circumstances,

the entire plasma volume passes the vascular membranes to the extravascular space and back to the circulation at least once a day, and even more often under pathophysiological conditions such as after trauma or during systemic inflammatory response syndrome (SIRS) and sepsis.

This means that accumulation of plasma fluid and proteins in the interstitium resulting in hypovolemia and tissue edema is not only a question of microvascular permeability to fluid and proteins, but also a question of the capacity of the lymphatic system. As discussed below, other factors may also be involved, such as hydrostatic capillary pressure, types of plasma volume expanders, and the infusion strategy. The present chapter is an attempt to explain the mechanisms controlling microvascular fluid exchange under physiological and pathophysiological conditions, and the importance of the relationship between the volumes of the intravascular and the interstitial spaces. This knowledge is essential not only for an adequate treatment of hypovolemia, but also to reduce side effects of the fluid treatment.

Transvascular fluid exchange outside the brain

Fluid exchange across the capillary membrane has been described by the classical Starling fluid equation for transcapillary fluid exchange:

$$Jv = Lp \times S(\Delta P - \sigma \Delta \pi)$$

where Lp represents hydraulic permeability (fluid conductivity), S is the surface area available for fluid exchange, reflecting the number of perfused capillaries, ΔP is the net transcapillary hydrostatic force for filtration, σ is the reflection coefficient for

---

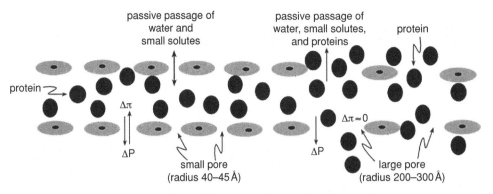

Figure 10.1 A schematic illustration of the principles used in control of transvascular exchange of fluid and macromolecules according to the two-pore theory. Absence of an oncotic absorbing force across the large pore means that the hydrostatic transcapillary force (ΔP) is the main force creating a "jet" stream of protein-rich fluid through each large pore, mainly via convection from the intravascular to the extravascular space. An increase in the number and the area of large pores and an increase in the hydrostatic transcapillary pressure will increase the loss of proteins.

macromolecules (plasma proteins), and $\Delta\pi$ is the transcapillary oncotic absorbing pressure force.

The reflection coefficient for plasma proteins describes the effective part of the transcapillary oncotic pressure counteracting fluid filtration, and represents the difficulty (relative to water) with which the proteins pass the exchange vessels. The reflection coefficient is 1.0 when the membrane is impermeable to the molecules and 0 when the molecules pass through the membrane without any hindrance.

The reflection coefficient for proteins is below 1.0 in all organs of the body except the brain. For albumin it is 0.90–0.95 in skeletal muscle, 0.50–0.65 in the lung, and 0.8 in the intestine and in the subcutis. A reflection coefficient below 1.0 means a continuous leakage of proteins to the interstitium. A system with recirculation of proteins between blood vessels and tissue and back to the intravascular space is essential to allow access of antibodies, protein-bound hormones, cytokines, and other macromolecules to the interstitial space. The reflection coefficient can be reduced significantly under a state of inflammation, leading to increased loss of albumin and other macromolecules to the interstitium. Tissue edema is formed when the leakage of plasma fluid is greater than the net recirculating capacity involving the lymphatic system, and hypovolemia develops in parallel.

The Starling formula, however, gives no information about the mechanisms responsible for the protein leakage. There has been a general belief for decades that active (energy-consuming) transcytosis (vesicle transport) across the endothelial membrane of the capillaries is responsible for a large part of the protein loss to the interstitium.[2] However, it is unlikely that the relatively small capacity of an active vesicle transporting mechanism would be responsible for transport of as much as 5–6% per hour of all intravascular plasma proteins – and even more than that under inflammatory states. The capacity of an energy-consuming process is also reduced by inflammation. Furthermore, blockade of transcytosis by cooling or pharmacological inhibition in the rat was not found to reduce TER.[3,4] Therefore, transport of proteins across the capillary membrane should be mainly a *passive process* independent of energy-consuming activities, as discussed below.

The two-pore theory

By the alternative two-pore theory for transcapillary fluid and protein exchange,[5] the large loss of proteins from the intravascular to the extravascular space can be explained by passive mechanisms. According to this theory, fluid and small solutes pass the capillary membrane through all the pores along the entire capillary bed and in venules, whereas proteins pass the membrane mainly through the much less abundant (by a factor of 10–30 thousand) large pores on the venous side of the capillary network, and in the venules (Figure 10.1).

Whereas the small pores with their radius of 40–45 Å are freely permeable to electrolytes and other small molecules and much less permeable to proteins, the large pores with their radius of about 250 Å are also freely permeable to proteins. This means that the oncotic pressure gradient across the large pore is low. The protein loss to the interstitium via the large pores can partly be explained by diffusion, but the main mechanism is *convection* when the proteins follow the large-pore fluid stream with the transcapillary/transvenular hydrostatic pressure as the major driving force. This means that the protein loss depends on both the number and size of large pores (large-pore permeability) and the transcapillary/transvenular hydrostatic pressure.

The lymphatic system

The capacity of the lymphatic system is of great importance for maintenance of a balance between the intravascular and the interstitial space. A normal TER of 5–6% of plasma volume per hour, corresponding to 150–200 ml plasma per hour for an adult, is in the range of the capacity of the lymphatic system under normal circumstances.[1] The capacity of the lymphatic drainage increases with increase in skeletal muscle activity and it can be reduced by inactivity, such as in immobile patients.

If TER is increased, such as after trauma and during sepsis/SIRS, the capacity of the lymphatic system may be too low to transfer enough leaking plasma fluid back to the circulation, and *tissue edema* in combination with *hypovolemia* develops. The situation will be aggravated in immobile patients by the reduced recirculating capacity of the lymphatic system.

Physiotherapy might improve this capacity and help to counteract tissue edema, hypovolemia, and the need for plasma volume expanders in critically ill patients.

Transvascular fluid exchange in the brain

The volume regulation of the brain is more effective than that of other organs of the body. This is of importance as there is no room for expansion in volume of the brain when it is tightly enclosed in the cranium. The brain also lacks a lymphatic drainage system.[6] The sophisticated regulation of the brain volume can be ascribed to the low permeability of cerebral capillaries, which creates the so-called *blood–brain barrier* (BBB). The cerebrospinal fluid system may also be involved to maintain a normal intracranial pressure.

The intact BBB means that the cerebral capillaries are impermeable to passive transport of all molecules except water. Thus, neither macromolecules such as proteins nor small solutes such as sodium or chloride ions can pass the cerebral capillary passively. This means that a disturbed balance between the hydrostatic and the oncotic pressures will result in transfer of only water across the cerebral capillaries, and the subsequent dilution/concentration of the crystalloid osmotic pressure of brain interstitium will result in immediate interruption of further fluid exchange.[6]

In the injured brain with a disrupted BBB – in the sense that it has also become passively permeable for small solutes – there will be much less dilution during filtration. The filtration will continue for a longer time, creating a vasogenic brain edema, and it will finally be balanced by the increase in intracranial pressure (ICP).[7]

Crystalloids and colloids as plasma volume expanders

While the healthy patient is normovolemic and needs no extra plasma volume expansion, most critically ill patients develop hypovolemia due to increased leakage of plasma fluid that exceeds the capacity of the absorbing effect and the lymphatic system. However, there is still debate regarding which plasma volume expander should be used to maintain or achieve normovolemia. In this chapter we attempt to describe the advantages and drawbacks of using crystalloids and various colloids as plasma volume expanders.

Because of the small radius of electrolytes (<2–3 Å) relative to the radius of the small pores (40–45 Å), the reflection coefficient of electrolytes is very small. The infused *crystalloid solution* is therefore distributed relatively quickly over the whole extracellular space, and more or less independently of the prevailing microvascular permeability, also resulting in reduction in plasma and interstitial oncotic pressure. As plasma volume is only about 20–25% of total extracellular volume, only 20–25% of the infused solution can be used for plasma volume expansion and the rest will result in tissue edema. A simultaneous increase in urine production must be compensated by further infusions to maintain normovolemia.

Tissue edema not only has cosmetic consequences, but it can also be a real drawback in terms of pulmonary edema, acute respiratory distress syndrome (ARDS), and increased intercapillary distances. It may also compromise perfusion because of an increased tissue pressure, and there is a risk of compartment syndrome. Reduction in plasma oncotic pressure may also result in further filtration according to the Starling formula. Distribution of a crystalloid solution to the interstitium will not occur in the normal brain because of the intact BBB, but it may occur to some extent in the injured brain if the cerebral capillaries have become permeable to small solutes, aggravating a vasogenic brain edema.[7,8] Crystalloid solutions with high concentrations of chloride ions may cause hyperchloremic acidosis. This can be avoided by using balanced crystalloid solutions instead.

Albumin is the predominant protein in plasma and the only natural colloid solution recommended for plasma volume expansion today, as transfusion with plasma is justified mainly to compensate for coagulation disturbances. The albumin molecule is monodisperse with a molecular weight of 69 kDa and the solutions are available in various concentrations (3.5%, 4%, 5%, 20%, and 25%, preferably in an isotonic solution). The albumin molecule is negatively charged, and this may moderate its distribution to the interstitium. It is transported back to the intravascular compartment via the lymphatic system. In contrast to synthetic colloids, it is degraded very slowly, which can be of advantage by acting as a plasma volume expander for a longer time; but this can also be a disadvantage when it accumulates in the interstitium. The effectiveness of albumin as a plasma volume expander has been questioned, however, as some studies could not demonstrate better outcome with albumin than with saline.[9] It is suggested that the beneficial absorbing effect of albumin has been overestimated, especially during states of inflammation. At a general increase in permeability, more plasma fluid and proteins will leak to the interstitium, and the effectiveness of albumin as a plasma volume expander will be reduced. Further, a revision of the classical Starling principles incorporating the endothelial glycocalyx layer means reduced absorption effect of transcapillary oncotic pressure in favor of the hydrostatic capillary pressure.[10] This hypothesis, however, is highly controversial and has still not been confirmed.[11] These mechanisms taken together may explain why the plasma expanding effect of albumin is not as good as expected. The effectiveness of albumin as a plasma volume expander can be improved and side effects reduced by adhering to specific rules in its administration, as will be described below. Allergic reactions are rare.

The *synthetic colloids* available today are dextran, hydroxyethyl starch (HES), and gelatin – and they are all cheaper than albumin. In contrast to albumin, which is monodisperse, they are all polydisperse with molecular weights ranging from low to higher values, and with the majority of molecules concentrated in the range of the average molecular weight. They are degraded in plasma and in the interstitium. Their recirculation back to the intravascular space via the lymphatic system is less effective than for albumin. When degraded to molecules with weights below their renal threshold, they are also lost via the kidneys.

Dextran solutions are produced by hydroxylation of polysaccharides. The predominant dextran solution is dextran 70, with an average molecular weight of 70 kDa. It is slowly degraded to CO_2 and water or lost via the kidneys. It improves the microcirculation and has the most effective and long-lasting plasma volume-expanding effect of all colloids available for clinical use today.[12,13] The risk of anaphylaxis is very low on pretreatment with 1 kDa dextran molecules (hapten competitor dextran 1), and therefore this should be obligatory. By its influence on platelet function, dextran can exacerbate an underlying coagulopathy, which limits its use in larger volumes during surgery or other situations with risk of bleeding. In larger volumes, the beneficial effect on microcirculation, therefore, should be weighed against the risk of increased tendency of bleeding. It is of great value preferentially in intensive care through its good and long-lasting plasma volume-expanding effect, through improving microcirculation, and through its prophylactic effect against thrombosis.

Owing to side effects with HES solutions of higher molecular weights, the third generation of *HES solutions* – with mean molecular weight of 130 kDa and molar substitution of approximately 0.4 – now predominate. The HES molecules are degraded relatively rapidly by amylase to smaller molecules below the renal threshold and cleared from the circulation via the kidney. The half-time of the plasma concentration of HES130 after a bolus infusion is 1.5 to 2 hours, and it is almost totally eliminated after 4 hours.[14] This has made the third generation of HES solutions less effective as plasma volume expanders, but this can be compensated for by repeating the infusion. Allergic reactions to the modern HES solutions are less common. The coagulopathic effect appears to be smaller with HES than with dextran. The use of HES solutions as plasma volume expanders to septic patients, however, was recently questioned after publication of a multicentre study, showing increased frequency of renal failure and increased mortality in septic patients given HES.[15]

Gelatin solutions are derived from bovine collagen. The mean molecular weight of molecules in gelatin solutions is only 35 kDa, which means that it is on the borderline to be defined as a crystalloid solution. This fact in combination with the relatively fast degradation of gelatin molecules and loss via the kidneys explains their relatively poor and short-lasting plasma volume-expanding effect. Gelatin has no or only moderate effects on coagulation, but anaphylactic reactions are more common with gelatin than with other synthetic colloids.

How to reduce the need for colloids?

Maintenance of normovolemia by infusion of plasma volume expanders in critically ill patients is always associated with interstitial accumulation of fluid due to the increased TER, the reduced capacity of lymphatic recirculation in these patients, and the fluid distribution to the extracellular space. The accumulation is associated with side effects in terms of tissue edema, compromised perfusion, and respiratory insufficiency. This also explains why normovolemia often is short-lasting after infusion of a plasma volume expander.

Increased amounts of macromolecules in the interstitium reduce the transcapillary oncotic pressure, resulting in further tissue edema. Besides maintenance of normovolemia by giving plasma volume expanders, an optimal strategy in the treatment of these patients must therefore be to simultaneously minimize accumulation of fluid and proteins in the interstitial space.

There are no evidence-based measures to reduce the amount of fluid accumulated in the interstitium, and thereby reduce the need for colloids to maintain normovolemia. However, based on the two-pore theory and other well-established physiological principles of hemodynamic vascular control, a few quite simple measures may help to maintain normovolemia with a relatively small amount of colloids infused. For example, high concentrations of albumin may be more effective as plasma volume expanders than low concentrations, as a result of their higher oncotic absorbing pressure and the smaller amount of fluid given for the same plasma expanding effect.

As shown both experimentally in the rat and clinically in patients,[16,17] the plasma volume is better preserved at a *normal arterial pressure* than at a high one. Increase in blood pressure by vasopressors may therefore increase the plasma volume loss, and avoidance of high arterial pressures by avoidance of vasopressors or by the use of antihypertensive treatment can be an effective alternative to reduce the need for plasma volume expanders.

Owing to the transient increase in arterial pressure by bolus infusions and the fact that a bolus infusion may result in an atrial natriuretic peptide-induced (ANP-induced) increase in microvascular permeability and increase in urine production,[18] a more effective long-term plasma expansion may be obtained by giving the colloid slowly rather than using a faster infusion rate.[19] Stimulation of the lymphatic system with physiotherapy may also reduce the interstitial fluid accumulation by improving the recirculating capacity of leaking plasma fluid.

There is controversy regarding the lowest acceptable hemoglobin concentration,[20] but arguments can be made that maintenance of a relatively normal hemoglobin concentration may be beneficial. The red blood cells do not pass the capillary membrane and remain intravascularly, thus contributing to preservation of the blood volume. Owing to the relatively smaller volume of plasma at a normal compared with a low hemoglobin concentration, the leakage and the need of intravascular volume to substitute may be smaller – a hypothesis supported by an experimental study in dogs.[21]

Side effects with blood transfusion can be reduced by using leukocyte-depleted and recently stored blood, which is highly recommended.[22] Blood cell transfusion has also been shown to be associated with improved outcome after subarachnoid hemorrhage [23] and increases local cerebral oxygenation.[24]

This chapter describes physiological hemodynamic principles of fluid exchange that form the basis of normovolemia, hypovolemia, and edema formation, and are fundamental for fluid therapy and for optimization of microcirculation and oxygenation. In view of the lack of appropriate evidence-based clinical studies in this field, such principles may be used as a guide in the use of colloids, crystalloids and erythrocytes in intensive care.

References

1. Haskell A, Nadel ER, Stachenfeld NS, Nagashima K, Mack GW. Transcapillary escape rate of albumin in humans during exercise-induced hypervolemia. *J Appl Physiol* 1997; 83: 407–13.

2. Predescue D, Vogel SM, Malik AB. Functional and morphological studies of protein transcytosis in

continuous endothelia. *Am J Physiol Cell Mol Physiol* 2004; 287: L895–901.

3. Rippe B, Kamiya A, Folkow B. Is capillary micropinocytosis of any significance for the transcapillary transfer of plasma proteins? *Acta Physiol Scand* 1977; 100: 258–60.

4. Rosengren BI, Al Rayyes O, Rippe B. Transendothelial transport of low-density lipoprotein and albumin across the rat peritoneum *in vivo*: effects of the transcytosis inhibitors NEM and filipin. *J Vasc Res* 2002; 39: 230–7.

5. Rippe B, Haraldsson B. Transport of macromolecules across microvascular walls: the two-pore theory. *Physiol Rev* 1994; 74: 163–219.

6. Fenstermacher JD. *Volume Regulation of the Central Nervous System*. In: Staub NC, Taylor AE, eds. New York: Raven Press, 1984: 383–404.

7. Gründe PO. The Lund concept for treatment of a severe brain trauma – a physiological approach. *Intensive Care Med* 2006; 32: 1475–84.

8. Jungner M. Gründe PO, Mattiasson G, Bentzer P. Effects on brain edema of crystalloid and albumin fluid resuscitation after brain trauma and hemorrhage in the rat. *Anesthesiology* 2010; 112: 1194–203.

9. The SAFE Study Investigators. Saline or albumin for fluid resuscitation in patients with traumatic brain injury. *N Engl J Med* 2007; 357: 874–84.

10. Woodcock TE, Woodcock TM. Revised Starling equation and glycocalyx model of transvascular fluid exchange: an improved paradigm for prescribing intravenous fluid therapy. *Br J Anaesth* 2012; 108: 384–94.

11. Rippe B. Does an endothelial surface layer contribute to the size selectivity of the permeable pathways of the three-pore model? *Perit Dial Int* 2008; 28: 20–4.

12. Lamke LO, Liljedahl SO. Plasma volume changes after infusion of various plasma expanders. *Resuscitation* 1976; 5: 93–102.

13. Persson J, Gründe PO. Plasma volume expansion and transcapillary fluid exchange in skeletal muscle of albumin, dextran, gelatin, hydroxyethyl starch, and saline after trauma in the cat. *Crit Care Med* 2006; 34: 2456–62.

14. Waitzinger J, Bepperling F, Pabst G, *et al.* Pharmacokinetics and tolerability of a new

hydroxyethyl starch (HES) specification [HES (130/0.4)] after single-dose infusion of 6% or 10% solutions in healthy volunteers. *Clin Drug Investig* 1998; 16: 151–60.

15. Perner A, Haase N, Guttormsen AB, *et al.* Hydroxyethyl starch 130/0.42 vs. Ringer's acetate in severe sepsis. *N Engl J Med* 2012; 367: 124–34.

16. Dubniks M, Persson J, Gründe PO. Effect of blood pressure on plasma volume loss in the rat under increased permeability. *Intensive Care Med* 2007; 33: 2192–8.

17. Nygren A, Redfors B, Thoren A, Ricksten SE. Norepinephrine causes a pressure-dependent plasma volume decrease in clinical vasodilatory shock. *Acta Anaesthesiol Scand* 2010; 54: 814–20.

18. Curry FR, Rygh CB, Karlsen T, *et al.* Atrial natriuretic peptide modulation of albumin clearance and contrast agent permeability in mouse skeletal muscle and skin: role in regulation of plasma volume. *J Physiol* 2010; 588: 325–39.

19. Bark B, Persson J, Gründe PO. Importance of the infusion rate for the plasma expanding effect of 5% albumin, 6% HES130/0.4, 4% gelatin, and 0.9% NaCl in the septic rat. *Crit Care Med* 2013; 41: 857–66.

20. Hébert PC, Wells G, Blajchman A, *et al.* A multicenter, randomized, controlled clinical trial of transfusion requirements in critical care. *N Eng J Med* 1999; 340: 409–18.

21. Valeri CR, Donahue K, Feingold HM, Cassidy GP, Altschule MD. Increase in plasma volume after the transfusion of washed erythrocytes. *Surg Gynecol Obstet* 1986; 162: 30–6.

22. Hébert PC, Fergusson D, Blajchman MA, *et al.* Leukoreduction Study Investigators. Clinical outcomes following institution of the Canadian Universal Leukoreduction Program for red blood cell transfusions. *JAMA* 2003; 289: 1941–9.

23. Naidech A, Jovanovic B, Wartenberg K, *et al.* Higher hemoglobin is associated with improved outcome after subarachnoid hemorrhage. *Crit Care Med* 2007; 35: 2383–9.

24. Smith M, Stiefel M, Magge S, *et al.* Packed red blood cell transfusion increases local cerebral oxygenation. *Crit Care Med* 2005; 33: 1104–8.

The glycocalyx layer

Anna Bertram, Klaus Stahl, Jan Hegermann, and Hermann Haller

Summary

Endothelial cells cover the inner surface of the vasculature and are essential for vascular homeostasis with regulation of vasodilation and vasoconstriction, permeability, inflammation, and coagulation. The endothelium is not a barren surface but is covered by a thick layer of so-called glycocalyx. The glycocalyx is built of heavily glycosylated proteins such as syndecans which are anchored in the cell membrane, freely associating proteoglycans such as hyaluronidase, and also a multitude of plasma molecules that bind and interact with the proteoglycans.

The glycoproteins collectively organize into the glycocalyx, which plays a vital role in several important vascular functions. It serves as a mechanotransductor mediating information on blood flow and cellular movement to the endothelium, it regulates permeability via its physical properties, it regulates binding of vascular factors to the endothelium, and it is the "habitat" of the resident components of the complement system and the coagulation cascade. In addition, the glycocalyx serves as a sink for small molecules and electrolytes in the plasma and generates chemokine gradients to guide leukocytes to sites of inflammation. The delicate structures of the glycocalyx can be easily disturbed and damaged by acute disease such as sepsis or ischemia, as well as chronic disease such as diabetes or hypertension. The proteoglycans and/or its sugar moieties can be shed by specific enzymes. Novel tools have been developed to better visualize the glycocalyx both *in vitro* and *in vivo*. An understanding and, possibly, a molecular manipulation of the glycocalyx will be important to improve our therapeutic strategies in patients.

Over the past decade we have learnt that the endothelium is not a passive cellular layer of the vessel wall but has important functions in the communication between the blood and the vessel wall. Several important functions such as vascular permeability, vasodilation and -constriction, the regulation of inflammation via adhesion molecules and cytokines as well as coagulation and the complement system are important mechanisms regulated by the endothelial cells. We have coined the rather vague term "endothelial dysfunction" to describe damaged and/or dysfunctional endothelium under pathophysiological conditions such as hypertension, diabetes, sepsis, and/or ischemia. It has only recently been recognized that the interaction between the bloodstream and the endothelial cell surface is even more complicated. It seems that the endothelium is covered with a thick layer of heavily glycosylated protein, a structure that has been called the glycocalyx.[1,2]

The glycocalyx is situated at the luminal side of all blood vessels and covers the surface receptors and other membrane-bound molecules of the endothelium. The volume of the glycocalyx depends on the balance between biosynthesis and the enzymatic or shear-dependent shedding of its components.[3] Historically, the glycocalyx has been described as a thin mucous layer of <100 nm.[4] However, it is notoriously difficult to visualize.[5,6] It is mostly destroyed upon conventional tissue fixation and optically transparent in most light microscopic examinations. Using electron microscopy and different staining methods, it

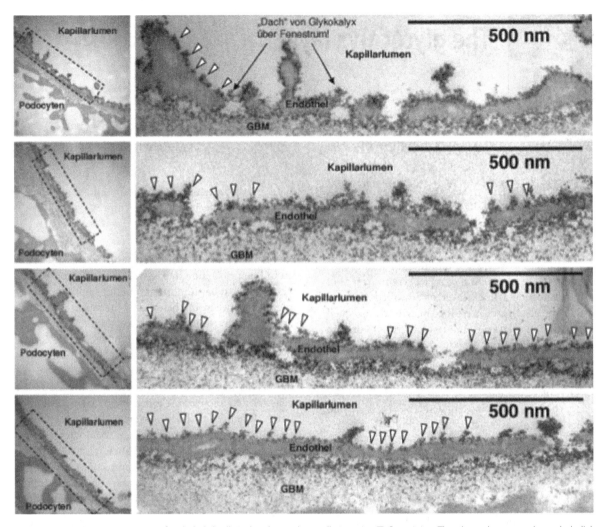

Figure 11.1 Electron microscopy of endothelial cells in the glomerular capillaries using ThO$_2$ staining. The glycocalyx covers the endothelial cell surface in regularly distributed focal structures. The glycocalyx "bridges" the endothelial cell fenestrations. GBM, glomerular basement membrane. (Kapillarlumen = capillary lumen, podocyten = podocytes, Dach von Glykokalyx uber Fenestrum = roof of glycocalyx above fenestrations.)

has been demonstrated to reach up to 0.5–3 μm intra-luminally (Figure 11.1).[7]

The glycocalyx is a negatively charged, organized mesh of membranous glycoproteins, with core proteoglycans of the syndecan and glypican family carrying highly sulfated, linear glycosaminoglycan attachments (mostly of the heparan, chondroitin, and dermatan sulfate families). Hyaluronic acid and the negatively charged heparan sulfate proteoglycans are its major constituents.[1,2,3,5] This structure of core proteins "decorated" with long glycosaminoglycans provides a sea-grass-like surface where components of functional systems such as the coagulation cascade or the complement system can be located and plasma constituents may interact intensely and dynamically. This "habitat" on the surface of the endothelium has also been named an endothelial surface layer (ESL) and may attain a thickness up to 1 μm in certain blood vessels (Figure 11.2).

It is obvious that this glycocalyx or ESL, whatever nomenclature we use, plays an important role both under physiological and under pathophysiological conditions. In this chapter we will briefly review the contribution of the glycocalyx for vascular permeability, as a mechanotransducer, and its role in inflammation. We will also discuss the methods to assess

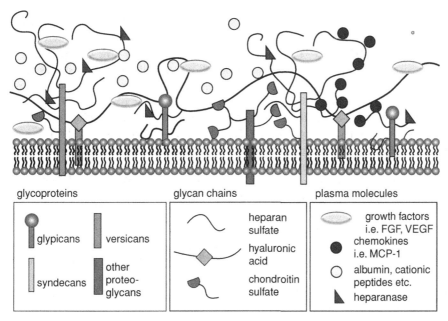

Figure 11.2 Schematic diagram showing the components and spatial organization of the endothelial glycocalyx. FGF, fibroblast growth factor; VEGF, vascular endothelial growth factor; MCP-1, monocyte chemoattractant protein-1.

the glycocalyx in humans and describe under which pathophysiological conditions the glycocalyx is damaged and disturbed.

Glycocalyx and vascular permeability

The glycocalyx influences vascular permeability. The importance of the loss of glycocalyx barrier functions leading to increased vascular permeability was suggested from experiments showing that glycocalyx degradation is associated with a reduction in the exclusion of anionic dextrans, with an increased protein permeability, with an increased glomerular clearance of albumin, and with the formation of perivascular edema. The phenomenon has been mostly investigated in glomerular capillaries.[8] Under physiological perfusion conditions, albumin is confined to the glomerular capillary lumen and endothelial fenestrae, implying resistance at the level of glomerular endothelial surface.[9] Chappell *et al.* have demonstrated that shedding of the glycocalyx induced by the inflammatory cytokine tumor necrosis factor-alpha (TNF-α), or by ischemia-reperfusion, causes a substantial increase in vascular permeability to both plasma and colloids.[10] Selective removal of endothelial glycocalyx from coronary vessels increases permeability, which provides evidence that it constitutes a barrier to macromolecular permeability.[11]

This association between loss of glycocalyx and an increase in vascular permeability has been shown in animal models other than that of Chappell. Once removed, recovery of the hydrodynamically relevant glycocalyx required 5–7 days. It seems that the composition of the glycocalyx can be modulated by different factors. Salmon *et al.* have used angiopoietin-1 (Ang-1), a ligand for the tyrosine kinase receptor Tie-2, and were able to demonstrate that the increased permeability after digestion of glycocalyx was mitigated by pre-perfusion with Ang-1.[12] In addition, perfusion with Ang-1 nearly doubled glycocalyx thickness. Mice treated with glycocalyx-degrading enzymes show reduction in thickness of glomerular endothelial glycocalyx coinciding with increased albumin excretion. Therefore, the presence of a significant endothelial glycocalyx contributes significantly to the barrier to macromolecules. Loss or alterations of the glycocalyx may contribute to states of edema associated with endothelial dysfunction such as in infections and/or sepsis. Whether this is a property of the physicochemical characteristics of the glycocalyx, or whether an intact glycocalyx improves the barrier function of the endothelium, is as yet unclear.[5]

Glycocalyx as a mechanotransducer

To maintain vascular homeostasis, endothelial cells are endowed with a complex set of mechanisms to sense mechanical forces imparted by blood flow.[13] The concept that the glycocalyx contributes to the regulation of microvascular perfusion was originally hypothesized by the group of Duling in 1990, when they showed that the adenosine-induced increase in capillary tube hematocrit in hamster cremaster muscle vessels was diminished after enzymatic glycocalyx degradation.[14]

Based on the structure of the glycocalyx, with its regular grass-like distribution of the core proteoglycans, it has been assumed that these core proteoglycans bend under the influence of the bloodstream velocity and transmit signals to the intracellular cytoskeleton and/or other signaling complexes. The evidence that supports a central role for the glycocalyx in mechanotransduction comes from experiments involving degrading specific components of the glycocalyx, followed by a reassessment of function, mostly nitric oxide synthase (NOS) activation and/or NO production. Several glycosamine-degrading enzymes have been used.[15] Heparinase (which selectively degrades heparan sulfates), neuramidase (degrading sialic acid), and hyaluronidase (affecting hyaluronic acid) have been shown to reduce NO production and flow-dependent vasodilation significantly. Because flow-dependent vasodilation is mediated by NO release in many arteries, these studies suggest that glycosaminoglycans contributes to shear-induced production of NO. The core proteoglycans may also contribute to the mechano-sensing properties of the glycocalyx.

The different proteoglycans and their location on the cell mebrane seem to influence erent intracellular pathways. Both syndecan-1, a transmembrane proteoglycan that is linked to the cytoskeleton and mediates endothelial cell remodeling in response to shear stress, and the membrane-bound but not transmembranous proteoglycan glypican-1 that is enriched in caveolae near the intracellular endothelial nitric oxide synthase (eNOS) mediate vasodilation with shear-induced eNOS activation and cytoskeletal remodeling.[16] However, gene knockdown of glypican-1 blocked only eNOS activation, not remodeling, and knockdown of syndecan-1 blocked only remodeling, not eNOS activation, demonstrating that the glycocalyx can convert the mechanical signal shear stress into diverse cellular responses through distinct proteoglycans. Another possible mechanism for how the glycocalyx regulates vasodilation is the binding of substrates such as arginine to heparan sulfates. Heparan sulfates may play a role in the availability of arginine to its transporters close to the endothelial cell surface, thereby providing eNOS with its necessary substrate.[17]

Glycocalyx as a storage system

Heparan sulfates display high affinities for polycationic molecules. In addition, they provide a significant storage volume which is easily accessible from the fluid phase. Oberleithner *et al.* suggested that plasma sodium is stored in the glycocalyx, partially neutralizing the negative surface charges.[18] A "good" glycocalyx has a high sodium store capacity, but still maintains sufficient surface negativity at normal plasma sodium. A "bad" glycocalyx shows the opposite. Thus, proteoglycans and glycosaminoglycans (i.e. mainly extracellular polyanions) may provide potential sinks for sodium and may serve as a means of concentrating cations close to the plasma membrane.

Heparan sulfates adsorbed to a surface undergo a conformational change when exposed to flow: their core proteins unfold from a random coil to an extended filament, and their heparan sulfate chains elongate significantly. This finding was used to illustrate how sodium ions bound to heparan sulfates could not only be stored, but be delivered by the stretched glycosaminoglycan to their transporter channels. Such a concept of "storage space" in an intact glycocalyx has important implications for the binding of other cations to the heparan sulfates of the glycocalyx. Nucleic acids bind to the glycocalyx, and incorporation of DNA increases markedly in cells that lack the major anionic components of the glycocalyx, sialic acid and glycosaminoglycans, and anionic oligosaccharides may provide a barrier to the uptake of nucleic acids by mammalian cells. This phenomenon could also play an important role in the development of crystalloid solutions.

Glycocalyx and inflammation

The vascular endothelium is one of the earliest sites of injury during inflammation.[19] The glycocalyx and its glycosaminoglycans play an important role in various aspects of inflammation and in the physiological functioning of a range of inflammatory mediators, including chemokines, growth factors, endothelial adhesion molecules, and inflammatory cell emigration. A multitude of studies suggest that at least two mechanisms of the glycocalyx, a change in glycosamine composition as well as enzymatic disruption of the proteoglycans, may have a strong effect on inflammatory responses.[20]

A change in glycosamine composition of the glycocalyx affects the early inflammatory mechanisms in several ways: van der Vlag and his group have demonstrated that an early response of the glycocalyx to inflammatory stimuli is a change in the N-deacetylase-N-sulfotransferase-mediated composition of the heparan sulfate. They have argued that modulation of heparan sulfates in the endothelial glycocalyx significantly reduces or enhances the inflammatory response in inflammatory kidney disease.[20]

The binding properties of the glycosaminoglycans play a second important role in inflammation. A hallmark of immune cell trafficking is directional guidance via gradients of soluble or surface-bound chemokines. Vascular endothelial cells produce, transport, and deposit either their own chemokines or chemokines produced by the underlying stroma. Endothelial heparan sulfate has been suggested to be a critical scaffold for these chemokine pools. Stoler-Barak et al. have shown that the blood vasculature creates steep gradients of heparan sulfate scaffolds between the luminal and basolateral endothelium, and that inflammatory processes can further enrich the heparan sulfate content near inflamed vessels.[21] They proposed that chemokine gradients between the luminal and abluminal sides of vessels could be generated by these sharp heparan sulfate scaffold gradients in the glycocalyx. In addition, certain chemokines require interactions with glycosaminoglycans for their in vivo function. Proudfoot has shown that chemokines oligomerize on immobilized glycosaminoglycans, and this ability to form higher-order oligomers has also been shown to be essential for the activity of certain chemokines in vivo.[22]

The binding properties of the glycocalyx also play a role in the regulation of the complement system, which is a major player in innate immunity. One of the most important regulators of the complement cascade is complement factor H (CFH). The surface-bound glycocalyx glycosaminoglycan constituent heparan sulfate is crucial for CFH binding and function, both in recognition of host tissue and prevention of spontaneous complement activation via the alternative pathway.[23] Most of the clinically relevant genetic mutations in CFH result in incorrect binding to heparan sulfate. Loss of the heparan sulfate binding site will results in impaired binding of CFH, thereby reducing inhibitory signals to the complement system, which increases its local activation.[24]

A second mechanism whereby glycocalyx affects and influences the complement system is via thrombomodulin (TM).[24] TM is a cell-surface-expressed transmembrane glycoprotein which was originally identified on vascular endothelium, and is by definition a part of the glycocalyx. It is a co-factor for thrombin binding that mediates protein C activation and inhibits thrombin activity. In addition to its anticoagulant activity, recent evidence has revealed that TM, especially its lectin-like domain, has potent anti-inflammatory function through a variety of molecular mechanisms. The lectin-like domain of TM plays an important role in suppressing inflammation independent of the TM anticoagulant activity. Loss of the glycocalyx proteoglycan TM is therefore associated with increased complement activity and enhanced inflammatory response.

The loss of constituents of the endothelial glycocalyx has been termed "shedding." Shedding can range from selective cleavage of heparan sulfates to major alterations with removal of entire syndecan and glypican core proteins together with the attached glycosaminoglycan side chains. The shedding of the glycocalyx in response to inflammatory mediators such as cytokines and chemoattractants was found to occur in arterioles, capillaries, and venules under various experimental models of inflammation. The major enzyme responsible for shedding of proteoglycans is heparanase, which is the only known mammalian endoglycosidase capable of degrading heparan sulfate glycosaminoglycan. Enzymatic degradation of glycocalyx by heparanase profoundly affects numerous physiological and pathological processes.[25]

Besides heparinase, there are other molecules that can affect glycocalyx composition and shedding.[26] Based on mechanism of action, inflammatory mediators can directly affect endothelial cells that, in response, alter glycocalyx structures. Additionally, under inflammatory conditions, activated subsets of leukocytes, such as polymorphonuclear leukocytes, macrophages, and mast cells, release enzymes which then can contribute to degradation of the glycocalyx. Upon activation, inflammatory cells release a wide range of enzymes and reactive species that can contribute to glycocalyx damage. In particular, activated neutrophil granulocytes, the most abundant blood leukocytes in humans, can induce glycocalyx damage by producing reactive oxygen and nitrogen species and releasing proteases from their storage granules. Moreover, mast cells, a less abundant leukocyte subset, can release heparanase directly with a significant potential to disturb glycocalyx structure through the degradation of heparan sulfates.

The cleavage of heparan sulfates due to reactive oxygen, and the subsequent increase in macromolecular permeability, follows a similar pattern to that seen after treatment with glycocalyx-degrading enzymes. This suggests common pathways in the degradation of the glycocalyx. Moreover, the protein core of proteoglycans can also be subject to oxidation/nitrosation and these oxidative and nitrosative modifications at the level of proteoglycans could negatively affect glycocalyx integrity.

The loss of the glycocalyx uncovers membrane surface adhesion molecules providing a direct contact area between leukocytes and the endothelium, and thereby potentiating leukocyte adhesion to the vessel wall. It should also be appreciated that degradation of the glycocalyx by inflammatory mediators, and the release of its fragments into the circulation, can significantly contribute to the potentiation of inflammatory processes, starting and maintaining a potentially destructive feedback mechanism. The glycocalyx fragments that have been shed, which may be released after glycocalyx damage, are suggested to act as pro-inflammatory molecules with significant chemotactic properties.[27]

How to assess glycocalyx in patients

Visualization of the glycocalyx is no easy task. Recent advances in staining techiques and advanced electron microscopy techniques (serial block face scanning electron microscopy [SBF], focused ion beam milling scanning electron microscopy [FIB-SEM], transmission electron tomography [Tom-TEM]) have made a better analysis of the glycocalyx under experimental conditions possible.[6,7] However, to analyze the glycocalyx in patients is still a challenge. Basically two approaches are feasible. One can either try to visualize the glycocalyx by determining the area between the capillary wall and circulating blood cells in capillaries,[6,28,29] or one can measure the constituents of the glycocalyx in the bloodstream, assuming that an increase in glycocalyx components such as hyaluronan or syndecan reflect damge to the glycocalyx in patients.[30,31] Both methods have been used by several groups.

The first method to measure glycocalyx health *in vivo* is intravital microscopy utilizing the property of the endothelial glycocalyx to function as a barrier to maintain a certain distance between red blood cells and the endothelial cell membrane.[6,28,29] The method measures these features in sublingual capillaries and depends on the hypothesis that impaired glycocalyx barrier properties in the sublingual microcirculation are associated with changes in microvascular perfusion capacity in other vascular beds (Figure 11.3). The camera uses green light-emitting diodes (LED; 540 nm) to detect the hemoglobin of passing red blood cells. To determine the spatio-temporal variation in radial displacement of individual red blood cells into the endothelial glycocalyx in microvessels, sidestream dark field (SDF) imaging is used.

SDF imaging is a non-invasive technique which visualizes hemoglobin within the red blood cells by reflected LED light from the microvasculature. With this technique, it has been shown that the red blood cells with a diameter of 7 to 8 µm maintain a certain distance from the endothelium of capillaries (diameter of 5 µm), and this was postulated to be due to the barrier function of the glycocalyx against the red blood cells. Using software which automatically identifies all available measurable microvessels (below 30 µm thickness) during the acquisition by contrast between the red blood cells and the background, the longitudinal and radial distribution of red blood cells in sublingual microvessels could be measured, and information about the *in vivo* endothelial glycocalyx barrier properties in humans can be obtained. This method has recently been tested in various patient groups with cardiovascular disease or risk factors, such as end-stage renal disease, stroke, premature coronary artery disease, and critically ill patients (septic and non-septic). It could be shown that a perturbed glycocalyx allowed the erythrocytes to penetrate deeper towards the endothelium, resulting in an increase in the perfused boundary region.[6]

The second method to assess glycocalyx in patients is measuring circulating, "shed" constituents of the glycocalyx.[30,31] Several markers of "glycocalyx

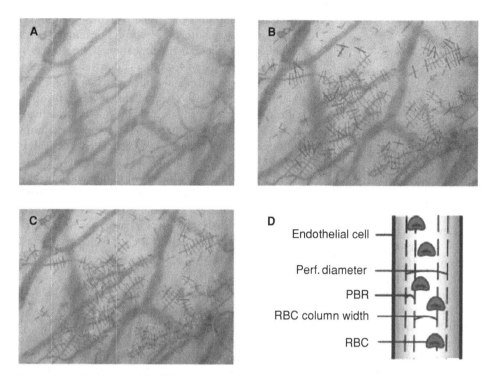

Figure 11.3 Sidestream dark field (SDF) imaging and data assessment in sublingual microvessels. **A**: Typical example of a single SDF image of the sublingual capillary bed. **B, C**: During each period a large number of capillaries are assessed. **D**: Cartoon depicting the median RBC column width, perfused diameter, and the PBR in a blood vessel. PBR, perfused boundary region; RBC, red blood cell.

degradation" such as syndecan-1, thrombomodulin, von Willebrand factor, intercellular adhesion molecule-1, E-selectin, protein C, tissue factor pathway inhibitor (TFPI), tissue-type plasminogen activator (tPA), urokinase-type plasminogen activator (uPA), soluble uPA receptor, and plasminogen activator inhibitor-1 have been used.[31–34]

In trauma patients, Rahbar *et al.* demonstrated that high levels of circulating syndecan-1, as a marker of endothelial glycocalyx degradation, was associated with inflammation, coagulopathy, and increased mortality.[32] In patients with sepsis, levels of interleukin-6(IL-6) correlated with circulating syndecan-1 levels.[34] After major abdominal surgery, glycocalyx markers in human plasma were found to be at levels comparable to those of patients with sepsis. Several groups have used hyaluronan as a measure of glycocalyx breakdown and have found that hyaluronan levels were increased in chronic disease, such as in diabetes, as well as in acutely ill patients.[32] Measurement of syndecan-1 and/or serum hyaluronan may therefore supplement the assessment of disease severity in patients. It has also been suggested, as described above, that these breakdown products might have implications in the pathogenesis of critical illness and sepsis.

Recently, Schmidt *et al.* have refined this diagnostic approach by using a novel methodology for the analysis of glycosaminoglycan-derived disaccharides.[31] This method is based on specific polysaccharide digestion and labeling of the disaccharides, followed by mass spectroscopy detection. Using this method they could show that circulating heparan sulfate fragments were significantly elevated in patients with indirect lung injury, while circulating hyaluronic acid concentrations were elevated in patients with direct lung injury. They concluded that circulating glycosaminoglycans are elevated in patterns characteristic of the etiology of respiratory failure and may serve as diagnostic and/or prognostic biomarkers of critical illness.

It is uncertain which of these methods reflects the true state of the glycocalyx, and this needs to be shown in other studies. Interestingly, the elevations in circulating glycosaminoglycans persisted for several days after the onset of respiratory failure in the last study. Time course and differences in the damage to the glycocalyx as well as possible repair has yet to be analyzed.

Glycocalyx in disease

Sepsis and surgery

Several studies have investigated the deterioration of the vascular glycocalyx in patients with sepsis or after major abdominal surgery, and compared these findings with healthy volunteers.[35,36] Within these, it has been demonstrated that in patients either with severe sepsis or after major abdominal surgery, the plasma concentrations of glycocalyx markers (syndecan-1, heparan sulfate) increased by the same extent. This implies that under both situations, the glycocalyx is shed off the endothelium.

In sepsis, the glycocalyx marker syndecan-1 correlates with concentrations of inflammatory markers (intercellular adhesion molecule-1 [ICAM-1], vascular cell adhesion molecule-1 [VCAM-1], and mainly with IL-6), which were significantly higher than after abdominal surgery.[33] During sepsis and after abdominal surgery, the plasma leaks out into the interstitial space, and this has great impact on the development of edema and impaired oxygen and nutrient supply to tissues. The deterioration of the endothelial glycocalyx seems to be one of the earliest steps within this scenario that triggers the loss of endothelial barrier function. The degradation of the glycocalyx during sepsis and major abdominal surgery has a great impact on fluid balance and the development of edema.[35,37] However, so far, no methods exist to evaluate endothelial dysfunction and vascular leakage during sepsis and during the postoperative period; therefore, diagnosis of fluid distribution during these scenarios is very difficult. The findings of Steppan *et al.* that the glycocalyx is damaged during major abdominal surgery and sepsis can explain the large fluid shifts into the interstitial space.[30] During impaired endothelial barrier function, colloidal solutions also distribute into the interstitial space and can aggravate edema. Monitoring of glycocalyx compounds in the bloodstream might be employed for longer periods in order to determine further endothelial barrier damage or amelioration of endothelial function. This will possibly reduce vascular leaking, with its fateful impact on organ functions, and improve the outcome of patients after abdominal surgery and sepsis.

An important role of the glycocalyx in sepsis has been demonstrated by Schmidt *et al.* in an animal model of TNF-α-induced sepsis and lung injury.[38] They tested the hypothesis that sepsis-associated lung injury is initiated by degradation of the pulmonary endothelial glycocalyx, leading to neutrophil adherence and inflammation. Using intravital microscopy, they found that endotoxemia in mice rapidly induced pulmonary microvascular glycocalyx degradation. Glycocalyx degradation involved the specific loss of heparan sulfate and coincided with activation of the endothelial heparanase. Heparanase inhibition prevented endotoxemia-associated glycocalyx loss and neutrophil adhesion and, accordingly, attenuated sepsis-induced acute lung injury and mortality in mice. These findings are in an experimental model. Nonetheless they demonstrate how powerful a "glycocalyx-based" therapeutic strategy can be in a disease that is often deleterious and for which few therapeutic options exist.

References

1. Pries AR, Secomb TW, Gaehtgens P. The endothelial surface layer. *Pflugers Arch* 2000; 440: 653–66.

2. Reitsma S, Slaaf DW, Vink H, van Zandvoort MA, oude Egbrink MG. The endothelial glycocalyx: composition, functions, and visualization. *Pflugers Arch* 2007; 454: 345–59.

3. Haraldsson B, Nyström J, Deen WM. Properties of the glomerular barrier and mechanisms of proteinuria. *Physiol Rev* 2008; 88: 451–87.

4. Danielli JF. Capillary permeability and edema in the perfused frog. *J Physiol (London)* 1940; 98: 109–29.

5. Weinbaum S, Tarbell JM, Damiano ER. The structure and function of the endothelial glycocalyx layer. *Annu Rev Biomed Eng* 2007; 9: 121–67.

6. Dane MJ, van den Berg BM, Lee DH, *et al.* A microscopic view on the renal endothelial glycocalyx. *Am J Physiol Renal Physiol* 2015; 308: F956–66.

7. Arkill KP, Qvortrup K, Starborg T, *et al.* Resolution of the three dimensional structure of components of the glomerular filtration barrier. *BMC Nephrol* 2014; 15: 24.

8. Salmon AH, Satchell SC. Endothelial glycocalyx dysfunction in disease: albuminuria and increased microvascular permeability. *J Pathol* 2012; 226: 562–74.

9. Satchell S. The role of the glomerular endothelium in albumin handling. *Nat Rev Nephrol* 2013; 9: 717–25.

10. Chappell D, Jacob M. Role of the glycocalyx in fluid management: small things matter. *Best Pract Res Clin Anaesthesiol* 2014; 28: 227–34.

11. Garsen M, Rops AL, Rabelink TJ, Berden JH, van der Vlag J. The role of heparanase and the endothelial

glycocalyx in the development of proteinuria. *Nephrol Dial Transplant* 2014; 29: 49–55.

12. Salmon AH, Neal CR, Sage LM, *et al.* Angiopoietin-1 alters microvascular permeability coefficients *in vivo* via modification of endothelial glycocalyx. *Cardiovasc Res* 2009; 83: 24–33.

13. Tarbell JM, Simon SI, Curry FR. Mechanosensing at the vascular interface. *Annu Rev Biomed Eng* 2014; 16: 505–32.

14. Desjardins C, Duling BR. Heparinase treatment suggests a role for the endothelial cell glycocalyx in regulation of capillary hematocrit. *Am J Physiol* 1990; 258: H647–54.

15. Fu BM, Tarbell JM. Mechano-sensing and transduction by endothelial surface glycocalyx: composition, structure, and function. *Wiley Interdiscip Rev Syst Biol Med* 2013; 5: 381–90.

16. Ebong EE, Lopez-Quintero SV, Rizzo V, Spray DC, Tarbell JM. Shear-induced endothelial NOS activation and remodeling via heparan sulphate, glypican-1, and syndecan-1. *Integr Biol (Camb)* 2014; 6: 338–47.

17. Yen W, Cai B, Yang J, *et al.* Endothelial surface glycocalyx can regulate flow-induced nitric oxide production in microvessels *in vivo. PLoS One* 2015; 10: e0117133.

18. Oberleithner H. Vascular endothelium: a vulnerable transit zone for merciless sodium. *Nephrol Dial Transplant* 2014; 29: 240–6.

19. Rops AL, Loeven MA, van Gemst JJ, *et al.* Modulation of heparan sulphate in the glomerular endothelial glycocalyx decreases leukocyte influx during experimental glomerulonephritis. *Kidney Int* 2014; 86: 932–42.

20. Rops AL, van den Hoven MJ, Baselmans MM, *et al.* Heparan sulphate domains on cultured activated glomerular endothelial cells mediate leukocyte trafficking. *Kidney Int* 2008; 73: 52–62.

21. Stoler-Barak L, Moussion C, Shezen E, *et al.* Blood vessels pattern heparan sulphate gradients between their apical and basolateral aspects. *PLoS One* 2014; 9: e85699.

22. Proudfoot AE. Chemokines and glycosaminoglycans. *Front Immunol* 2015; 6: 246.

23. Boels MG, Lee DH, van den Berg BM, *et al.* The endothelial glycocalyx as a potential modifier of the hemolytic uremic syndrome. *Eur J Intern Med* 2013; 24: 503–9.

24. Clark SJ, Ridge LA, Herbert AP, *et al.* Tissue-specific host recognition by complement factor H is mediated by differential activities of its glycosaminoglycan-binding regions. *J Immunol* 2013; 190: 2049–57.

25. Goldberg R, Rubinstein AM, Gil N, *et al.* Role of heparanase-driven inflammatory cascade in pathogenesis of diabetic nephropathy. *Diabetes* 2014; 63: 4302–13.

26. Becker BF, Jacob M, Leipert S, Salmon AH, Chappell D. Degradation of the endothelial glycocalyx in clinical settings: searching for the sheddases. *Br J Clin Pharmacol* 2015; 80: 389–402.

27. Goodall KJ, Poon IK, Phipps S, Hulett MD. Soluble heparan sulphate fragments generated by heparanase trigger the release of pro-inflammatory cytokines through TLR-4. *PLoS One* 2014; 9: e109596.

28. Lee DH, Dane MJ, van den Berg BM, *et al.* Deeper penetration of erythrocytes into the endothelial glycocalyx is associated with impaired microvascular perfusion. *PLoS One* 2014; 9: e96477.

29. Dane MJ, Khairoun M, Lee DH, *et al.* Association of kidney function with changes in the endothelial surface layer. *Clin J Am Soc Nephrol* 2014; 9: 698–704.

30. Steppan J, Hofer S, Funke B, *et al.* Sepsis and major abdominal surgery lead to flaking of the endothelial glycocalix. *J Surg Res* 2011; 165: 136–41.

31. Schmidt EP, Li G, Li L, *et al.* The circulating glycosaminoglycan signature of respiratory failure in critically ill adults. *J Biol Chem* 2014; 289: 8194–202.

32. Rahbar E, Cardenas JC, Baimukanova G, *et al.* Endothelial glycocalyx shedding and vascular permeability in severely injured trauma patients. *J Transl Med* 2015; 13: 117.

33. Ostrowski SR, Sørensen AM, Windeløv NA, *et al.* High levels of soluble VEGF receptor 1 early after trauma are associated with shock, sympathoadrenal activation, glycocalyx degradation and inflammation in severely injured patients: a prospective study. *Scand J Trauma Resusc Emerg Med* 2012; 20: 27.

34. Sallisalmi M, Tenhunen J, Yang R, Oksala N, Pettilä V. Vascular adhesion protein-1 and syndecan-1 in septic shock. *Acta Anaesthesiol Scand* 2012; 56: 316–22.

35. Burke-Gaffney A, Evans TW. Lest we forget the endothelial glycocalyx in sepsis. *Crit Care* 2012; 16: 121.

36. Henrich M, Gruss M, Weigand MA. Sepsis-induced degradation of endothelial glycocalix. *Sci World J* 2010; 10: 917–23.

37. Wiesinger A, Peters W, Chappell D, *et al.* Nanomechanics of the endothelial glycocalyx in experimental sepsis. *PLoS One* 2013; 8: e80905.

38. Schmidt EP, Yang Y, Janssen WJ, *et al.* The pulmonary endothelial glycocalyx regulates neutrophil adhesion and lung injury during experimental sepsis. *Nat Med* 2012; 18: 1217–23.

Chapter

12 Monitoring of the microcirculation

Atilla Kara, Şakir Akin, and Can Ince

Summary

Perioperative fluid management requires comprehensive training and an understanding of the physiology of oxygen transport to tissue. Administration of fluids has a limited window of efficacy. Too little fluid reduces organ perfusion and too much fluid causes organ dysfunction from edema. In addition, isotonic saline carries the danger of hyperchloremia, whereas balanced crystalloid solutions are pragmatic choices of fluid in the majority of perioperative resuscitation settings.

The prime aim of fluid therapy is to improve tissue perfusion so as to provide adequate oxygen to the tissues. Macrohemodynamical parameters and/or surrogates of tissue perfusion do not always correspond to microcirculatory functional states, and especially not in states of inflammation. Even when targets for macrohemodynamics are reached, the microcirculation may still remain damaged and dysfunctional.

Observation of the microcirculation in the perioperative setting provides a more physiologically based approach for fluid therapy by possibly avoiding the unnecessary and inappropriate administration of large volumes of fluids.

Hand-held videomicroscopy is able to visualize microcirculatory perfusion sublingually. It can be used to monitor the functional state of the microcirculation by assessment and quantification of sublingual microvascular capillary density, and thus to guide fluid therapy. The Cytocam-IDF device might provide the needed clinical platform because of its improved imaging capacity in terms of density and perfusion parameters as well as providing on-line quantification of the microcirculation.*

Perioperative fluid management is an essential component of successful surgical outcome. It is also a highly controversial issue, with much debate concerning the type and amount of fluids (restrictive versus liberal) and whether the administration of fluids should be guided by hemodynamic goals.[1,2] Although the debate is ongoing, the major factor that determines the type and amount of fluid is the preference of the practitioner. A retrospective observational study on intraoperative fluid therapy practiced at two US medical centers, on 5,912 patients undergoing different types of abdominal surgery, found considerable variability in the amounts of crystalloid solutions being administered, with the average infusion rate being 7.1 (SD 4.9) ml/kg per hour at both institutions. In addition, this study confirmed that by far the most important predictor of the amount of fluid being administered was the individual anesthetist.[3]

The aim of fluid therapy during surgery is to ensure normal hemodynamics, with the main purpose of providing adequate perfusion and oxygenation to the tissue cells by replacing losses of fluid with appropriate fluid types.[4] The physiological basis by which this is achieved can be divided into three parts. The first part concerns the systemic circulation, consisting of blood pressure, cardiac output, and vascular resistance. The second part concerns the peripheral microvasculature, transporting oxygen-carrying red blood cells within each organ. The final pathway of oxygen transport is from the microcirculation to the mitochondria where oxygen is utilized by the respiratory chain. Summarized, there are two main determinants of oxygen

---

* Summary compiled by the Editor.

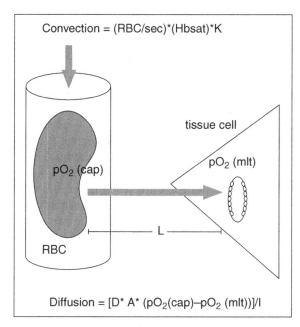

Convection = (RBC/sec)*(Hbsat)*K

tissue cell

pO_2 (cap)

pO_2 (mlt)

L

RBC

Diffusion = [D* A* (pO_2(cap)–pO_2 (mlt))]/l

Figure 12.1 The convective and diffusive determinants of oxygen transport from the microcirculation to the tissue cell. The convective flow is defined by the product of the oxygen-carrying saturation (Hbsat, in %) of the red blood cells (RBC), the rate at which red blood cells enter the capillary (RBC/sec), and the oxygen-carrying capacity of a RBC at 100% saturation ($K = 0.0362$ picoliters O_2/RBC). The diffusive movement of oxygen from the RBC to the mitochondria is defined by Fick's law of diffusion where the flux of oxygen shown above is the product of the oxygen gradient from RBC to mitochondria and the diffusion distance D times the exchange surface area (A), divided by the diffusion distance (l) from the RBC to the mitochondria.

transport to tissue, the first being convective transport of oxygen-carrying red blood cells to the capillaries, and the second the passive diffusion of oxygen leaving the red blood cells to the respiring mitochondria to achieve ATP production by oxidative phosphorylation (Figure 12.1).

Hemodynamic targets are conventionally aimed at the promotion of convective flow, on the assumption that hypovolemia is mainly associated with decreased blood flow. In daily practice, when hypovolemia and tissue hypoperfusion is suspected, fluids are given with the expectation that tissue perfusion and oxygenation will be restored. For this purpose, clinicians use various systemic hemodynamic parameters, such as heart rate, venous pressure, blood pressure, cardiac output, stroke volume variation, and pulse pressure variation to guide the amount of administered fluid. Recent randomized controlled trials suggest that goal-directed therapy aimed at optimizing systemic oxygen

transport fails to improve survival.[5,6] Hence, simply correcting global systemic variables is ineffective in promoting microcirculatory and tissue oxygen perfusion. Pottecher and co-workers observed that changes in cardiac output and microvascular variables after fluid administration did not follow each other, suggesting that mechanisms other than changes in cardiac output may affect the microvascular perfusion.[7] Ospina-Tascon *et al.* [8] and Pranskunas *et al.* [9] reported similar results when analyzing simultaneously systemic and microcirculatory effects of fluid administration. Both studies showed that improvement of microcirculatory perfusion was not coherently related to increases in cardiac output. Similar results were reported by Silva and co-workers when using gastric mucosal pCO_2 as a surrogate for tissue perfusion.[10] De Backer *et al.* reported that the relation between systemic hemodynamics and the microcirculation is not fixed, even though cardiac output and blood pressure values may be within normal ranges.[11]

This shows that apparent adequate systemic hemodynamics may be accompanied by derangements in the microcirculation. The persistence of such a condition has been shown to be related to adverse outcome, especially in sepsis.[11] These studies suggest that organ function is more directly related to the success of perfusion and oxygenation of the microcirculation than simply the restoration of systemic hemodynamic variables. Achievement of good microcirculatory function can, in this context, be considered to be the primary target of cardiovascular resuscitation.

Administrating fluids to hypovolemic patients with the aim of achieving an increase in global flow by optimizing systemic hemodynamics can actually result in a decrease of oxygen availability at the cellular level, owing to several mechanisms. Firstly, important reductions in the oxygen-carrying capacity of blood due to hemodilution can cause a decrease in oxygen availability to the parenchymal cells. A second condition might occur in the presence of capillary leak. Tissue edema occurring in this manner can be aggravated when fluids are infused, greatly worsening the diffusive component of the oxygen transport to the tissue cells. A third condition is when fluid administration targeting elevated central venous pressure results in impaired microcirculatory blood flow because of venous tamponade.[12] This detrimental effect might be amplified when using fluid therapy strategies targeting raised venous pressures, as currently recommended in some international guidelines.[13] A fourth condition can be caused by heterogeneous microcirculatory blood flow alterations due, for example, to endothelial and red blood cell dysfunction and leukocyte activation as occurs in sepsis; this can result in the shunting of microcirculatory weak units and lead to regional tissue hypoxia.[14]

These issues indicate that the effects of fluid administration are indeed complex, and that improvement of the macrocirculatory perfusion does not necessarily result in a coherent optimization of the microcirculation. From a physiological point of view, the integration of microcirculatory parameters to hemodynamic monitoring would provide a helpful complement to conventional systemic hemodynamic monitoring. This could allow us to optimize tissue perfusion and to identify conditions where there is a loss of hemodynamic coherence between systemic and microcirculatory determinants of oxygen delivery during resuscitation. To this end, a functional microcirculatory approach has been proposed to optimize fluid administration based on the concept of microcirculatory fluid-responsiveness balancing convective flow to diffusive microcirculatory capacity with the aim of achieving optimal oxygen transport to the cells.[4]

The microcirculation consists of a complex network of small blood vessels (<100 μm diameter) such as arterioles (responsible for modulating local arterial tone to match local metabolic demands), capillaries (acting as the primary exchange place for supplying oxygen and transporting metabolic cell waste products), and the outflow venules (where leukocyte interactions take place and vascular permeability changes largely take place). This complex system consists of different cell types such as endothelial cells inside microvessels, smooth muscle cells (mostly in arterioles), red blood cells, leukocytes, and plasma components in blood. These cellular systems interact with each other and are regulated by different complex mechanisms to optimize microcirculatory perfusion with the aim of providing adequate oxygen transport to the tissue cells.[15]

Microvascular perfusion can be monitored directly by various methods. It can be evaluated indirectly by indices of tissue perfusion and oxygenation such as skin mottling/capillary refill time, mixed-venous and central-venous O_2 saturation, lactate, laser Doppler, tissue pCO_2, and near infrared spectroscopy.[16] Direct monitoring of the microcirculation can be accomplished by hand-held videomicroscopy.

Several systems have been introduced. The first such device clinically introduced by us was orthogonal polarizing spectral (OPS) imaging, followed by its technical successor sidestream dark field (SDF) imaging. These first and second generations require video capture and storage of movies followed by off-line analysis of images to quantify abnormalities.[17,18] These devices emit green light with a wavelength (530 nm) which is absorbed by hemoglobin, thereby identifying erythrocytes as dark moving cells through the microcirculation. The area of visualization is about 1 mm^2.[19] Software-assisted analysis can be used to give several indices related to microcirculatory function. These include the microvascular flow index (MFI), providing information about convective flow of blood, functional capillary density (FCD; that portion of functional capillaries in which there is flow), and proportion of perfused vessels (PPV), which provides information on diffusion distance of oxygen from the capillary vessels to the tissue cells.[20,21]

The use of hand-held vital microscopy has gone through a number of technological developments with the ultimate aim of introducing these devices for routine clinical use. A third-generation device has recently been introduced, called Cytocam incident dark field (IDF) imaging, based on a computer-controlled imaging sensor which allows automatic quantification of images. This development has been made possible by a new hardware platform, consisting of a high-density pixel imaging sensor illuminated by short green light-emitting diode (LED) pulses. Computer-controlled synchronization of illumination and image acquisition allows semi-automatic image analysis. The device is a pen-like probe incorporating IDF illumination with a set of high-resolution microscope lenses projecting images on to the image sensor. The probe is covered by a sterilizable cap.

Cytocam-IDF imaging is based on IDF, a principle originally introduced by Sherman *et al.*[22] The recent study by Aykut *et al.* validated this device and showed that 30% more capillaries could be visualized with Cytocam-IDF imaging than with its predecessors.[23] Now that it has been validated, Cytocam-IDF imaging may provide a new improved imaging modality fit for routine use for clinical assessment of microcirculatory alterations in patients.[23] Results obtained from hand-held videomicroscopy has contributed to the understanding that microvascular dysfunction can occur despite optimization of systemic hemodynamic parameters. Several studies have in addition shown that the persistence of such microcirculatory alterations is associated with postoperative complications, increased length of ventilation, and even increased mortality.[24–26]

Besides the correct physiological compartment being targeted when monitoring the effects of fluid therapy, the composition of the type of fluid is also an essential component for optimizing fluid therapy. The chloride content of normal saline is 154 mmol/l, which is much higher than that found in plasma (101 to 110 mmol/l) and also higher than in the so-called balanced solutions such as (modified) Ringer's or Hartmann's solution which contain other anions than chloride (for instance, bicarbonate precursors such as lactate, acetate, or gluconate).[27] The difference in chloride concentrations accounts for strong ion difference of these latter solutions, which is closer to the value of plasma (-42 mEq/l). For this reason administration of balanced salt solutions causes less dilution acidosis than does administration of saline.

Saline, however, is still by far the most commonly used fluid for resuscitation. It has the lowest price of all fluids, is relatively safe, and clinicians have an extended experience with its use at the bedside. In a recent trial on the association between saline and postoperative complications associated with hyperchloremic acidosis, McCluskey et al. [28] found that about 35,000 liters of crystalloid solution was used at their institution per year, of which more than 55% was saline. Ince et al. [29] reported that 11,800 liters of saline was used for resuscitation during 12,857 treatment days in their 36-bed mixed intensive care department in 2012, in comparison to 1,630 liters of Ringer's lactate (RL), the only balanced crystalloid solution used in their department. Unfortunately, over the past decade, evidence is accumulating concerning the deleterious effects of saline. One of the most important problems is thought to be the high chloride content of saline, resulting in hyperchloremic dilutional acidosis.[30]

Hyperchloremia has been shown to be the cause of various adverse effects including afferent renal arterial vasoconstriction in animal models and in volunteers, possibly contributing to kidney dysfunction.[31,32] Three separate studies in pigs comparing 0.9% saline with RL after 30 min of uncontrolled hemorrhage have been described.[33–35] All showed that 0.9% saline required significantly greater volumes to reach hemodynamic targets than RL (256 ± 145 ml/kg saline vs. 126 ± 67 ml/kg RL, $p < 0.04$).[35] Hyperchloremic acidosis and dilutional coagulopathy were also found with saline.[35] Hypercoagulability and low blood loss were noted with RL.[33] Extravascular lung water index increased with both fluid types, but this occurred earlier and to a greater degree in the saline group.[34] In a hemodilution study in pigs comparing colloids (0.6% hydroxyethyl starch [HES]) with crystalloids, using hematocrit as a target for hemodilution, Konrad et al. [36] showed that much less colloid than crystalloid was required to reach similar targets, demonstrating the effectiveness of colloids for volume expansion. Similarly in a rat hemorrhagic shock study, where blood pressure was targeted as a resuscitation endpoint, much less of a balanced crystalloid solution was required to reach target in comparison with the unbalanced crystalloid solution.[37]

In 30 patients undergoing major surgery, randomized to receive either 0.9% saline or Plasma-Lyte 148 at 15 ml/kg per hour, those receiving saline had significantly increased chloride concentrations ($\Delta[\text{Cl}^-]$ $+6.9$ vs. $+0.6$ mmol/l, $p < 0.01$), decreased bicarbonate concentrations ($\Delta[\text{HCO}_3^-]$ -4.0 vs. -0.7 mmol/l, $p < 0.01$), compared with those receiving Plasma-Lyte 148.[38] There are two randomized controlled double-blind trials ($n = 66$ and $n = 51$) comparing 0.9% saline with RL in the perioperative period, with both showing that the use of 0.9% saline resulted in more adverse events than RL.[39,40] In patients undergoing abdominal aortic aneurysm repair, those receiving saline needed significantly greater volumes of packed red blood cells (780 vs. 560 ml), platelets (392 vs. 223 ml), and bicarbonate therapy (30 vs. 4 ml) than those receiving RL.[39] Hyperchloremic acidosis was found in the saline group, but this did not result in a difference in outcome.[39]

Recent large observational studies [28, 41–43] have suggested that the high chloride content of 0.9% saline may cause adverse events, especially when renal outcomes are considered. Assessment of outcomes in a propensity-matched study of 2,788 adults undergoing major open abdominal surgery who received only 0.9% saline, and in 926 patients who received only a balanced crystalloid on the day of surgery, showed that unadjusted in-hospital mortality (5.6 vs. 2.9%) and the percentage of patients developing complications (33.7 vs. 23%) were significantly greater ($p < 0.01$) in those receiving 0.9% saline than in those receiving the balanced crystalloid.[41] Although mortality in the saline group remained higher after correction for confounding variables, the difference ceased to be significant. Patients in the 0.9% saline group also received an average of 316 ml more fluid ($p < 0.001$), had a greater need for blood transfusion (odds ratio [95% CI]: 11.5 [10.3 to 12.7] vs. 1.8 [1.2 to 2.9]%, $p < 0.001$), and had more infectious complications ($p < 0.001$), and were 4.8 times more likely to require dialysis ($p < 0.001$) than those in the balanced crystalloid group. Overall complications were fewer in the balanced crystalloid group (odds ratio [95% CI]: 0.79 [0.66 to 0.97]).

Another study on 22,851 surgical patients with normal preoperative serum chloride concentration and renal function showed that 22% incidence of acute postoperative hyperchloremia.[28] Of the 4,955 patients with hyperchloremia after surgery, 4,266 (85%) patients were propensity matched with an equal number of patients who had normochloremia postoperatively. Patients with hyperchloremia were at increased risk of 30-day postoperative mortality (3.0 vs. 1.9%; odds ratio [95% CI]: 1.58 [1.25 to 1.98]) and had a longer median hospital stay (7.0 days [interquartile range 4.1–12.3] vs. 6.3 days [interquartile range 4.0–11.3], $p < 0.01$) than those with normal postoperative serum chloride concentrations.[28] Patients with postoperative hyperchloremia were also more likely to have postoperative renal dysfunction as defined by a 25% decrease in glomerular filtration rate (12.9 vs. 9.2%, $p < 0.01$). All these studies have shown that hyperchloremic acidosis is not a benign, self-limiting metabolic disturbance. It can be stated that 0.9% saline is neither "normal" nor "physiological" and that its high chloride content can lead to many pathophysiological changes, especially in renal function. These negative changes were not seen after infusion of balanced crystalloids.

A further topic of controversy concerns the effect of balanced and unbalanced solutions on immune suppression and modulation of coagulation.[27] It has been assumed that normal, unbalanced saline has proinflammatory properties relating to neutrophil activation.[44,45] This could contribute to detrimental effects in trauma and sepsis resuscitation. Balanced solutions such as RL may also be proinflammatory, although it has been shown that the D-lactate form was responsible for such effects.[45,46] Nevertheless, on the basis of current literature there is adequate evidence to suggest that the effects of balanced crystalloids are less detrimental than those of 0.9% saline, especially in relation to renal function.

Although balanced solutions have some advantages over 0.9% saline, normal saline is a better choice of fluid than RL in certain clinical scenarios such as brain injury where its isotonicity is of benefit.[47,48] A subset analysis of the SAFE trial showed the superiority of saline over albumin for brain injury patients where the hypo-osmolality of the albumin solutions was thought to contribute to increased intracranial pressures.[49] The plasma osmolality of the albumin used in that study was in the range of 280–300 mosmol/kg H_2O whereas saline osmolality is 286 mosmol/kg H_2O, which can be considered isotonic. RL, on the other hand, is hypo-osmolar (257 mosmol/kg H_2O) and can potentially promote tissue edema and cause cells to swell, especially in conditions where there is a damaged vascular endothelial barrier such as can occur in brain injury.[50] However, Roquilly et al., who used a balanced solution in head injury patients, found that its use was comparable to 0.9% saline, with patients showing no difference in intracranial pressure increases following fluid therapy.[51] Finally, some of the acetate-based solutions contain calcium, which is contraindicated for blood tranfusions where blood has been preserved in citrate-based solutions.[52]

The most important impact of fluid therapy is determined by the amount of fluid administered.[4] Although fluid therapy is essential in the treatment of hypovolemia and tissue hypoperfusion, overhydration and a positive fluid balance are considered harmful and contribute to organ dysfunction.[4,53–56] Fluids dilute blood and can decrease its oxygen-delivering capacity. Less than 3% of oxygen transported by blood is dissolved in plasma and fluids. Fluids transport hardly any oxygen in themselves and are only effective in promoting blood flow. This means that fluid therapy has a limited window of efficacy: excess fluids cause a reduction in the oxygen-carrying capacity of blood by causing too much hemodilution while having limited effects on cardiac output and microcirculatory blood flow.[4,36,57,58] In a clinical study, Arikan et al. showed that fluid overload causes a reduction in the oxygenation index associated with adverse outcomes in pediatric patients.[59] Crystalloid fluids can decrease mortality in hypovolemic patients, but optimal type and dose of fluids remain to be defined.

Colloids have three- to four-fold greater plasma volume-expanding and hemodynamic effects compared with crystalloids and are the fluid of choice when volume expansion is indicated as a result of hypovolemia.[60–63] The Colloids versus Crystalloids for the Resuscitation of the Critically Ill (CRISTAL) trial was designed to compare colloids and crystalloids in need of volume expansion due to hypovolemia. The trial included 1,443 patients in the crystalloid group and 1,414 patients in the colloid group. Hypovolemic shock was the primary diagnosis in each group. The trial showed that the use of colloids vs. crystalloids did not result in a significant difference in 28-day mortality, although 90-day mortality was lower among patients in the colloid group. Additionally, no evidence of an increased risk of renal replacement therapy was detected in the colloid group.[64] Another study, Crystalloid versus Hydroxyethyl Starch Trial (CHEST), involved 7,000 adults in the ICU. In that study, the use of 6% HES (130/0.4), as compared with saline, was not associated with a significant difference in 90-day mortality (relative risk, 1.06; 95% CI, 0.96 to 1.18; $P = 0.26$). Although not an endpoint, the use of HES was associated with a slight increase in the rate of renal replacement therapy in a subset of the initial included patient group. However, there was a lower vasopressor requirement for the patients with HES.[65] Even though starches have been brought into disrepute in two large randomized control trial studies (the CHEST and 6S trials), it is important to realize that these colloid fluids were administered to patients who were not hypovolemic and in need of volume expansion, and their results should be interpreted with reservation. Indeed, in the CRISTAL trial where patients were truly hypovolemic and in need of volume expansion, colloid, of which the majority was starches, resulted in an outcome benefit. In a microcirculation trial in septic shock patients, Edul and coworkers compared 6% HES 130/0.4 to saline solution targeting mean arterial pressure. They found that fluid resuscitation with 6% HES 130/0.4 needed less volume than saline solution to normalize sublingual microcirculation.[66]

Atasever et al. [67] compared red blood cell transfusion to gelatin solutions and to no infusion after cardiac surgery, and studied the effect on microvascular perfusion, vascular density, hemoglobin, and oxygen saturation. They found no difference in changes in systemic delivery O_2, O_2 uptake, and extraction between the groups. Relative to gelatin or control, however, red blood cell transfusion increased perfused microcirculatory vessel density, hemoglobin content, and saturation in the microcirculation, while microcirculatory blood flow remained unchanged. Restricted fluid policy (usually defined as <7 ml/kg per hour), on the other hand, has been suggested in randomized studies in surgical patients to result in fewer complications than standard or more liberal fluid strategy, regardless of the type of solution used.[53–55,68–71] From this point of view, colloid administration offers advantages since less volume is needed, although care should be taken to protect vulnerable organs such as the kidney.

Microcirculatory-guided fluid resuscitation would provide a more physiologically based approach and possibly avoid fluid overload.[4] Targeting the microcirculation in this way may provide an important complement to targeting systemic hemodynamic variables. Functional microcirculatory hemodynamics (FMH), in parallel to the concepts underlying functional hemodynamics, may provide a new approach because observing the microcirculation allows verification of whether administration of fluids is successful in promoting convective flow. It can also establish the presence of microcirculatory fluid responsiveness.[4,7,9] The conceptual framework underlying FMH for optimal administration of fluids, introduced by Ince [4], is shown in Figure 12.2. The diagram is adapted from the work by Bellamy [72] and Peng and Kellum [73] who demonstrated the dilemma over how to decide the optimal volume of fluid to be administered to a specific patient. Shown on the x-axis of Figure 12.2 is the amount of fluid administered, and on the y-axis the risk of developing complications. This figure illustrates that in states of hypovolemia both too little and too much fluid are associated with clinical complications. In the concept of FMH, position A in Figure 12.2 is defined as true hypovolemia where, in the presence of clinical signs of hypovolemia, there is slow microcirculatory convective flow. This situation in FMH indicates the need for fluid administration.

Microcirculatory fluid responsiveness is the observation that convective microcirculatory blood flow increases as a result of fluid administration and signals the success of fluid therapy. This view also means that, despite the presence of clinical symptoms of hypoperfusion, if normal microcirculatory flow is observed, then there is no physiological rationale for administering fluids.[9] The optimal fluid volume is defined as that needed to achieve normalized convective flow with an optimal density of perfused capillaries (position B in Figure 12.2).[4] If too much fluid is given, then a loss of FCD is measured and the transport of oxygen to the cells is compromised. Such a condition is signaled by a reduction in FCD accompanied by an

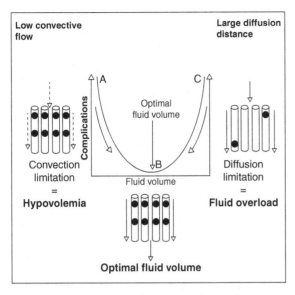

FIGURE 12.2 The conceptual framework of functional microcirculatory hemodynamics. The relation is shown between fluid volume administration on the x-axis and the chances of developing clinical complication on the y-axis (adapted from [72] and [73]). The left side of the diagram indicates hypovolemia, where position A defines the condition in which clinical indicators of organ hypoperfusion coincide with reduced convection, indicating the need for fluid administration. Microcirculatory fluid responsiveness is indicated by improvement in flow (from A to B). Optimal convection and optimal diffusion (conserved FCD) define the optimal amount of fluid volume administration shown in position B. A diffusive limitation, which signals that too much fluid has been administrated, develops as a result of prolonged diffusion distance when RBC-filled capillaries are lost.

increase in the distances between red-blood-cell-filled capillaries and indicates the development of diffusion limitation, shown by position C in Figure 12.2. Thus, observation of a loss of FCD during fluid therapy indicates that enough fluid has been administered. A conservative strategy is then advised.

References

1. Bundgaard-Nielsen M, Secher NH, Kehlet H. 'Liberal' vs. 'restrictive' perioperative fluid therapy – a critical assessment of the evidence. *Acta Anaesthesiol Scand* 2009; 53: 843–51.

2. Chappell D, Jacob M, Hofmann-Kiefer K, Conzen P, Rehm M. A rational approach to perioperative fluid management. *Anesthesiology* 2008; 109: 723–40.

3. Lilot M, Ehrenfeld JM, Lee C, *et al.* Variability in practice and factors predictive of total crystalloid administration during abdominal surgery: a retrospective two-center analysis. *Br J Anaesth* 2015; 114: 767–76.

4. Ince C. The rationale for microcirculatory-guided fluid therapy. *Curr Opin Crit Care* 2014; 20: 301–8.

5. Yealy DM, Kellum JA, Huang DT, *et al.* A randomized trial of protocol-based care for early septic shock. *N Engl J Med* 2014; 370: 1683–93.

6. Pearse RM, Harrison DA, MacDonald N, *et al.* Effect of a perioperative, cardiac output-guided hemodynamic therapy algorithm on outcomes following major gastrointestinal surgery: a randomized clinical trial and systematic review. *JAMA* 2014; 311: 2181–90.

7. Pottecher J, Deruddre S, Teboul JL, *et al.* Both passive leg raising and intravascular volume expansion improve sublingual microcirculatory perfusion in severe sepsis and septic shock patients. *Intensive Care Med* 2010; 36: 1867–74.

8. Ospina-Tascon G, Neves AP, Occhipinti G, *et al.* Effects of fluids on microvascular perfusion in patients with severe sepsis. *Intensive Care Med* 2010; 36: 949–55.

9. Pranskunas A, Koopmans M, Koetsier PM, *et al.* Microcirculatory blood flow as a tool to select ICU patients eligible for fluid therapy. *Intensive Care Med* 2013; 39: 612–19.

10. Silva E, De Backer D, Creteur J, Vincent JL. Effects of fluid challenge on gastric mucosal pCO_2 in septic patients. *Intensive Care Med* 2004; 30: 423–9.

11. De Backer D, Ortiz JA, Salgado D. Coupling microcirculation to systemic hemodynamics. *Curr Opin Crit Care* 2010; 16: 250–4.

12. Vellinga NAR, Ince C, Boerma EC. Elevated central venous pressure is associated with impairment of microcirculatory blood flow in sepsis: a hypothesis generating post hoc analysis. *BMC Anesthesiol* 2013; 13: 17.

13. Dellinger RP, Levy MM, Rhodes A, *et al.* The Surviving Sepsis Campaign Guidelines Committee including The Pediatric Subgroup. Surviving Sepsis Campaign: international guidelines for management of severe sepsis and septic shock, 2012. *Intensive Care Med* 2013; 39: 165–228.

14. Ince C, Sinaasappel M. Microcirculatory oxygenation and shunting in sepsis and shock. *Crit Care Med* 1999; 27: 1369–77.

15. Gruartmoner G, Mesquida J, Ince C. How can we monitor microcirculation in sepsis? Does it improve outcome? In: Deutschman CS, Neligan PJ, eds. *Evidence-Based Practice of Critical Care*. 2nd edn. Philadelphia: Saunders, 2010: 291–6.

16. De Backer D, Ospina-Tascon G, Salgado D, *et al.* Monitoring the microcirculation in the critically ill patient: current methods and future approaches. *Intensive Care Med* 2010; 36: 1813–25.

17. Arnold RC, Parrillo JE, Dellinger RP, *et al.* Point-of-care assessment of microvascular blood flow in critically ill patients. *Intensive Care Med* 2009; 35: 1761–6.

18. Goedhart PT, Khalilzada M, Bezemer R, *et al.* Sidestream dark field (SDF) imaging: a novel stroboscopic LED ring-based imaging modality for clinical assessment of the microcirculation. *Optics Express* 2007; 15: 15101–14.

19. Groner W, Winkelman JW, Harris AG, *et al.* Orthogonal polarization spectral imaging: a new method for study of the microcirculation. *Nat Med* 1999; 5: 1209–12.

20. De Backer D, Hollenberg S, Boerma C, *et al.* How to evaluate the microcirculation: report of a round table conference. *Crit Care* 2007; 11: R101.

21. Boerma EC, Mathura KR, van der Voort PHJ, *et al.* Quantifying bedside-derived imaging of microcirculatory abnormalities in septic patients: a prospective validation study. *Crit Care* 2005; 9: R601–6.

22. Sherman H, Klausner S, Cook WA. Incident dark-field illumination: a new method for microcirculatory study. *Angiology* 1971; 22: 295–303.

23. Aykut G, Veenstra G, Scorcella C, Ince C, Boerma C. Cytocam-IDF (incident dark field illumination) imaging for bedside monitoring of the micro-circulation. *Intensive Care Med Exp* 2015; 3: 40.

24. Jhanji S, Lee C, Watson D, *et al.* Microvascular flow and tissue oxygenation after major abdominal surgery: association with postoperative complications. *Intensive Care Med* 2009; 35: 671–7.

25. De Backer D, Dubois MJ, Schmartz D, *et al.* Microcirculatory alterations in cardiac surgery: effects of cardiopulmonary bypass and anesthesia. *Ann Thorac Surg* 2009; 88: 1396–403.

26. Karliczek A, Benaron DA, Baas PC, *et al.* Intraoperative assessment of microperfusion with visible light spectroscopy for prediction of anastomotic leakage in colorectal anastomoses. *Colorectal Dis* 2010; 12: 1018–25.

27. Guidet B, Soni N, Della Rocca G, *et al.* A balanced view of balanced solutions. *Crit Care* 2010; 14: 325.

28. McCluskey SA, Karkouti K, Wijeysundera D, *et al.* Hyperchloremia after noncardiac surgery is independently associated with increased morbidity and mortality: a propensity-matched cohort study. *Anesth Analg* 2013; 117: 412–21.

29. Ince C, Groenveld AB. The case for 0.9% NaCl: is the undefendable, defensible? *Kidney Int* 2014; 86: 1087–95.

30. Handy JM, Soni N. Physiological effects of hyperchloraemia and acidosis. *Br J Anaesth* 2008; 101: 141–50.

31. Wilcox CS. Regulation of renal blood flow by plasma chloride. *J Clin Invest* 1983; 71: 726–35.

32. Bullivant EM, Wilcox CS, Welch WJ. Intrarenal vasoconstriction during hyperchloremia: role of thromboxane. *Am J Physiol* 1989; 256: F152–7.

33. Kiraly LN, Differding JA, Enomoto TM, *et al.* Resuscitation with normal saline (NS) vs. lactated Ringers (LR) modulates hypercoagulability and leads to increased blood loss in an uncontrolled hemorrhagic shock swine model. *J Trauma* 2006; 61: 57–64.

34. Phillips CR, Vinecore K, Hagg DS, *et al.* Resuscitation of haemorrhagic shock with normal saline vs. lactated Ringer's: effects on oxygenation, extravascular lung water and haemodynamics. *Crit Care* 2009; 13: R30.

35. Todd SR, Malinoski D, Muller PJ, *et al.* Lactated Ringer's is superior to normal saline in the resuscitation of uncontrolled hemorrhagic shock. *J Trauma* 2007; 62: 636–9.

36. Konrad FM, Mik EG, Bodmer SIA, *et al.* Acute normovolemic hemodilution in the pig is associated with renal tissue edema, impaired renal microvascular oxygenation and functional loss. *Anesthesiology* 2013; 119: 256–69.

37. Aksu U, Bezemer R, Yavuz B, *et al.* Balanced vs. unbalanced crystalloid resuscitation in a near-fatal model of hemorrhagic shock and the effects on renal oxygenation, oxidative stress, and inflammation. *Resuscitation* 2012; 83: 767–73.

38. McFarlane C, Lee A. A comparison of Plasmalyte 148 and 0.9% saline for intra-operative fluid replacement. *Anaesthesia* 1994; 49: 779–81.

39. Waters JH, Gottlieb A, Schoenwald P, *et al.* Normal saline versus lactated Ringer's solution for intraoperative fluid management in patients undergoing abdominal aortic aneurysm repair: an outcome study. *Anesth Analg* 2001; 93: 817–22.

40. O'Malley CM, Frumento RJ, Hardy MA, *et al.* A randomized, double-blind comparison of lactated Ringer's solution and 0.9% NaCl during renal transplantation. *Anesth Analg* 2005; 100: 1518–24.

41. Shaw AD, Bagshaw SM, Goldstein SL, *et al.* Major complications, mortality, and resource utilization after open abdominal surgery: 0.9% saline compared to Plasma-Lyte. *Ann Surg* 2012; 255: 821–9.

42. Yunos NM, Bellomo R, Hegarty C, *et al.* Association between a chloride-liberal vs. chloride-restrictive intravenous fluid administration strategy and kidney injury in critically ill adults. *JAMA* 2012; 308: 1566–72.

43. Yunos NM, Kim IB, Bellomo R, et al. The biochemical effects of restricting chloride-rich fluids in intensive care. Crit Care Med 2011; 39: 2419–24.

44. Rhee P, Wang D, Ruff P, et al. Human neutrophil activation and increased adhesion by various resuscitation fluids. Crit Care Med 2000; 28: 74–8.

45. Khan R, Kirschenbaum LA, Larow C, Astiz ME. The effect of resuscitation fluids on neutrophil-endothelial cell interactions in septic shock. Shock 2011; 36: 440–4.

46. Wu BU, Hwang JQ, Gardner TH, et al. Lactated Ringer's solution reduces systemic inflammation compared with saline in patients with acute pancreatitis. Clin Gastroenterol Hepatol 2011; 9: 710–17.

47. Brain Trauma Foundation; American Association of Neurological Surgeons; Congress of Neurological Surgeons. Guidelines for the management of severe traumatic brain injury. J Neurotrauma 2007; 24: S1–106.

48. Bederson JB, Connolly ES, Batjer HH, et al. Guidelines for the management of aneurysmal subarachnoid hemorrhage: a statement for healthcare professionals from a special writing group of the Stroke Council, American Heart Association. Stroke 2009; 40: 994–1010.

49. Cooper DJ, Myburgh J, Heritie S, et al. Albumin resuscitation for traumatic brain injury: is intracranial hypertension the cause of increased mortality? J Neurotrauma 2013; 30: 512–18.

50. Tommassino C, Moore S, Todd MM. Cerebral effects of isovolemic hemodilution with crystaloid or colloid solutions. Crit Care Med 1988; 16: 862–71.

51. Roquilly A, Loutrel O, Cinotti R, et al. Balanced versus chloride-rich solutions for fluid resuscitation in brain-injured patients: a randomized double-blind pilot study. Crit Care 2013; 17: R77.

52. Morgan TJ. The ideal crystalloid – what is 'balanced'? Curr Opin Crit Care 2013; 19: 299–307.

53. Doherty M, Buggy DJ. Intraoperative fluids: how much is too much? Br J Anaesth 2012; 109: 69–79.

54. Holte K, Sharrock NE, Kehlet H. Pathophysiology and clinical implications of perioperative fluid excess. Br J Anaesth 2002; 89: 622–32.

55. Stewart RM, Park PK, Hunt JP, et al. National Institutes of Health/National Heart, Lung, and Blood Institute Acute Respiratory Distress Syndrome Clinical Trials Network. Less is more: improved outcomes in surgical patients with conservative fluid administration and central venous pressure monitoring. J Am Coll Surg 2009; 208: 725–35.

56. Ley EJ, Clond MA, Srour MK, et al. Emergency department crystalloid resuscitation of 1.5 L or more is associated with increased mortality in elderly and nonelderly trauma patients. J Trauma 2011; 70: 398–400.

57. Van Bommel J, Siegenund M, Henny CP, Trouwborst A, Ince C. Critical hematocrit in intestinal tissue oxygenation during severe normovolemic hemodilution. Anesthesiology 2001; 94: 152–60.

58. Vermeer H, Teerenstra S, de Sevaux RGL. The effect of hemodilution during normothermic cardiac surgery on renal physiology and function: a review. Perfusion 2008; 23: 329–33.

59. Arikan AA, Zappitelli M, Goldstein SL, et al. Fluid overload is associated with impaired oxygenation and morbidity in critically ill children. Pediatr Crit Care Med 2012; 13: 253–8.

60. Perel P, Roberts I. Colloids versus crystalloids for fluid resuscitation in critically ill patients. Cochrane Database Syst Rev 2007; 4: CD000567.

61. Jones SB, Whitten CW, Monk TG. Influence of crystalloid and colloid replacement solutions on hemodynamic variables during acute normovolemic hemodilution. J Clin Anesth 2004; 16: 11–17.

62. Lobo DN, Stanga Z, Aloysius MM, et al. Effect of volume loading with 1 liter intravenous infusions of 0.9% saline, 4% succinylated gelatin (Gelofusine) and 6% hydroxyethyl starch (Voluven) on blood volume and endocrine responses: a randomized, three-way crossover study in healthy volunteers. Crit Care Med 2010; 38: 464–70.

63. James MFM, Michell WL, Joubert IA, et al. Resuscitation with hydroxyethyl starch improves renal function and lactate clearance in penetrating trauma in a randomized controlled study: the FIRST trial (fluids in resuscitation of severe trauma). Br J Anaesth 2011; 107: 693–702.

64. Annane D, Siami S, Jaber S, et al. CRISTAL Investigators. Effects of fluid resuscitation with colloids vs. crystalloids on mortality in critically ill patients presenting with hypovolemic shock: the CRISTAL randomized trial. JAMA 2013; 310: 1809–17.

65. Myburgh JA, Finfer S, Bellomo R, et al. Hydroxyethyl starch or saline for fluid resuscitation in intensive care. N Engl J Med 2012; 367: 1901–11.

66. Edul VS, Enrico C, Laviolle B, et al. Quantitative assessment of the microcirculation in healthy volunteers and in patients with septic shock. Crit Care Med 2012; 40: 1443–8.

67. Atasever B, van der Kuil M, Boer C, et al. Red blood cell transfusion compared with gelatin solution and no infusion after cardiac surgery: effect on microvascular perfusion, vascular density, hemoglobin, and oxygen saturation. Transfusion 2012; 52: 2452–8.

68. Nisanevich V, Felsenstein I, Almogy G, *et al.* Effect of intraoperative fluid management on outcome after intraabdominal surgery. *Anesthesiology* 2005; 103: 25–32.

69. de Aguilar-Nasciamento JE, Diniz BN, Do Carmo AV, Silveira EAO, Silva RM. Clinical benefits after the implementation of a protocol of restricted perioperative intravenous crystalloid fluids in major abdominal operations. *World J Surg* 2009; 33: 925–30.

70. Melis M, Marcon F, Masi A, *et al.* Effect of intra-operative fluid volume on perioperative outcomes after pancreaticoduodenectomy for pancreatic adenocarcinoma. *J Surg Oncol* 2012; 105: 81–4.

71. Abraham-Nordling M, Hjern F, Pollack J, *et al.* Randomized clinical trial of fluid resuscitation in colorectal surgery. *Br J Surg* 2012; 99: 186–91.

72. Bellamy MC. Wet, dry or something else? *Br J Anaesth* 2006; 97: 755–7.

73. Peng Z, Kellum J. Perioperative fluids: a clear road ahead? *Curr Opin Crit Care* 2013; 19: 353–8.

Pulmonary edema

13

Göran Hedenstierna, Claes Frostell, and João Batista Borges

Summary

Pulmonary edema can be either hydrostatic (cardiac) or high-permeability (non-cardiac). In the first type, therapy should focus on a reduction of hydrostatic pressure. Pain relief and anxiety relief reduces vascular pressures by bringing down sympathetic nervous system drive. Treatment also consists in oxygen supplementation, furosemide, continuous positive airway pressure (CPAP) on a tight-fitting face-mask, and possibly venesection.

High-permeability pulmonary edema implies that the barrier function of the vasculature to larger molecules and cells is no longer intact. The permeability increase leads to a rapid and profound fluid leakage, followed by inflammation and destruction of lung parenchymal structure. Treatment consists of fluid restriction while maintaining adequate organ perfusion. Extracorporeal membrane oxygenation (ECMO) may be used in patients with severe non-cardiac pulmonary edema. Adequate treatment of the primary etiology of the condition is essential.

Resolution of pulmonary edema might include local reabsorption, clearance through the lymphatic system, clearance via the pleural space, or clearance through the airway. Maintaining spontaneous breathing, whenever possible, cannot be over-emphasized. Spontaneous breathing with CPAP both counteracts atelectasis formation in the lung and facilitates the ability to clear secretions with the re-emergence of cough.*

---

* Summary compiled by the Editor.

The lung may react with edema and consolidation in response to various insults. The morphological changes are accompanied by functional disturbances signified by impaired ventilation-perfusion matching and shunt, with subsequent impediment to oxygenation of blood and carbon dioxide removal. This chapter will review clinical and theoretical aspects of pulmonary edema formation and treatment.

As a clinician, the prime question arising in facing pulmonary edema patients is, "What is the rational approach that gives a patient the optimum chance to heal?" First of all, a probable cause needs to be established. It is practical and traditional to divide pulmonary edema into at least two main groups: hydrostatic (cardiac) pulmonary edema (HPE), and high-permeability (non-cardiac) pulmonary edema (HPPE).[1]

The division into two main types of edema rests on the knowledge that even a perfectly healthy lung may react with a rapid and dangerous increase in extravascular lung water (EVLW) if pulmonary capillary pressure is elevated and maintained above 25 mmHg.[2]

However, if pressure is reduced, reabsorption will take place and we will see rapid clearing of the fluid from lung parenchyma. The main safety factor involved is lymphatic drainage. Any process that retards or obstructs lung lymph flow will thus predispose for pulmonary edema formation and slow down reabsorption. In addition, patients with reduced plasma oncotic pressure will react with edema formation at a lower threshold hydrostatic pressure.

Clinical aspects

Treatment of hydrostatic (cardiac) pulmonary edema (HPE). From this introduction, it is obvious that effective therapy should focus on a reduction

---

Clinical Fluid Therapy in the Perioperative Setting, Second Edition, ed. Robert G. Hahn. Published by Cambridge University Press. © Cambridge University Press 2016.

of hydrostatic pressure as soon as HPE is suspected. Relieving pain and anxiety (IV administration of morphine) reduces vascular pressures by bringing down sympathetic nervous system drive; oxygen supplementation releases hypoxic pulmonary vasoconstriction, which adds to a reduction in pulmonary artery pressure; furosemide redistributes intravascular fluid to the periphery even before enhancing diuresis, all of which reduce filling pressures. Venesection or a form of phlebotomy can be achieved by occluding venous return from the legs, thus reducing central venous pressure and favoring reabsorption of lung fluid. Breathing a continuous positive airway pressure (CPAP) on a tight-fitting face-mask should offer immediate improvement in arterial oxygen saturation. This can be explained by a reduction in shunting through redistribution of edema in the lung at the same level of EVLW, similar to applying positive end-expiratory pressure (PEEP) during mechanical ventilation (MV).[3]

Treatment of high-permeability (non-cardiac) pulmonary edema (HPPE). HPPE is the hallmark of acute lung injury (ALI) and its severe forms, acute respiratory distress syndrome (ARDS).[4] For years, intensive care unit meetings have been flooded with information on etiology, therapeutic approaches, and treatment strategies. We have seen expensive molecular targeted therapies yield disappointing efficacy results in one randomized study after another.

The crucial point to consider is that the barrier function of the vasculature to larger molecules and cells is no longer intact in HPPE. The permeability increase leads to a rapid and profound fluid leakage followed by inflammation and destruction of lung parenchymal structure over a period of a few weeks. Furthermore, the process is not completely irreversible, and patients displaying even the most severe forms of disease are known to have pulled through and progressed to an impressive recovery of lung function, as tested up to a year after the acute illness.[5] Thus, there is little room for therapeutic nihilism even in life-threatening circumstances.

An important part of therapy in HPPE is fluid restriction while maintaining adequate organ perfusion. A recent study of patients treated with extracorporeal membrane oxygenation (ECMO) reported a fairly good outcome.[6] A combined approach was used, aiming at a strongly negative fluid balance, by applying continuous veno-venous hemofiltration when necessary, as well as early reestablishment of

spontaneous breathing (SB) efforts on continuing ECMO support of gas exchange (Dr K. Palmér, personal communication). Their overall aim is to optimize pulmonary edema resolution capacity, where SB is thought to pump out extravasated fluid through the lymphatic system. A further advantage of ECMO is that the low central venous pressure does not oppose lymph drainage. The clinical hypothesis is based, among other observations, upon animal studies discussed earlier.[7] Therapy of HPPE threatens to fail if the primary etiology of ALI/ARDS is not treated adequately, such as correct antibiotics in sepsis, surgery for an abdominal compartment syndrome, drainage of septic foci, stabilization of fractures, administration of steroids if rheumatoid-type cause is suspected, and much more.

Spontaneous breathing. The importance of maintaining SB cannot be over-emphasized. In addition to the above, SB at CPAP may both counteract atelectasis formation basally in the lung and facilitate the ability to clear secretions with the re-emergence of cough. Restricted use of sedatives brings a more awake patient, who can move around in the bed a little, and allows the patient to participate in physiotherapy. It should be mentioned that pulmonary edema might be seen in a few additional and more unusual circumstances. Among them, we recognize pulmonary edema due to extreme negative intrapleural pressures (occluded upper airway and breathing efforts), pulmonary edema after re-expansion of collapsed lung, and high-altitude pulmonary edema.

Theoretical aspects of pulmonary edema

About a century has passed since Starling presented experiments demonstrating that hydrostatic and oncotic factors balanced each other over the capillary membrane, determining the rate of fluid moving from the circulation to an extravascular region. A later modification of his work led to the equation now named after him:[8]

$$Q = K_f(P_{mv} - P_{pmv}) - \delta(\pi_c - \pi_t)$$

where Q is the net fluid filtration from the pulmonary microvascular (intravascular) capillary system to the peri-microvascular (extravascular) pulmonary tissue, K_f is the capillary filtration coefficient, P is the hydrostatic pressure, given as P_{mv} and P_{pmv} in the microvascular and peri-microvascular compartments, respectively, δ is the protein reflection coefficient –

varying between 0 (freely permeable) and 1 (non-permeable to proteins) – and π is the protein colloid osmotic pressure in the microvascular (π_c) and peri-microvascular (π_t) tissue. The expression K_f reflects the surface area available for fluid and the hydraulic conductance for fluid.

It is obvious from this expression that edema may form in a tissue for a variety of reasons or combination of factors. In the lung, we recognize HPE as opposed to HPPE. The idea here is that the former may be a result of mainly extrapulmonary factors, such as left heart failure. In contrast, the latter type of edema is mainly caused by an alteration of the permeability of the capillary membranes in the lung, permitting fluid and large molecules to extravasate even with normal vascular pressures. Naturally, the therapeutic approach, apart from symptomatic support, differs according to the etiology of edema formation.

Experimental studies on pulmonary edema

Edema may accumulate because of a combination of altered hydrostatic and permeability factors. This can, for example, be seen in early experimental septicemia caused by injecting live bacteria or lipopolysaccharides. Sheep typically react with both a sharp increase in pulmonary artery pressure and an increased permeability in lung capillaries.[9] Both these factors, therefore, contribute to edema formation in the lung.

To what degree the maintenance of a high airway pressure is detrimental has been the subject of considerable debate. We have experienced an era where the idea of "super PEEP" was advocated by some groups in the treatment of ALI. Because MV was introduced in the treatment of ALI, it was obvious that barotrauma, with or without pneumothorax, was an adverse effect to consider when using intermittent positive-pressure ventilation.[10] The Kolobow group studied sheep treated with MV that had their lungs overexpanded by the application of peak airway pressures at 50 cmH$_2$O.[11] With this ventilator setting, the clinical picture of ARDS could be produced by MV alone.

Webb and Tierney created impressive alveolar edema in rats by ventilating with high airway pressures for only 20 min.[12] This work was confirmed and extended by Dreyfuss and Saumon [13], suggesting the term "volotrauma" as opposed to

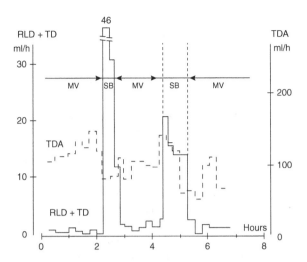

Figure 13.1 Pulmonary lymph flow (RLD + TD) and abdominal lymph flow (TDA) during mechanical ventilation (MV) and spontaneous breathing (SB) in a 30 kg anesthetized dog. Note the considerable increase in lung lymph flow during SB, suggestive of impeded lymph drainage during MV. Note also the decrease in abdominal lymph flow during SB. Whether this reflects decreased capillary leakage remains to be shown. From Ref. [7].

"barotrauma." This latter study offered evidence that overexpansion of the lung tissue by volume alterations is more damaging than overexpansion by pressure alterations. We can conclude that severe lung damage with edema can be caused by airway-mediated mechanical factors, resulting in repeated tearing of tissue due to overexpansion by volume. West and Mathieu-Costello have published impressive electron microscopic evidence of how "overexpansion by pressure release" of either the airway or the capillary vessels (increased blood pressure) will result in "stress failure" of these structures.[14] The damaged structures allow fluid, larger molecules, and sometimes whole blood corpuscular elements to exit the circulation and participate in edema formation.

Our group measured lung lymph flow in anesthetized dogs ventilated with or without PEEP. During MV with PEEP 10 cmH$_2$O, the lymphatic flow from the lung was reduced by almost 50% compared with that occurring with zero end-expiratory pressure. On the other hand, during SB, lung lymph flow was markedly elevated (Figure 13.1).[7] This indicates that intra-pulmonary pressure can influence lung fluid balance, and that SB considered in relation to lung lymph flow might have an advantage when compared with MV.

Summary of factors that promote pulmonary edema

A number of factors contribute to edema formation in the early stages of lung injury:

1. Increased capillary pressure (fluid overloading, left heart failure);
2. Elevated airway pressure causing barotrauma (MV, PEEP, and need for higher tidal volumes due to intra-pulmonary shunting);
3. Elevated airway pressure impeding lymphatic drainage of lung tissue and possibly pleural cavities;
4. Increased permeability of the capillary or alveolo-capillary membranes;
5. Impeded active transport of water from the alveoli back to the interstitium and circulation;
6. Extravasation of activated neutrophils and macrophages, which further lowers permeability after releasing inflammatory mediators locally and into the bloodstream;
7. Microthrombotization of lung blood or lymph capillaries by local activation of platelets, reducing the functional area of the lung capillary bed, which contributes to an elevated microvascular (hydrostatic) pressure (flow limitation) and possibly impedes the lymphatic flow.

Clearance of pulmonary edema

When discussing clearance of extravasated fluid from the lung, the situation becomes very complex. From a clinical point of view, it seems advisable on the basis of the above discussion to keep vascular pressures low (pulmonary artery pressure and central venous pressure). We attempted to optimize Starling factors by using a hyperoncotic, hypertonic infusion during pulmonary edema in dogs, but found to our surprise that this manipulation did not increase the rate of reduction of EVLW.[15] Obviously, other factors limited the maximum rate of all relevant factors that determine lung fluid balance.

An illustration of the need to take additional factors into account is the demonstration that the pleural cavities may act as safety factors delaying and minimizing edema formation. It is now known that a significant portion of interstitial fluid during edema formation is excreted into the pleural cavities and cleared from the parietal pleura.[16] Experiments on dogs demonstrate

to what extent this animal is dependent on an intact lymphatic system to clear the pleural cavity of protein-rich, extravasated fluids. This was shown by ligating the lymphatic vessels draining the pleural cavity and measuring the rate of removal of indicator-labeled protein from a pleural effusion.[17] The dog could not remove such an effusion after lymphatic ligation. Our conclusion must be that a number of factors concerning clearance of edema, and safety factors against edema formation, have to be taken into consideration when discussing the fluid balance of lung tissue. We have previously suggested the calculation of "net fluid leakage" per time unit as a more relevant parameter to use for such an analysis.[18]

Summary of factors that facilitate the clearance of pulmonary edema

Our understanding today is that there exist several ways by which the lung can rid itself of edema. Fluid can be:

1. Locally reabsorbed through the capillary membrane by Starling-type mechanisms, or actively pumped out of the alveoli;[19]
2. Cleared through the lymphatic system as lymph and returned to the circulation;[8]
3. Excreted to the pleural space directly from the lung tissue and from there taken up into parietal pleural lymphatics for return to the circulation;[16]
4. Transported to the lung hilus interstitially and from there migrate into the mediastinum and be absorbed;[20]
5. Cleared through the airway.

Different pathways of fluid transport in the lung are shown schematically in Figure 13.2.[21]

Ventilator-induced lung injury and pulmonary edema

A concept that has emerged during the past few years is lung damage caused by the ventilator *per se*, so called ventilator-induced lung injury (VILI). Positron emission tomography (PET) studies have shown that measures of barrier function are a nonspecific index of lung injury indicating functional, not structural, lung injury.[22,23] PET imaging methods can measure

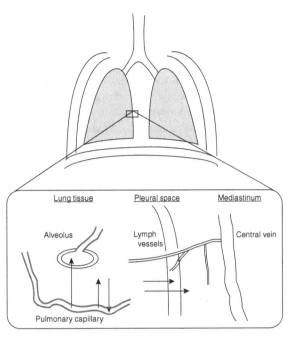

Figure 13.2 Pathways of filtered fluid from the intravascular to the extravascular spaces in the lung. From Ref. [21].

the rate at which proteins move across the endothelial barrier, from vascular to extravascular compartments, the so-called pulmonary transcapillary escape rate (PTCER). Palazzo *et al.* [24] used PET imaging to measure PTCER in an *in vivo* canine model of unilateral pulmonary ischemia-reperfusion injury and found it to be increased in the ischemic lung. Interestingly, both lungs had an increased PTCER when compared with control non-ischemic lungs, suggesting that injury in one lung can lead to similar injury in the contralateral lung, a finding that has been observed in an analogous clinical setting such as acute unilateral pneumonia.

Calandrino *et al.* described that, while PTCER and extravascular density (a close correlate to EVLW) were both elevated in patients with ARDS, they correlated poorly with one another on a regional basis.[22] Moreover, even as extravascular density returned to normal, PTCER remained elevated suggesting that lung tissue injury might be "subclinical" but still present, even after pulmonary edema has actually resolved. This was further confirmed by Sandiford *et al.* [25] who examined the regional distribution of PTCER and extravascular density more closely in ARDS patients and found ventral–dorsal gradients only for extravascular density but not for PTCER. Once more, functional injury was

detected even in lung regions that appeared to be free of structural injury.

The finding that the lungs of patients with ARDS are more diffusely involved than what might otherwise be assumed from just structural radiological imaging, such as computed tomography, helps explain why ARDS lungs are so vulnerable to VILI: radiographically "normal" lung, i.e. lung with a normal EVLW content, in non-dependent lung regions may still be abnormal and vulnerable to mechanical stresses caused by MV. These data tell us that non-dependent regions of ARDS lungs are "at risk" because they demonstrate subclinical evidence of injury, which can be made manifest by inappropriate ventilator use. Jones *et al.* [26] evidenced a surprisingly high pulmonary uptake of [^{18}F]-fluorodeoxyglucose (^{18}F-FDG) in patients with head injury, at risk of developing ARDS but without lung symptoms at the time of the scan. This signal may reflect sequestration of primed neutrophils in lung capillaries. *In vitro* studies in isolated human neutrophils have demonstrated that the uptake of deoxyglucose is increased to the same extent in cells that are only primed, or primed and stimulated.[27] This indicates the vulnerability of these patients while on ventilatory support, because, even though neutrophils remain in a primed state, any additional stimulus precipitates actual tissue damage.

PET with ^{18}F-FDG, which is a glucose-analog tracer, offers the opportunity to study regional lung inflammation *in vivo*. ^{18}F-FDG is taken up predominantly by metabolically active cells and has been recognized as a key marker of neutrophilic inflammation in the inflamed non-tumoral lung.[28,29] There is a theoretical concern that in ALI ^{18}F-FDG might leak to the alveolar spaces, becoming a major and non-specific determinant of the ^{18}F-FDG signal, and potentially causing a false, non-inflammation-related increase in the measured uptake (K_i). The presence of edema, however, does not seem to affect the measurement of K_i, as suggested by Chen *et al.* [30] who measured glucose uptake with ^{18}F-FDG in anesthetized dogs after intravenous oleic acid-induced ALI or after low-dose intravenous endotoxin followed by oleic acid. The rate of ^{18}F-FDG uptake was significantly elevated in both endotoxin-treated groups, but not in the group treated only with oleic acid, leading the authors to conclude that pulmonary vascular leak, and consequently edema, does not significantly contribute to the K_i in ARDS lungs.

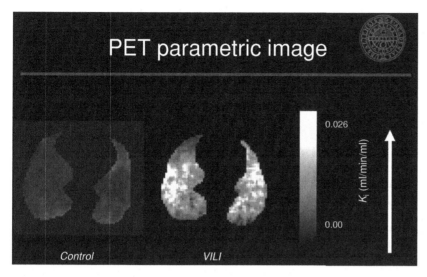

Figure 13.3 Representative positron emission tomography and X-ray computed tomography images of net [^{18}F]-fluoro-2-deoxy-D-glucose uptake rate in an experimental model of ventilator-induced lung injury. Note the predominance of the activity in the normal and poorly aerated regions as seen in the corresponding X-ray computed tomography image.

We studied the location and magnitude of early inflammatory changes using PET imaging of ^{18}F-FDG in a porcine experimental model of ARDS.[31] We evaluated the individual contributions of regional injurious mechanisms during early stages of VILI. We found the highest uptake in the normal and poorly aerated regions, while the hyperinflated and non-aerated regions were similar to the control group (Figure 13.3). These findings challenge the current notion that hyperinflation and/or repeated collapse and re-expansion of alveolar units play the major role in early VILI. Instead, our data suggest that tidal stretch was highest in the poorly and normally aerated regions, and that this mechanism is the most important trigger of inflammation in these conditions. They also support the concept that the smaller the ventilated lung, the higher the VILI-triggering forces will be, as a larger fraction of tidal volume V_T is delivered to a smaller lung volume.

Ventilatory support and abdominal edema

Although this chapter deals with pulmonary edema, a short note will also be made on abdominal edema formation since it can be heavily influenced by lung disease and, in particular, ventilator support with positive-pressure ventilation. Any impedance of lymph drainage will promote edema formation, and the mechanisms described for the lung in this chapter will also apply for the abdomen. Thus, MV can obstruct or increase the lymph vessel resistance, mainly the thoracic duct that drains the abdomen and passes through the thorax to drain into innominate veins. Similarly, increased central venous pressure by the MV or by other means will also elevate the systemic capillary pressure and cause an increased leakage into the abdominal extravascular bed.[32]

ARDS has a high mortality of 30–40%, and the mortality is caused more frequently by multi-organ failure than by lung failure.[33] Thus, abdominal edema formation may be as important as, or more important than, lung edema in ARDS. Attempts have been made to compare edema formation with inflammation in the abdomen, but whether it is the edema *per se* or reduced perfusion pressure of abdominal organs that is important is not fully clear. Hypoperfusion is most likely an important mechanism, but it may also be that the edema formation *per se* impedes the perfusion.[34]

These observations may shed further light on the concept of "lung protective ventilation." Low "driving pressure" has recently been shown to be beneficial for outcome and may reduce intrathoracic pressure,[35] although the level of PEEP is an additional factor with impact on lymph drainage. One may ask to what extent low tidal volumes during ventilator treatment improve outcome by lung protection or by abdomen protection.

References

1. Prichard JS. Pulmonary edema. In: Weatherhall DJ, Ledingham JGG, Warrel DA, eds. *Oxford Textbook of Medicine*. 3rd edn. Oxford/New York/Tokyo: Oxford University Press, 1996: 2495–505.

2. Guyton AO, Lindsey AW. Effect of elevated left atrial pressure and decreased plasma protein concentration upon the development of pulmonary edema. *Circ Res* 1959; 7: 649–57.

3. Blomqvist H, Wickerts CJ, Berg B, *et al*. Does PEEP facilitate the resolution of extravascular lung water after experimental hydrostatic pulmonary edema? *Eur Respir J* 1991; 4: 1053–9.

4. Bernard GR, Artigas A, Brigham KL, *et al*. and the Consensus Committee. The American-European Consensus Conference on ARDS: definitions, mechanisms, relevant outcomes and clinical trial coordination. *Am J Respir Crit Care Med* 1994; 149: 818–24.

5. Luhr O, Aardal S, Nathorst-Westfelt U, *et al*. Pulmonary function in adult survivors of severe acute lung injury treated with inhaled nitric oxide. *Acta Anaesthesiol Scand* 1998; 42: 391–8.

6. Linden V, Palmer K, Reinhard J, *et al*. High survival in adult patients with acute respiratory distress syndrome treated by extracorporeal membrane oxygenation, minimal sedation, and pressure supported ventilation. *Intensive Care Med* 2000; 26: 1630–7.

7. Frostell C, Blomqvist H, Hedenstierna G, Pieper R. Thoracic and abdominal lymph drainage in relation to mechanical ventilation and PEEP. *Acta Anaesthesiol Scand* 1987; 31: 405–12.

8. Staub NC. State of the art review. Pathogenesis of pulmonary edema. *Am Rev Respir Dis* 1974; 109: 358–72.

9. Brigham KL, Meyrick B. Endotoxin and lung injury. *Am Rev Respir Dis* 1986; 133: 913–27.

10. Slutsky AS. Consensus Conference on mechanical ventilation – Jan 28–30, 1993 at Northbrook, Illinois, USA. Part 2. *Intensive Care Med* 1994; 20: 150–62.

11. Kolobow T, Moretti MP, Fumagalli R, *et al*. Severe impairment in lung function induced by high peak airway pressure during mechanical ventilation. An experimental study. *Am Rev Respir Dis* 1987; 135: 312–15.

12. Webb HH, Tierney DF. Experimental pulmonary edema due to intermittent positive pressure ventilation with high inflation pressures. Protection by positive end-expiratory pressure. *Am Rev Respir Dis* 1974; 110: 556–65.

13. Dreyfuss D, Saumon G. Lung overinflation. Physiologic and anatomic alterations leading to pulmonary edema. In: Zapol WM, Lemaire F, eds. *Adult Respiratory Distress Syndrome*. New York: Marcel Dekker Inc, 1991: 433–49.

14. West JB, Mathieu-Costello O. Stress failure of pulmonary capillaries: role in lung and heart disease. *Lancet* 1992; 340: 762–7.

15. Wickerts CJ, Berg B, Frostell C, *et al*. Influence of hypertonic-hyperoncotic solution and furosemide on extravascular lung water resorption in canine hydrostatic pulmonary edema. *J Physiol* 1992; 458: 425–38.

16. Matthay MA, Wiener-Kronish JP. Pleural effusions associated with hydrostatic and increased permeability pulmonary edema. *Chest* 1988; 93: 852–8.

17. Miniati M, Parker JC, Pistolesi M, *et al*. Reabsorption kinetics of albumin from pleural space of dogs. *Am J Physiol* 1988; 255: H375–85.

18. Blomqvist H, Berg B, Frostell C, Wickerts C-J, Hedenstierna G. Net fluid leakage (LN) in experimental pulmonary edema in the dog. *Acta Anaesthesiol Scand* 1990; 34: 377–83.

19. Matthay MA, Wiener-Kronish JP. Intact epithelial barrier function is critical for the resolution of alveolar edema in humans. *Am Rev Respir Dis* 1990; 142: 1250–7.

20. Staub NC. What's new in pulmonary edema research? In *Recent Advances in Anaesthesia, Pain, Intensive Care and Emergency*. APICE 1987, Trieste: 3–9.

21. Blomqvist H, Frostell C, Pieper R, Hedenstierna G. Measurement of dynamic lung fluid balance in the mechanically ventilated dog. Theory and results. *Acta Anaesthesiol Scand* 1990; 34: 370–6.

22. Calandrino FSJ, Anderson DJ, Mintun MA, Schuster DP. Pulmonary vascular permeability during the adult respiratory distress syndrome: a positron emission tomographic study. *Am Rev Respir Dis* 1988; 138: 421–8.

23. Schuster DP. What is acute lung injury? What is ARDS? *Chest* 1995; 107: 1721–6.

24. Palazzo R, Hamvas A, Shuman T, *et al*. Injury in nonischemic lung after unilateral pulmonary ischemia with reperfusion. *J Appl Physiol* 1992; 72: 612–20.

25. Sandiford P, Province MA, Schuster DP. Distribution of regional density and vascular permeability in the adult respiratory distress syndrome. *Am J Respir Crit Care Med* 1995; 151: 737–42.

26. Jones HA, Clark JC, Minhas PS, *et al*. Pulmonary neutrophil activation following head trauma (abstract). *Am J Respir Crit Care Med* 1998; 157: A349.

27. Jones HA, Cadwallader KA, White JF, *et al*. Dissociation between respiratory burst activity and deoxyglucose uptake in human neutrophil

granulocytes: implications for interpretation of (18)F-FDG PET images. *J Nucl Med* 2002; 43: 652–7.

28. de Prost N, Costa EL, Wellman T, *et al.* Effects of surfactant depletion on regional pulmonary metabolic activity during mechanical ventilation. *J Appl Physiol* 2011; 111: 1249–58.

29. Costa ELV, Musch G, Winkler T, *et al.* Mild endotoxemia during mechanical ventilation produces spatially heterogeneous pulmonary neutrophilic inflammation in sheep. *Anesthesiology* 2010; 112: 658–69.

30. Chen DL, Schuster DP. Positron emission tomography with [18F]fluorodeoxyglucose to evaluate neutrophil kinetics during acute lung injury. *Am J Physiol Lung Cell Mol Physiol* 2004; 286: L834–40.

31. Borges JB, Costa ELV, Suarez-Sipmann F, *et al.* Early inflammation mainly affects normally and poorly aerated lung in experimental ventilator-induced lung injury*. *Crit Care Med* 2014; 42: e279–87.

32. Lattuada M, Hedenstierna G. Abdominal lymph flow in an endotoxin sepsis model: influence of spontaneous breathing and mechanical ventilation. *Crit Care Med* 2006; 34: 2792–8.

33. Zambon M, Mont GI, Landoni G. Outcome of patients with acute respiratory distress syndrome: causes of death, survival rates and long-term complications. In: Vincent JL, ed. *Annual Update in Intensive Care and Emergency Medicine*. Berlin: Springer, 2014: 245–53.

34. Lattuada M, Bergquist M, Maripuu E, Hedenstierna G. Mechanical ventilation worsens abdominal edema and inflammation in porcine endotoxemia. *Crit Care* 2013; 17: R126.

35. Amato MB, Meade MO, Slutsky AS, Brochard L. Driving pressure and survival in the acute respiratory distress syndrome. *N Engl J Med* 2015; 372: 747–55.

Chapter

14

Invasive hemodynamic monitoring

Jonathan Aron and Maurizio Cecconi

Summary

The aim of hemodynamic monitoring is to enable the optimization of cardiac output and therefore improve oxygen delivery to the tissues, avoiding the accumulation of oxygen debt, in the perioperative period. Instigating goal-directed therapy based on validated optimization algorithms has been shown to reduce mortality in high-risk patients and complications in moderate- to high-risk patients.

A number of devices are available to facilitate this goal. The pulmonary artery catheter was the first hemodynamic monitor, but its invasive nature precludes its routine use in today's clinical practice. More recently, devices that continuously analyze the arterial pressure waveform to calculate various flow parameters have been developed and validated. These devices have facilitated the introduction of hemodynamic monitoring to the wider surgical population, providing useful clinical information that enables the judicious use of fluid therapy whilst avoiding hypervolemia.

This chapter explores the role that hemodynamic optimization plays in perioperative care, describes some of the commonly used invasive hemodynamic monitors, and explains how to use the information produced effectively. Used correctly, any monitor can be useful to improve outcome if applied to the right population, at the right time, and with the right strategy.

Hemodynamic monitoring refers to continuous measurement of a hemodynamic variable. Cardiac output (CO) monitoring enables the clinician to guide hemodynamic management and improve oxygen delivery (DO_2). It began 50 years ago with the pulmonary artery catheter (PAC) and has evolved to the latest minimally invasive and non-invasive devices. The use of these monitors to optimize CO and tissue perfusion may positively influence the outcome for patients in the perioperative setting. Implementing this strategy successfully is dependent on correct interpretation of the information produced so that the appropriate interventions can be administered at the appropriate time.

This chapter will analyze the role of hemodynamic monitoring in the perioperative setting, describe some of the most commonly used invasive devices and how to use the information obtained from them in clinical practice.

Evidence for hemodynamic monitoring and optimization in the perioperative period

Patients who achieve a higher CO, oxygen delivery, and oxygen consumption after high-risk surgery have long been observed to have a greater chance of survival.[1,2] This led to the concept that an "oxygen debt" accumulated within patients who were unable to mount a sufficient cardiorespiratory response to meet the increased metabolic demands that occur during and after surgery. In an important study, the use of fluid and inotrope administration to achieve supranormal hemodynamic targets, guided by the PAC, resulted in a decrease in mortality and morbidity in a cohort of high-risk surgical patients.[1] Other investigators subsequently studied goal-directed therapy

Clinical Fluid Therapy in the Perioperative Setting, Second Edition, ed. Robert G. Hahn. Published by Cambridge University Press. © Cambridge University Press 2016.

(GDT) in the perioperative period and demonstrated similar results.[3,4] Unsurprisingly, using invasive monitoring was associated with increased resource utilization and complications.[5] Subsequent development of less-invasive technologies allowed the safe implementation of hemodynamic optimization to be applied to a wider surgical population.

The use of GDT to improve patient outcome has been repeatedly reproduced in a variety of clinical settings.[6–8] Recently published meta-analyses [9–11] and a Cochrane review [12] in perioperative patients have demonstrated that GDT reduces postoperative morbidity, length of hospital stay, and mortality. In particular, mortality was reduced in patients undergoing high-risk surgery, and morbidity was reduced in all patient groups.[9,10] The most successful GDT protocols involved optimization of DO_2 or CO, and this was most effectively achieved if inotropes in addition to fluid therapy were used to meet these targets in the highest-risk group of patients.[9,10]

More recently, however, a number of studies have found no benefit in using GDT.[13,14] It is likely that after the introduction of initiatives that improve the overall standard of perioperative care, such as Enhanced Recovery After Surgery (ERAS), a single change in management has less of a demonstrable impact than it once did. The recent OPTIMISE trial [15] also failed to demonstrate an improvement in outcome when using GDT; however, in a sub-analysis in which the first 10 patients managed at each center were removed, the reduction in postoperative complications became significant. This suggests that optimization bundles are likely to require a period of familiarization before they are used to their full potential. Timing is also likely to be important: when GDT was used later after surgery (within 48 hours of ICU admission), it was not found to improve outcome and was even shown to harm some patients.[16]

In summary, it should be emphasized that a CO monitor is most effective in improving patient care if it is used to facilitate a validated hemodynamic optimization protocol. Used together correctly, hemodynamic monitoring and appropriate therapy have the potential to reduce mortality in high-risk patients, and morbidity in moderate- to high-risk patients. It is important to remember that any monitor can be useful to improve outcome only if applied to the right population, at the right time, and with the right strategy.

Assessing a cardiac output monitor

Apart from safety and efficacy considerations, there are likely to be institutional and financial factors that may influence the choice of a particular CO monitor. The clinician must be aware of the limitations of a device with particular reference to the accuracy, the precision, and the ability to track changes in physiology in the specific patient population used.

Despite limitations in clinical use, the PAC has become the gold standard by which most CO monitoring devices are assessed. The most frequently used statistical method for comparing the accuracy of two CO monitoring devices is the Bland–Altman method. Critchley et al. defined an acceptable percentage error of less than 30% for a clinical CO device.[17] However, comparison studies are not homogeneous, the statistical methods used for analysis have been questioned, and acceptable performance limits remain debatable.[18]

The role of echocardiography

Trans-thoracic and trans-esophageal echocardiography provide an immediate point-of-care assessment of fluid status, myocardial function, cardiac structure, and response to treatment. Many hemodynamic measurements are possible, including measures of right heart function. However, its use as a continuous monitor remains impractical apart from in specific settings such as cardiac surgery, as the availability of equipment and trained personnel may limit the widespread implementation for perioperative monitoring. Trans-esophageal echocardiography is used routinely during cardiac operations where its role has been well established in guiding and changing perioperative management.[19] The use of echocardiography to manage the shocked patient is recommended by an expert panel in recent guidelines.[20]

Intra-pulmonary thermodilution: the pulmonary artery catheter

The PAC was introduced in the 1970s and was the first clinical hemodynamic monitor. Initially used for patients with cardiac dysfunction, it rapidly became the standard of care for perioperative monitoring in high-risk patients for the subsequent 20 years and has been extensively investigated in this context.

The PAC is a balloon-tipped catheter that is available in a range of lengths and sizes for adults and

Table 14.1 Accepted indications for using a pulmonary artery catheter (PAC) in current clinical practice

Category	Example
Cardiac (medical) especially in the context of right ventricular failure	Complicated acute myocardial infarction Left ventricular failure Right ventricular failure
Shock especially in the context of right ventricular failure	Differentiating between different types of shock (for example cardiogenic, septic, hypovolemic, obstructive)
Pulmonary edema	Differentiating between cardiogenic edema and non-cardiogenic edema
Monitoring and titrating therapy	Fluids Inotropes Vasoconstrictors Vasodilators Mechanical assist devices
Pulmonary hypertension	Primary and secondary pulmonary hypertension Intra-cardiac shunts

children. In addition to the balloon there are three lumina, two of which terminate in the right atrium and one that terminates distal to the balloon. A thermistor wire is 4 cm from the tip, proximal to the balloon, and measures blood temperature used in the calculation of cardiac output.

See Table 14.1 for accepted indications for using a PAC in current clinical practice.

Originally, an intermittent value for CO was produced using manual thermodilution, requiring a 10 ml bolus of cold fluid to be rapidly injected into a proximal port of the PAC at the end of expiration. The temperature of blood in the pulmonary artery is plotted against time, and the area under the curve is calculated (see Figure 14.1) to produce CO. The addition of a heating element that automatically semi-continuously warms the blood in the pulmonary artery allows more continuous CO monitoring and is the basis of the Vigilance™ system. The mean CO is calculated over several minutes to improve the accuracy, resulting in a delay in the display of any acute changes.

Complications

The rate of complications when using the PAC may be inversely related to user experience. Complications related to insertion are observed in 6% of cases. Cardiac arrhythmias also occur frequently (12.5%) but are usually transient (including atrial and ventricular ectopic beats, ventricular tachycardia, and right bundle branch block). Rare complications include catheter malposition or knotting, valve trauma, and pulmonary

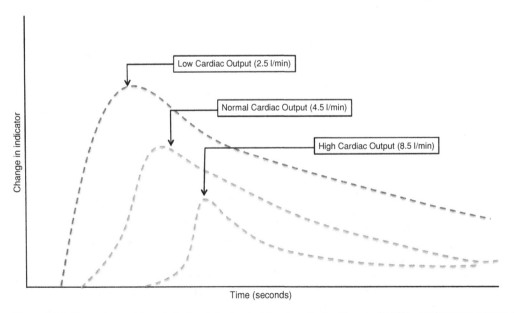

Figure 14.1 Change in an arbitrary indicator plotted against time in patients with normal and low cardiac output states. A high cardiac output state results in a greater dispersal of indicator resulting in a lower peak concentration and a prolonged wash-out curve. Flow is inversely proportional to the rate of indicator change, and cardiac output is inversely proportional to the area under the curve (Stewart–Hamilton calculation).

arterial rupture. Late complications are infrequent if the catheter is removed within 72 hours and include infection, thrombosis, and pulmonary infarction.[21]

Limitations

Reliable results depend on correct catheter position, injection technique, and thermistor accuracy. The presence of intra-cardiac shunts, tricuspid or mitral valve regurgitation, and mitral valve stenosis affects accuracy. High ventilator pressures may also result in falsely high CO readings. The avoidance of complications and the successful interpretation of the PAC data are user-dependent.

Validation

Outcome studies are conflicting. As discussed previously, when the PAC was used to guide therapy in high-risk surgical patients, a mortality and morbidity benefit was found by several investigators.[1,3,4] However, subsequent studies have demonstrated potential harm by using the PAC and increased resource utilization.[5,22,23] Some studies found that despite guiding therapy, no outcome benefit could be demonstrated.[22–24] In addition, the insertion and subsequent interpretation is heavily user-dependent, and experience of the operator is likely to be important. A Cochrane review concluded that PACs did not alter hospital length of stay, mortality, or cost.[21] Importantly, complications occurring as a result of catheter insertion did not result in harm or death.[21,22]

Summary of the PAC

PAC use may still be beneficial in a select group of patients as discussed above and only if the operator and the institution have experience in the insertion, interpretation, and subsequent care of these catheters. In this context it is still an important monitoring tool and provides unique clinical information not easily obtained from other modalities.

Arterial waveform analysis

These devices use an arterial pressure trace to continuously calculate the CO. Compared with the PAC, they are less invasive and require less expertise to insert, maintain, and interpret. Continuous stroke volume (SV) analysis allows the prediction of fluid responsiveness (discussed later), an advantage over intermittent measurements provided by the PAC.

To calculate flow from the pressure trace, the device must calculate the overall vascular impedance, based on the measurement or prediction of vascular resistance and compliance. This may be achieved by using a calibrated technique or by using an uncalibrated technique based on normograph data.

Calibrated devices using pulse-contour analysis or pulse-power analysis

A calibrated device will use an intermittent transpulmonary dilution technique. An indicator injected into venous blood will dissipate through cardiac and pulmonary blood volumes before reaching the systemic circulation where it is measured. The change in indicator is plotted against time, and the area under the curve is calculated by the modified Stuart–Hamilton equation as for the PAC. Once calibrated, the device will utilize pulse-contour or pulse-power analysis to provide continuous SV and CO data.

PiCCO™ (Pulsion Medical Systems, Munich, Germany)

The PiCCO™ family of devices (PiCCO$_{plus}$™ and PiCCO$_{O2}$™) use a rapid bolus of cold fluid as the indicator, injected through a central venous catheter. A proprietary thermistor-tipped catheter, which detects the change in temperature, is inserted into the femoral or axillary artery. The proprietary algorithm calculates the aortic impedance and subsequently uses pulse-contour analysis to continuously calculate the SV every 3 seconds. A number of static values of preload such as global end-diastolic volume (GEDV) and intrathoracic blood volume (ITBV) are also produced, discussed later.

The VolumeView™ set EV1000™ platform (Edwards Life Sciences, Irvine, USA)

The VolumeView™ using the EV1000™ platform software is calibrated with cold-bolus thermodilution (as above) and uses pulse-contour analysis to measure similar values to the PiCCO™ system. A proprietary thermistor-tipped femoral arterial cannula is also required, and an optional PreSep™ catheter for continuous central venous oxygenation monitoring is available. The unique feature is the software package, which presents the hemodynamic data with a graphical interface facilitating interpretation by the operator.

The LiDCO™ system (LiDCO Ltd, Cambridge, UK)

LiDCO™ uses lithium as the indicator to calculate CO with the trans-pulmonary bolus technique. The peripheral arterial catheter is connected to a proprietary lithium-sensitive electrode which creates a voltage proportional to the lithium concentration in the blood. The algorithm assumes net power change is equal to net flow change and calibration creates a correction factor for vascular compliance. Pulse-power analysis (rather than the pulse-contour) is subsequently used for continuous flow monitoring. This system is less invasive as there is no need for a central arterial catheter or central venous access.

Validation of calibrated devices

The PiCCO™ in particular has been extensively validated in animal studies and in a variety of clinical conditions.[25] The use of GEDV to guide fluid administration in a cardiac ICU reduced duration of vasopressor and inotrope dependency, mechanical ventilation, and length of stay.[26] The EV1000/VolumeView™ monitor has demonstrated accuracy and reliability equal to that of PiCCO™, and superior accuracy in measurement of the GEDV.[27]

The LiDCO™ device has also been validated in numerous clinical situations, including in patients with impaired ventricular function after cardiac surgery and undergoing liver transplantation, with a wide variety of COs.[28,29] When used to facilitate GDT in postoperative patients to target a supranormal DO_2, a reduced rate of complications and length of hospital stay were demonstrated,[30] and this is used routinely in the author's institution.

Limitations

All pulse-contour devices, calibrated or not, depend on a good-quality arterial pressure trace. Severe arrhythmias and the use of intra-aortic balloon pump augmentation will result in unreliable data. A proprietary central arterial catheter and central venous access are required to calibrate the device, increasing the invasive nature of the technique. Owing to

changes in the vascular resistance, recalibration is required frequently if there is an obvious clinical change.

Summary of calibrated devices

These devices provide accuracy comparable to the PAC with the obvious benefits of being less invasive and less user-dependent, and allowing assessment of dynamic indices. The limitations include reliance of a good-quality arterial pressure trace and the need for recurrent calibrations over time. Each device has been validated for the use in perioperative clinical practice when used in conjunction with evidence-based optimization protocols, and they have found widespread clinical acceptance.

Uncalibrated devices using pulse-contour analysis

Devices without the need for external calibration are a more recent development to meet a need for a user-independent system to display trend data. This allows the assessment of dynamic indices to predict fluid responsiveness and protocol-guided optimization. Most devices use algorithms to calculate flow, which rely on databases containing information from laboratory or comparative studies. One newer system (MostCare™, Vytech) does not require calibration as it analyzes the arterial waveform to calculate the vascular impedance.

Vigileo/FloTrac System™ (Edward Life Sciences, Irvine, USA)

This device requires a proprietary transducer to be connected to a standard arterial catheter. Demographic data (age, height, sex, weight) are manually supplied to calculate the predicted vascular impedance. The arterial trace is sampled at 100 Hz over a 20 second period and compliance and resistance are estimated. The arterial pressure waveform is continually analyzed for changes, and SV, CO, stroke volume variation (SVV), and pulse pressure variation (PPV) are displayed.

Pulsioflex™ (Pulsion Medical Systems)

This system uses the same algorithm as the calibrated PiCCO™ devices without *in vitro* calibration, instead relying on normograph data and biometric information. The basic module will monitor SV, CO, SVV, PPV, and a contractility measurement. For greater accuracy, CO data for calibration can be supplied manually, for example from an esophageal Doppler device. The monitor is expandable and modules can be added that allow bolus thermodilution calibration and continuous SVO_2 monitoring.

LiDCOrapid™ (LiDCO Ltd, Cambridge, UK)

This un-calibrated system by LiDCO™ calculates the correction factor for SVR. Using normograph data produced by the manufacturer, aortic blood volume is calculated based on age, height, weight, and body surface area. Newer models also allow the escalation of monitoring with transpulmonary dilution calibration, if required.

MostCare™ System (Vytech, Padua, Italy)

The MostCare™ system is the latest evolution of CO monitor that des not require *in vitro* or external calibration using a pressure recording analytical method (PRAM) to calculate vascular impedance. The high sample rate of 1,000 Hz is able to identify subtle acceleration or deceleration changes in the arterial waveform produced by retrograde waves originating from the distal vascular tree. These changes are used to calculate the peripheral vascular impedance and therefore produce an extremely reactive system allowing calculation of SV, CO, and vascular resistance.

Validation of uncalibrated devices

A number of studies have been performed comparing the accuracy of the three pulse-contour systems described above.

The accuracy of the Vigileo/FloTrac™ device has been questioned despite several incremental updates. The first iteration showed poor agreement with PAC-derived values, and later generations remain unacceptably inaccurate, with published error rates of 40% in non-cardiac patients.[31] Detection of cardiac output changes due to fluid bolus administration and vasopressor therapy [32] was also unreliable. It has, however, been used successfully in protocols for fluid

administration in general surgical patients [33] and orthopedic patients.[34]

The uncalibrated LiDCO™ and PiCCO™ devices produce acceptably accurate results when compared to the PAC and are more able to track physiological changes than the FloTrac™ in a number of clinical situations.[35] The PiCCO™ device is able to accurately track the changes in the CO during fluid and vasopressors administration,[36] and both these devices have been successfully used to guide intravenous fluid therapy using GDT based on SV optimization and SVV in the perioperative period.

In patients undergoing cardiac interventional procedures and cardiac bypass surgery, PRAM performed well when compared to the PAC [37–39] and echocardiography.[39] In addition, it appears to be accurate in patients with low CO states, receiving inotropes or intra-aortic balloon pump augmentation. Although promising studies exist, larger validation studies are still required.

Summary of uncalibrated devices

These devices are useful for the perioperative patient as they are minimally invasive, do not require calibration and are not user-dependent. The use of these devices in conjunction with evidence-based GDT protocols has been shown to reduce complications following surgery. However, convenience is traded for accuracy, and it is likely that in a hemodynamically compromised patient, an alternative monitoring device may be more appropriate.

How to use these monitors to predict fluid responsiveness

The aim of perioperative care is to avoid the accumulation of oxygen debt by maintaining adequate oxygen delivery to the tissues. The first step is to identify patients who are not able to do this by themselves, by instigating the appropriate physiological monitoring. If augmentation is required, the clinician must determine whether this can be achieved with intravenous fluid therapy. Thus we need to predict which patients are likely to be fluid- or preload-responsive.

Static markers of preload status

Static markers of cardiac preload status include the central venous pressure (CVP), pulmonary artery

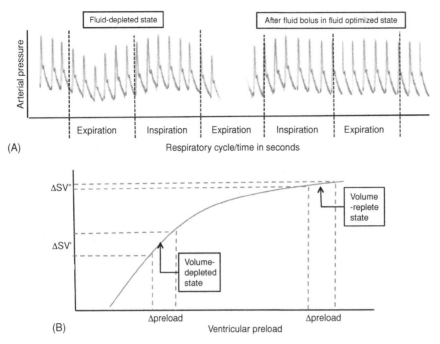

Figure 14.2 A: Positive intra-thoracic pressure reduces right ventricular (RV) filling. The reduced RV output flows through the pulmonary circulation resulting in reduced LV filling and a reduced SV, apparent 2–3 seconds later during expiration. After a fluid bolus the effect is less pronounced. **B**: The Starling curve. A change in ventricular preload due to positive-pressure ventilation has a marked effect on SV' in the volume-depleted state when the ventricle is operating on the steep position of the curve. This results in a large SV' variation over several cardiac cycles. In comparison, the same change in preload in the volume-replete state causes little variation in SV'.

occlusion pressure, ventricular end-diastolic volumes, GEDV, ITBV, and extravascular lung water (EVLW).

GEDV and ITBV are two static markers of preload provided by pulse-contour analysis devices (PiCCO^{TM} and VolumeView^{TM}). They have been incorporated successfully into a number of optimization protocols as discussed earlier and are superior to the CVP at identifying the fluid-responsive patient.[40] EVLW reflects the amount of pulmonary interstitial fluid. It does not correlate well with oxygenation or chest radiograph lung opacification but does reflect severity of illness and length of ventilation. Reducing the ITBV to normal levels may reduce the EVLW.

These values do not reliably predict the fluid-responsive state and are unable to identify which patients will benefit from fluid therapy. This is because the relationship between cardiac reserve, vascular reserve, and contractility is too complex to be adequately represented by one cardiac measurement.[40]

Dynamic markers of preload status

The application of a physiological change that alters ventricular preload allows the functional assessment of the cardiovascular system as a whole. Measuring changes in CO and SV before and after the preload change enables the reliable prediction of a fluid-responsive state.

Heart–lung interactions

In a patient who is undergoing mechanical positive-pressure ventilation, there is a cyclical (predictable) change in intrathoracic pressure. During inspiration, positive pressure impinges the right heart intermittently, reducing ventricular filling which is more affected in the volume-depleted state. Reducing right ventricular SV reduces left ventricular filling, and subsequently a decrease in left ventricular SV is seen 2–3 seconds later, during expiration (Figure 14.2). This delay is due to pulmonary flow transit time.

The variation in SV or pulse pressure over the respiratory cycle that occurs is due to the above phenomenon. A PPV or SVV of greater than 13–15% predicts that there will be an increase in CO in response to fluid administration. This has been validated in mechanically ventilated patients undergoing normal tidal ventilation (even as low as 8 ml/kg tidal volume) in a variety of clinical situations.[40] Most CO monitors calculate and display the PPV or SVV over a period of 10–20 seconds.

Limitations

Spontaneous ventilation results in varying intrathoracic pressure changes yielding uninterpretable results. Low-tidal-volume strategies do not provide the degree of intrathoracic pressure change required to produce discernible changes. Cardiac arrhythmia will cause beat-to-beat variation regardless of intrathoracic pressure conditions. Right ventricular failure is also a contraindication since the cyclical effect of the ventilation can affect the afterload of the right ventricle and generate falsely elevated PPV and SVV in the context of non-fluid-responsive patients (in whom fluid administration may actually be harmful).

Increasing cardiac preload with a passive leg raise, a fluid bolus, and an end-expiratory hold

To increase preload transiently and reversibly without administering fluid may be advantageous. In a mechanically ventilated patient a rapid Trendelenburg maneuver will provide an immediate 200–250 ml blood migration into the central circulation. An increase in CO of more than 10% is strongly predictive of a positive response to a 500 ml volume administration. The practical application of this maneuver may be challenging in the operating theater.

Using the CO monitor, the percentage change in SV before and immediately after a fluid challenge of sufficient volume (usually 250 ml) is calculated. An increase of greater than 10–15% in SV indicates a positive response and predicts a fluid-responsive state. The advantage of this technique is that it can be performed in spontaneously breathing, awake patients.

An end-expiratory pause of 15 seconds reduces intrathoracic pressure and allows increased ventricular filling. Studies have demonstrated that an increase in CO or PPV of more than 5% during this period is highly predictive of a positive response to fluid administration.

Using these indices in clinical practice

It is important to distinguish between predicting fluid responsiveness, performing a fluid challenge, and

treating with fluid therapy. The first is done without any fluid administration at all, which is the preferred method and avoids inappropriate administration of fluid. The second is using a minimal-volume fluid challenge as a diagnostic (and therapeutic) test to see whether the patient responds favorably.[41] The last is treatment of hypovolemia, which may be achieved using a number of different techniques.

Many algorithms exist that incorporate these concepts. The concept of SV optimization relies on administration of fluid as boluses until the SVV or PVV is less than 10%. Alternatively, a fluid bolus may be given as an assessment or when the CO increases by more than 10%, and repeated boluses may be given until no further response is detected. Use of these algorithms may allow a reduced volume of fluid to be administered, achieving hemodynamic optimization without over-administration of fluid therapy. These protocols should not be used without consideration of the individual patient and are therefore not a replacement for clinical judgment.

Conclusion

Cardiac output monitoring in the perioperative period is now safely available to a greater number of patients owing to the improved risk–benefit profile of modern devices. These devices allow the judicious use of intravenous fluid therapy to optimize oxygen delivery and avoid hypervolemia. When used in conjunction with an evidence-based GDT protocol it may improve the outcome of patients in the perioperative period. Adequate patient selection to identify moderate- to high-risk cases is probably one of the most important parts of these strategies.[10]

Each monitor has limitations that need to be considered by the clinician relying on the data provided. It is likely that the use of a particular monitor is less important than the implementation of a validated optimization protocol for the majority of patients. The monitoring tool may be escalated to a more invasive, accurate device and used in conjunction with echocardiography to manage the shocked perioperative patient.

References

1. Shoemaker WC, Appel PL, Kram HB, Waxman K, Lee TS. Prospective trial of supranormal values of survivors as therapeutic goals in high-risk surgical patients. *Chest* 1988, 94: 1176–86.

2. Ackland GL, Igbal S, Paredes LG, *et al.* for the POM-O (PostOperative Morbidity-Oxygen delivery) study group. Individualised oxygen delivery targeted hemodynamic therapy in high-risk surgical patients: a multicentre, randomised, double-blind, controlled, mechanistic trial. *Lancet Respir Med* 2015; 3: 33–41.

3. Boyd O, Grounds RM, Bennett ED. A randomized clinical trial of the effect of deliberate perioperative increase of oxygen delivery on mortality in high-risk surgical patients. *JAMA* 1993; 270: 2699–707.

4. Lobo SM, Salgado PF, Castillo VG, *et al.* Maximizing O_2 delivery in high-risk elderly surgery patients improves survivorship without altering O_2 consumption. *Crit Care Med* 2000; 28: 3396–404.

5. Connors AF Jr, Speroff T, Dawson NV, *et al.* for the SUPPORT Investigators. The effectiveness of right heart catheterization in the initial care of critically ill patients. *JAMA* 1996; 276: 889–97.

6. Pölönen P, Ruokonen E, Hippeläinen M, Pöyhonen M, Takala J. A prospective, randomized study of goal-oriented hemodynamic therapy in cardiac surgical patients. *Anesth Analg* 2000; 90: 1052–9.

7. Wakeling HG, McFall MR, Jenkins CS, *et al.* Intraoperative oesophageal Doppler guided fluid management shortens postoperative hospital stay after major bowel surgery. *Br J Anaesth* 2005; 95: 634–42.

8. Sinclair S, James S, Singer M. Intraoperative intravascular volume optimisation and length of hospital stay after repair of proximal femoral fracture: randomised controlled trial. *BMJ* 1997; 315: 909–12.

9. Hamilton MA, Cecconi M, Rhodes A. A systematic review and meta-analysis on the use of preemptive hemodynamic intervention to improve postoperative outcomes in moderate and high-risk surgical patients. *Anesth Analg* 2011; 112: 1392–402.

10. Cecconi M, Corredor C, Arulkumaran N, *et al.* Clinical review: Goal-directed therapy-what is the evidence in surgical patients? The effect on different risk groups. *Crit Care* 2013; 17: 209.

11. Kern JW, Shoemaker WC. Meta-analysis of hemodynamic optimization in high-risk patients. *Crit Care Med* 2002; 30: 1686–92.

12. Grocott MP, Dushianthan A, Hamilton MA, *et al.* Perioperative increase in global blood flow to explicit defined goals and outcomes following surgery, Optimisation Systematic Review Steering Group. *Cochrane Database Syst Rev* 2012; 11: CD004082.

13. Srinivasa S, Taylor MH, Singh PP, *et al.* Randomized clinical trial of goal-directed fluid therapy within an enhanced recovery protocol for elective colectomy. *Br J Surg* 2013; 100: 66–74.

14. McKenny M, Conroy P, Wong A, *et al.* A randomised prospective trial of intra-operative esophageal Doppler-guided fluid administration in major gynecological surgery. *Anaesthesia* 2013; 68: 1224–31.

15. Pearse RM, Harrison DA, MacDonald N, *et al.* for the OPTIMISE Study Group. Effect of a perioperative, cardiac output-guided hemodynamic therapy algorithm on outcomes following major gastrointestinal surgery: a randomized clinical trial and systematic review. *JAMA* 2014; 311: 2181–90.

16. Hayes MA, Timmins AC, Yau EH, *et al.* Elevation of systemic oxygen delivery in the treatment of critically ill patients. *N Engl J Med* 1994; 330: 1717–22.

17. Critchley LA, Critchley JA. A meta-analysis of studies using bias and precision statistics to compare cardiac output measurement techniques. *J Clin Monit Comput* 1999; 15: 85–91.

18. Cecconi M, Rhodes A, Poloniecki J, Della Rocca G, Grounds RM. Bench-to-bedside review. The importance of the precision of the reference technique in method comparison studies – with specific reference to the measurement of cardiac output. *Crit Care* 2009; 13: 201.

19. Fanshawe M, Ellis C, Habib S, Konstadt SN, Reich DL. A retrospective analysis of the costs and benefits related to alterations in cardiac surgery from routine intraoperative transesophageal echocardiography. *Anesth Analg* 2002; 95: 824–7.

20. Cecconi M, De Backer D, Antonelli M, *et al.* for the Task Force of the European Society of Intensive Care Medicine. Consensus on circulatory shock and hemodynamic monitoring. *Intensive Care Med* 2014; 40: 1795–815.

21. Rajaram SS, Desai NK, Kalra A, *et al.* Pulmonary artery catheters for adult patients in intensive care. *Cochrane Database Syst Rev* 2013; 2: CD003408.

22. Harvey S, Harrison DA, Singer M, *et al.* PAC-Man study collaboration. Assessment of the clinical effectiveness of pulmonary artery catheters in management of patients in intensive care (PAC-Man): a randomised controlled trial. *Lancet* 2005; 366: 472–7.

23. Sandham JD, Hulkl RD, Brant RF, *et al.* for the Canadian Critical Care Clinical Trials Group. A randomized, controlled trial of the use of pulmonary-artery catheters in high-risk surgical patients. *N Engl J Med* 2003; 348: 5–14.

24. Wheeler AP, Bernard GR, Thompson BT, *et al.* for the National Heart, Lung, and Blood Institute Acute Respiratory Distress Syndrome (ARDS) Clinical Trials Network. Pulmonary-artery versus central venous catheter to guide treatment of acute lung injury. *N Engl J Med* 2006; 354: 2213–24.

25. Goedje O, Hoeke K, Lichtwarck-Aschoff M, *et al.* Continuous cardiac output by femoral arterial thermodilution calibrated pulse contour analysis:

comparison with pulmonary arterial thermodilution. *Crit Care Med* 1999; 27: 2407–12.

26. Gepfert MS, Reuter DA, Akyol D, *et al.* Goal-directed fluid management reduces vasopressor and catecholamine use in cardiac surgery patients. *Intensive Care Med* 2007; 33: 96–103.

27. Kiefer N, Hofer CK, Marx G, *et al.* Clinical validation of a new thermodilution system for the assessment of cardiac output and volumetric parameters. *Crit Care* 2012; 16: R98.

28. Mora B, Ince I, Birkenberg B, *et al.* Validation of cardiac output measurement with the LiDCO™ pulse contour system in patients with impaired left ventricular function after cardiac surgery. *J Anesth* 2011; 66: 675–81.

29. Costa MG, Della Rocca G, Chiarandini P, *et al.* Continuous and intermittent cardiac output measurement in hyperdynamic conditions: pulmonary artery catheter vs. lithium dilution technique. *Intensive Care Med* 1008; 34: 257–63.

30. Pearse R, Dawson D, Fawcett J, *et al.* Early goal-directed therapy after major surgery reduces complications and duration of hospital stay. A randomised, controlled trial. *Crit Care* 2005; 9: 687–93.

31. Ostergaard M, Nielsen J, Nygaard E. Pulse contour cardiac output: an evaluation of the FloTrac method. *Eur J Anaesthesiol* 2009; 26: 484–9.

32. Phan TD, Wan C, Wong D, Padayachee A. A comparison of three minimally invasive cardiac output devices with thermodilution in elective cardiac surgery. *Anesthesiol Intensive Care* 2011; 39: 1014–21.

33. Penn A, Button D, Zollinger A, Hofer CK. Assessment of cardiac output changes using a modified FloTrac/Vigileo algorithm in cardiac surgery patients. *Crit Care* 2009; 13: R32.

34. Cecconi M, Fasano N, Langiano N, *et al.* Goal-directed hemodynamic therapy during elective total hip arthroplasty under regional anesthesia. *Crit Care* 2011; 15: R132.

35. Hadian M, Kim HK, Severyn DA, Pinsky MR. Cross-comparison of cardiac output trending accuracy of LiDCO, PiCCO, FloTrac and pulmonary artery catheters. *Crit Care* 2010; 14: R212.

36. Monnet X, Anguel N, Naudin B, *et al.* Arterial pressure-based cardiac output in septic patients: different accuracy of pulse contour and uncalibrated pressure waveform devices. *Crit Care* 2010; 14: R109.

37. Romano SM, Pistolesi M. Assessment of cardiac output from systemic arterial pressure in humans. *Crit Care Med* 2002; 30: 1834–41.

38. Giomarelli P. Cardiac output monitoring by pressure recording analytical method in cardiac surgery. *Eur J Cardiothorac Surg* 2004; 26: 515–20.

39. Calamandrei M, Mirabile L, Muschetta S, *et al.* Assessment of cardiac output in children: a comparison between the pressure recording analytical method and Doppler echocardiography. *Pediatr Crit Care Med* 2008; 9: 310–12.

40. Cecconi M, Parsons AK, Rhodes A. What is a fluid challenge? Current opinion in critical care. *Crit Care* 2011; 17: 290–5.

41. Cecconi M, Hofer C, Teboul JL, *et al.* Fluid challenges in intensive care: the FENICE study: a global inception cohort study. *Intensive Care Med* 2015; 41: 1529–37.

Chapter

15

Goal-directed fluid therapy

Timothy E. Miller and Tong J. Gan

Summary

Perioperative morbidity has been linked to the amount of fluid administered, with both insufficient and excess fluid leading to increased morbidity, resulting in a characteristic U-shaped curve. The challenge for us as clinicians is to keep our patients in the optimal range at all times during the perioperative period. Goal-directed therapy (GDT) is a term that has been used for nearly 30 years to describe methods of optimizing fluid and hemodynamic status. The arrival of a number of minimally invasive cardiac output monitors enables clinicians to guide perioperative volume therapy and cardiocirculatory support.

The most widely used monitor is the esophageal Doppler. There are several others that are able to analyze the arterial waveform to calculate stroke volume and cardiac output, and therefore use the "10% algorithm" in response to a fluid challenge. There are a number of studies that show improved outcomes with GDT-guided fluid optimization, as demonstrated by a faster return in gastrointestinal function, a reduction in postoperative complications, and reduced length of stay. The underlying mechanisms for the success of GDT are thought to relate to avoidance of episodes of hypovolemia, hypoxia, or decreased blood flow that may cause mitochondrial damage and subsequent organ dysfunction.*

_____
* Summary compiled by the Editor.

Over 310 million operations were performed worldwide in 2012. For most patients, the risks of surgery are thought to be low, and yet evidence increasingly suggests that morbidity and mortality are more common than expected. The recent European Surgical Outcomes Study (EuSOS) provided data for a population of more than 46,000 unselected patients undergoing non-cardiac in-patient surgery from 28 European countries, and found that 4% of included patients died before hospital discharge.[1]

High-risk surgery is associated with significant morbidity and mortality. From a database of over 4 million patients it has been shown that 80% of deaths occur in only 12.5% of surgical procedures.[2] In addition, patients who develop complications but survive to leave hospital often have reduced functional independence and long-term survival.[3]

Optimization of the high-risk surgical patient during the perioperative period aims to improve outcomes in this patient population. Goal-directed therapy (GDT) is a term that has been used for nearly 30 years to describe methods of optimizing fluid and hemodynamic status. Unfortunately the term GDT has not been standardized, and therefore can mean different things to people, causing a significant amount of confusion.

The term was first used to describe early oxygen-targeted GDT in the 1980s and 1990s which used the pulmonary artery catheter (PAC) to augment oxygen delivery (DO_2) to supranormal levels in high-risk surgical patients. More recently, GDT with fluid alone aims to maximize stroke volume (SV) and therefore cardiac output (CO), using a minimally invasive CO monitor. This review will concentrate on the evidence for the benefit of such GDT during major surgery.

Clinical Fluid Therapy in the Perioperative Setting, Second Edition, ed. Robert G. Hahn. Published by Cambridge University Press. © Cambridge University Press 2016.

Early GDT: supranormal oxygen delivery

The first major GDT study was conducted by Shoemaker and colleagues in 1988.[4] This landmark paper looked at patients undergoing high-risk surgery, and compared standard of care with supramaximal DO_2. The hypothesis was proposed that increased cardiac index (CI) and DO_2 are necessary circulatory compensations needed to cope with high postoperative metabolism. To do this in the protocol group a PAC was used to obtain targets of CI >4.5 liter/min/m^2, oxygen delivery index (DO_2I) >600 ml/min/m^2, and oxygen consumption index (VO_2I) >170 ml/min/m^2. This was achieved through a combination of fluids, inotropes (principally dobutamine), and vasopressors. Targets were based on physiological values that they had observed in survivors after high-risk surgery,[5] and the results showed a significant reduction in mortality.

This led to further studies of supranormal oxygen delivery in high-risk surgery, using the same oxygen delivery target of 600 ml/min/m^2. Boyd *et al.* in 1993 showed a reduction in mortality of 75% with GDT.[6] Mortality benefits were also seen with preoperative optimization,[7] as well as in cardiac [8] and general surgery patients.[9]

The underlying mechanisms for the success of GDT are thought to relate to avoidance of episodes of hypovolemia, hypoxia, or decreased blood flow that may cause mitochondrial damage and subsequent organ dysfunction. Therefore, adequate tissue oxygen supply throughout the perioperative period is the key to successful outcomes.

Despite these promising results, the technique was not widely adopted. The reasons for this are almost certainly multifactorial. Early GDT required significant resources, was very labor intensive, and most importantly was reliant on information from the PAC. Catheterization of the right heart began falling out of favor in intensive care units in the 1990s after the publication of several observational studies showing increased mortality.[10] As early GDT was linked so closely with the use of PAC, it became embroiled in this controversy.

Thus, despite the fact that numerous trials have shown that mortality, morbidity, and length of hospital stay can be reduced with early GDT, widespread use remained a pipedream for enthusiasts.

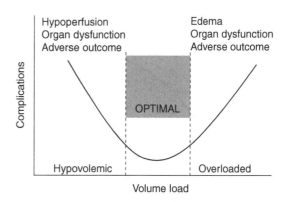

Figure 15.1 Fluid load versus complications (modified from Bellamy).[11]

Modern GDT: individualized volume optimization

The past 20 years have seen the arrival of a number of minimally invasive CO monitors that enable clinicians to guide perioperative volume therapy and cardiocirculatory support. GDT uses these monitors to depict a trend and optimize stroke volume and therefore CO.

Perioperative morbidity has been linked to the amount of fluid administered, with both insufficient and excess fluid leading to increased morbidity, resulting in a characteristic U-shaped curve (see Figure 15.1).[11] Episodes of hypovolemia during surgery can lead to organ hypoperfusion, ischemia, and adverse outcomes. Conversely, a number of studies have shown that perioperative fluid excess, particularly crystalloid, can result in tissue edema and increased complications.[12]

The challenge for us as clinicians is to keep our patients in the optimal range at all times during the perioperative period. Episodes of hypovolemia or edema if severe can cause major morbidity. More commonly, however, these changes can be subtle, with bowel mucosa ischemia or edema causing gastrointestinal tract dysfunction and prolonged postoperative ileus, with resultant inability to tolerate a normal diet, and increased length of hospital stay.[13]

Traditional monitoring techniques are not useful to accurately detect and optimize the volume status of patients. Healthy volunteers can lose 25% of their blood volume without any discernible change in heart rate or blood pressure, whilst at the same time advanced monitors show a significant reduction in

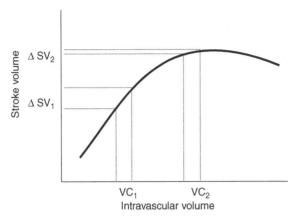

Figure 15.2 Frank–Starling-based stroke volume optimization.

stroke volume and gastric intramucosal pH, implying a degree of ischemia.[14] Central venous pressure (CVP) monitoring has also been shown to be a poor predictor of volume responsiveness.[15] A recent systematic review showed that CVP is not able to identify which patients need more fluid, and concluded that CVP should no longer be routinely measured in the ICU, operating room, or emergency department.[16]

Advanced monitors in GDT can be used to measure CO and SV non-invasively, and thereby allow the clinician to use fluid challenges to achieve SV optimization (see Figure 15.2). When a patient is hypovolemic and on the steep part of the Starling curve, an intravenous fluid challenge (VC_1 in Figure 15.2) will lead to a greater than 10% increase in SV. This patient has "recruitable" SV, and is in a fluid-responsive state. Fluid loading, typically with 250 ml boluses of

intravenous colloid, should continue until the increase in SV is less than 10% when the patient has reached the flat part of the Starling curve. This "Frank–Starling fluid challenge" provides a sophisticated method of titrating intravenous fluids to complex patients.

A crucial difference from the earlier Shoemaker concept for optimization is that the present approach is individualized to optimize flow-related parameters such as SV within the individual's cardiac capacity, as opposed to using predetermined supraphysiological goals.

Esophageal Doppler

There are a number of technologies that can be used for GDT. The most widely studied is undoubtedly the Esophageal Doppler Monitor (EDM, Deltex Medical, Chichester, UK). The Doppler probe is placed in the esophagus and focused at the descending thoracic aorta, where it uses the Doppler principle to measure blood flow and produce a waveform (Figure 15.3). This is then converted to SV using a nomogram of height, weight, and age to estimate the cross-sectional area of the descending aorta. EDM-derived SV measurements have been well validated in different environments and clinical scenarios.[17–22]

Another useful measurement is the corrected flow time (FTc), which is the width of the waveform, or length of systole in ms, corrected to a heart rate of 60. An FTc <350 ms is an additional indicator of recruitable SV.

There are a number of studies that show improved outcomes with EDM-guided fluid optimization, as

(A)

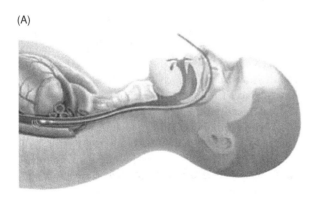

(B)

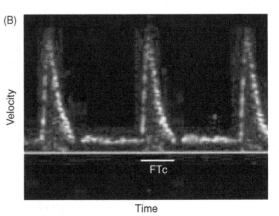

Figure 15.3 Esophageal Doppler. **A**: Schematic representation of esophageal Doppler probe in a patient, demonstrating the close relation between esophagus and descending thoracic aorta. **B**: Characteristic velocity waveform obtained in the descending aorta. FTc: corrected flow time.

Table 15.1 Summary of perioperative esophageal Doppler monitor-guided GDT studies

Reference	Surgical group	Patients (*n*)	Outcome
Mythen and Webb (1995) [28]	Cardiac	60	⇓ gastric acidosis in GDT ⇓ complications in GDT ⇓ LOS (3.5 days) in GDT
Sinclair *et al.* (1997) [30]	Neck of femur fracture	40	⇓ time FFD (5 days) in GDT ⇓ LOS (8 days) in GDT
Conway *et al.* (2002) [23]	Major bowel	57	⇑ ICU admissions in control, no difference in LOS
Gan *et al.* (2002) [24]	Major general	100	⇑ PONV in control ⇓ time to tolerating oral intake in GDT ⇓ LOS (2 days) in GDT
Venn *et al.* (2002) [31]	Neck of femur fracture	90	⇓ time FFD (6.2 days) in GDT (vs. control) ⇓ time FFD (3.9 days) in CVP (vs. control)
McKendry *et al.* (2004) [29]	Cardiac surgery	174	⇓ LOS (2.5 days) in GDT, no difference in complications
Wakeling *et al.* (2005) [25]	Colorectal	128	⇓ morbidity (GI and overall) in GDT ⇓ time to full diet (1 day) in GDT ⇓ LOS (1.5 days) in GDT
Noblett *et al.* (2006) [26]	Colorectal	108	⇓ morbidity in GDT ⇓ time to tolerating diet (2 days) in GDT ⇓ time FFD (3 days) in GDT ⇓ LOS (2 days) in GDT
Senagore *et al.* (2009) [27]	Laparoscopic colorectal	64	no difference in LOS no difference in complications

LOS, length of stay; FFD, fit for discharge; GI, gastrointestinal; PONV, postoperative nausea and vomiting.

demonstrated by a faster return in gastrointestinal function, a reduction in postoperative complications and reduced length of stay. Five studies were in a major general/colorectal study population,[23–27], two in cardiac surgery,[28,29], and two in patients scheduled for repair of fractured neck of femur [30,31] (see Table 15.1).

All of these studies used a 10% algorithm to optimize SV, often combined with assessment of FTc to predict fluid responsiveness. Although there are small differences between the studies, a typical algorithm is shown in Figure 15.4.

The major limitation of the EDM is the occasional need for repositioning of the probe to optimize the signal, which can be time-consuming. There is a learning curve for positioning the probe, and as such it is somewhat user-dependent. The use of electrocautery can also interfere with the signal.

Nevertheless, the evidence base behind its use is relatively strong, and its incorporation into Enhanced Recovery after Surgery (ERAS) programs is currently a strong driving force for increased interest.[32] Recently the Center for Medicare Services in the USA have reviewed the literature and supported a professional fee being paid to clinicians using EDM-guided perioperative volume optimization.[33] The Centre for Evidence-Based Purchasing division of the NHS Purchasing and Supply Agency in the UK has also recommended the EDM.[34]

Arterial pressure waveform analysis

The other major monitoring technique used in GDT is arterial pressure waveform analysis. There are several monitors available that are able to analyze the arterial waveform to calculate SV and CO, and therefore use the "10% algorithm" in response to a fluid challenge.

Arterial waveform analysis is also able to derive dynamic parameters of fluid responsiveness, based on cardiopulmonary interactions, such as stroke volume variation (SVV) and pulse pressure variation (PPV). These dynamic variables are superior to traditional static indices such as CVP in predicting volume responsiveness in mechanically ventilated patients.[35]

The physiology behind SVV and PPV is relatively simple. Positive-pressure ventilation induces cyclical changes in the loading conditions of the right ventricle,

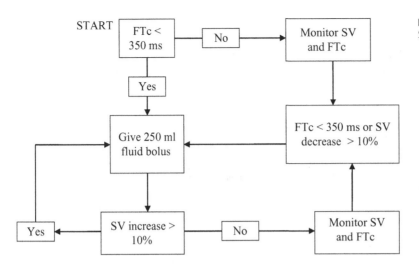

Figure 15.4 A typical combined FTc and SV optimization algorithm.

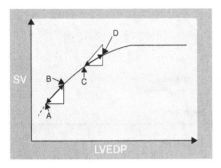

Figure 15.5 A Starling curve of left ventricular stroke volume (SV) against left ventricular end-diastolic pressure (LVEDP) demonstrating the change in SV that occurs with positive-pressure ventilation. The starting position on the curve determines the magnitude of the change in SV, and hence the SV variation. If the patient is hypovolemic the LVEDP will cycle between A and B, with respiration causing a cyclical change in SV and a swing in the arterial line. If the patient is euvolemic LVEDP will cycle between C and D, causing a much smaller change in SV.

with a reduction in preload during mechanical insufflation. This will lead to cyclical changes in SV. If the ventricle is operating on the steep part of the Starling curve, the magnitude of the change in SV and blood pressure will be greater, and will manifest itself as a characteristic "swing" in the arterial line pressure with respiration (Figure 15.5).

PPV and SVV represent "virtual" preload challenges occurring during each respiratory cycle in ventilated patients. There is no need to administer fluid to predict responders, with SVV or PPV greater than 10% accurately predicting a positive response to a fluid challenge.[36] As these metrics predict responders with more accuracy than CVP or pulmonary artery occlusion pressure (PAOP), there is less need for invasive central lines.

Targeting a PPV or SVV <10–13% has been shown to improve postoperative outcomes. At least eight randomized controlled trials have demonstrated that hemodynamic strategies based on PPV or SVV monitoring allow a significant reduction in postsurgical complications and hospital length of stay after major abdominal surgery.[37]

There are some important limitations to the use of the dynamic variables. The main limitation is that patients should be fully mechanically ventilated without any spontaneous breathing, and with a regular R:R interval. Fortunately in the operating room this is generally the case; less so in the intensive care unit. For optimal results the tidal volume should be 8 ml/kg with "normal" intrathoracic and intra-abdominal pressures. For example, during laparoscopic surgery after insufflation of the pneumoperitoneum, there will be an elevation of intra-abdominal pressure (IAP) that will decrease chest wall compliance, and consequently SVV and PPV will increase independently of changes in blood volume.[38,39] However, when IAP <15 mmHg, SVV and PPV still appear to predict fluid responsiveness fairly well, although the threshold may be raised (fluid responsive when PPV >15% rather than 10%).[38,40]

In practice, the limitations of each dynamic index should be taken into consideration and the dynamic variables used in combination with changes in SV to ensure that fluid boluses are given at the appropriate time to improve hemodynamics without any increase in risk.

Other technologies

An increasing number of new technologies that have recently been marketed have the ability to monitor CO non-invasively.

The NICOM (Cheetah Medical, Boston, MA) is a continuous non-invasive CO monitor based on chest bioreactance that is accurate when compared with the PAC.[41,42] It is totally non-invasive, comprising four surface electrodes that are placed across the chest. The NICOM has been shown to perform similarly to the EDM in guiding GDT, with no clinically significant differences in outcomes, and offers increased ease of use as well as fewer missing data points.[43]

The ClearSight system (Edwards Lifesciences, Irvine, CA) is another completely non-invasive method of measuring CO using an inflatable finger cuff. The cuff "clamps" the pulsating finger artery to a constant volume by applying a varying counterpressure equivalent to the arterial pressure. This results in a continuous pressure waveform that resembles an arterial line waveform, reliably tracks blood pressure,[44] and serves as the basis for determining continuous CO. There appears to be good correlation between ClearSight-derived CO and the PAC.[45]

The pleth variability index (PVI) is a similar value to SVV and PPV that is continuously calculated from the pulse oximeter tracing by the non-invasive Masimo monitor (Masimo Corporation, Irvine, CA). PVI-based goal-directed fluid management has been shown to reduce intraoperative and postoperative lactate levels.[46] As is the case with SVV and PVV, one should always bear in mind the same limitations before taking clinical decisions regarding the hemodynamic optimization of patients.

The BioZ (Cardiodynamics Intl. San Diego, CA) uses thoracic bioimpedance, which is less robust.[47] The Aesculon (Osypka Medical, La Jolla, CA) uses electrical velocimetry to interpret the maximal change in thoracic bioimpedance to calculate CO, and has been shown to be accurate.[48] The challenge for manufacturers is to produce not only a well-validated, reliable monitor, but to show an outcome benefit in this increasingly competitive field.

GDT within an Enhanced Recovery program

In the past few years, Enhanced Recovery programs are becoming standard of care for colorectal surgery, and are increasingly being applied to other major surgery.[49] Enhanced Recovery programs have been shown to reduce length of stay for colorectal surgery by 2.5 days, and decrease perioperative complications by 50%.[50] Such programs aim to avoid prolonged preoperative fasting, so that the patient is euvolemic upon arrival to the OR, potentially making intraoperative fluid management easier.

Single-center studies of GDT within an ERAS program have failed to find the same benefit on postoperative outcomes as the early studies.[51,52] This is perhaps not surprising, as care within the control group has significantly improved, making it harder to observe a difference versus GDT.

The multicenter POEMAS study randomized 142 patients undergoing major abdominal surgery within an Enhanced Recovery pathway to GDT using the NICOM or control, and found no difference in the incidence of overall complications or length of stay.[53]

In contrast, the larger multi-center OPTIMISE study focused on GDT using the LiDCO rapid system (LiDCO Ltd, Cambridge, UK) on 734 high-risk patient undergoing major abdominal surgery.[54] A significant proportion of these patients were managed within an ERAS pathway. In this high-risk population there was a non-significant trend towards decreased complications (36.6% vs. 43.4%, $p = 0.07$) and 180-day mortality (7.7% vs. 11.6%, $p = 0.08$) in the GDT group compared with usual care. The study was underpowered, as the complication rate in both groups was less than expected. However, inclusion of these data in an updated meta-analysis indicated that the intervention was associated with a reduction in complication rates.[54]

Therefore, whilst ERAS programs may have raised the threshold for benefit, current evidence suggests that there will still be many patients, whether expected or unexpected, for whom SV optimization will be beneficial. Many patients who are undergoing major surgery outside of ERAS pathways, such as vascular surgery, will also benefit from GDT.

Ultimately the need for GDT is specific to the patient, surgeon, procedure, and institution. Each institution needs to look at its outcomes and benchmark data for the benefitting population against other institutions before making an informed decision about appropriate implementation of GDT. This data should include length of stay, readmission rate, mortality, and costs. All patients should have an individualized plan for fluid management rather than a formulaic approach based on body weight and duration of surgical exposure. For patients undergoing colorectal surgery with limited blood loss within an ERAS pathway, minimal fluid may be required, and GDT may not offer additional benefits.[55] However, current evidence suggests that for the majority of patients undergoing major surgery, GDT remains the technique of choice for perioperative fluid and hemodynamic optimization.[56]

Which fluid should I use?

Although the need for maintenance fluids has recently been questioned, most GDT algorithms use a background infusion of a balanced crystalloid solution at 1–3 ml per kg per hour based on ideal body weight.

In addition, most GDT algorithms in the literature have used a colloid solution for fluid boluses. This is based on the principle that in the setting of hypovolemia a colloid will restore blood pressure and therefore organ perfusion faster and with less volume.[57] However, in clinical practice the superiority of colloids over crystalloids remains unresolved.[58] A recent study comparing crystalloids and colloids for fluid boluses within a GDT algorithm found no difference in the primary outcome of postoperative gastrointestinal morbidity.[59] Therefore, in practice, a combination of crystalloids and colloids are used for fluid challenges, with colloids typically reserved for definitive evidence of significant intravascular hypovolemia with blood loss.

Conclusion

As the population ages, the number of patients requiring high-risk non-cardiac surgery is only going to increase. The concept of individualized GDT for these patients seems to improve outcomes by ensuring adequate tissue perfusion at all times perioperatively. The underlying mechanism behind the success of GDT is related to the optimization of DO_2 to the tissues. This avoids an oxygen debt, which can cause mitochondrial damage and organ dysfunction.

Many authors have described how the use of GDT can reduce morbidity and length of stay in high-risk surgical patients, although most of the studies have been performed on small sample sizes from single centers. Two recent meta-analyses focusing on renal function [60] and gastrointestinal function [61] have also showed that surgical patients receiving perioperative

GDT are at decreased risk of renal and gastrointestinal impairment, which account for a significant proportion of postoperative morbidity. The largest study of GDT to date is the OPTIMISE study which showed a trend towards a reduction in complications that did not reach statistical significance. A larger OPTIMISE-2 study is planned.

Perioperative GDT has not become standard of care for a variety of reasons. It remains a challenge to implement GDT because of the significant commitment and resources needed. However, with an increasing number of studies being published on the clinical utility of non-invasive hemodynamic monitoring, the use of GDT should continue to gain popularity.

References

1. Pearse RM, Moreno RP, Bauer P, *et al.* Mortality after surgery in Europe: a 7 day cohort study. *Lancet.* 2012; 380[9847]: 1059–65.

2. Pearse RM, Harrison DA, James P, *et al.* Identification and characterisation of the high-risk surgical population in the United Kingdom. *Crit Care.* 2006; 10[3]: R81. Epub 2006/06/06.

3. Khuri SF, Henderson WG, DePalma RG, *et al.* Determinants of long-term survival after major surgery and the adverse effect of postoperative complications. *Ann Surg.* 2005; 242[3]: 326–41; discussion 41–3.

4. Shoemaker WC, Appel PL, Kram HB, *et al.* Prospective trial of supranormal values of survivors as therapeutic goals in high-risk surgical patients. *Chest.* 1988; 94[6]: 1176–86. Epub 1988/12/01.

5. Shoemaker WC, Montgomery ES, Kaplan E, *et al.* Physiologic patterns in surviving and nonsurviving shock patients. Use of sequential cardiorespiratory variables in defining criteria for therapeutic goals and early warning of death. *Arch Surg.* 1973; 106[5]: 630–6. Epub 1973/05/01.

6. Boyd O, Grounds RM, Bennett ED. A randomized clinical trial of the effect of deliberate perioperative increase of oxygen delivery on mortality in high-risk surgical patients. *JAMA.* 1993; 270[22]: 2699–707. Epub 1993/12/08.

7. Wilson J, Woods I, Fawcett J, *et al.* Reducing the risk of major elective surgery: randomised controlled trial of preoperative optimisation of oxygen delivery. *BMJ.* 1999; 318[7191]: 1099–103. Epub 1999/04/24.

8. Polonen P, Ruokonen E, Hippelainen M, *et al.* A prospective, randomized study of goal-oriented hemodynamic therapy in cardiac surgical patients. *Anesth Analg.* 2000; 90[5]: 1052–9. Epub 2000/04/27.

9. Lobo SM, Salgado PF, Castillo VG, *et al.* Effects of maximizing oxygen delivery on morbidity and mortality in high-risk surgical patients. *Crit Care Med.* 2000; 28[10]: 3396–404. Epub 2000/11/01.

10. Connors AF, Jr., Speroff T, Dawson NV, *et al.* The effectiveness of right heart catheterization in the initial care of critically ill patients. SUPPORT Investigators. *JAMA.* 1996; 276[11]: 889–97. Epub 1996/09/18.

11. Bellamy MC. Wet, dry or something else? *Br J Anaesth.* 2006; 97[6]: 755–7. Epub 2006/11/14.

12. Brandstrup B, Tonnesen H, Beier-Holgersen R, *et al.* Effects of intravenous fluid restriction on postoperative complications: comparison of two perioperative fluid regimens: a randomized assessor-blinded multicenter trial. *Ann Surg.* 2003; 238[5]: 641–8. Epub 2003/10/28.

13. Bennett-Guerrero E, Welsby I, Dunn TJ, *et al.* The use of a postoperative morbidity survey to evaluate patients with prolonged hospitalization after routine, moderate-risk, elective surgery. *Anesth Analg.* 1999; 89[2]: 514–19. Epub 1999/08/10.

14. Hamilton-Davies C, Mythen MG, Salmon JB, *et al.* Comparison of commonly used clinical indicators of hypovolaemia with gastrointestinal tonometry. *Intensive Care Med.* 1997; 23[3]: 276–81. Epub 1997/03/01.

15. Osman D, Ridel C, Ray P, *et al.* Cardiac filling pressures are not appropriate to predict hemodynamic response to volume challenge. *Crit Care Med.* 2007; 35[1]: 64–8. Epub 2006/11/03.

16. Marik PE, Baram M, Vahid B. Does central venous pressure predict fluid responsiveness? A systematic review of the literature and the tale of seven mares. *Chest.* 2008; 134[1]: 172–8. Epub 2008/07/17.

17. Davies JN, Allen DR, Chant AD. Non-invasive Doppler-derived cardiac output: a validation study comparing this technique with thermodilution and Fick methods. *Eur J Vasc Surg.* 1991; 5[5]: 497–500. Epub 1991/10/01.

18. Okrainec A, Bergman S, Demyttenaere S, *et al.* Validation of esophageal Doppler for noninvasive hemodynamic monitoring under pneumoperitoneum. *Surg Endosc.* 2007; 21[8]: 1349–53. Epub 2007/01/20.

19. Lafanechere A, Albaladejo P, Raux M, *et al.* Cardiac output measurement during infrarenal aortic surgery: echo-esophageal Doppler versus thermodilution catheter. *J Cardiothorac Vasc Anesth.* 2006; 20[1]: 26–30. Epub 2006/02/07.

20. Chytra I, Pradl R, Bosman R, *et al.* Esophageal Doppler-guided fluid management decreases blood lactate levels in multiple-trauma patients: a randomized controlled trial. *Crit Care.* 2007; 11[1]: R24. Epub 2007/02/23.

21. Rodriguez RM, Lum-Lung M, Dixon K, *et al.* A prospective study on esophageal Doppler hemodynamic assessment in the ED. *Am J Emerg Med.* 2006; 24[6]: 658–63. Epub 2006/09/21.

22. Dark PM, Singer M. The validity of trans-esophageal Doppler ultrasonography as a measure of cardiac output in critically ill adults. *Intensive Care Med.* 2004; 30[11]: 2060–6. Epub 2004/09/16.

23. Conway DH, Mayall R, Abdul-Latif MS, *et al.* Randomised controlled trial investigating the influence of intravenous fluid titration using oesophageal Doppler monitoring during bowel surgery. *Anaesthesia.* 2002; 57[9]: 845–9.

24. Gan TJ, Soppitt A, Maroof M, *et al.* Goal-directed intraoperative fluid administration reduces length of hospital stay after major surgery. *Anesthesiology.* 2002; 97[4]: 820–6.

25. Wakeling HG, McFall MR, Jenkins CS, *et al.* Intraoperative oesophageal Doppler guided fluid management shortens postoperative hospital stay after major bowel surgery. *Br J Anaesth.* 2005; 95[5]: 634–42.

26. Noblett SE, Snowden CP, Shenton BK, *et al.* Randomized clinical trial assessing the effect of Doppler-optimized fluid management on outcome after elective colorectal resection. *Br J Surg.* 2006; 93[9]: 1069–76.

27. Senagore AJ, Emery T, Luchtefeld M, *et al.* Fluid management for laparoscopic colectomy: a prospective, randomized assessment of goal-directed administration of balanced salt solution or hetastarch coupled with an enhanced recovery program. *Dis Colon Rectum.* 2009; 52[12]: 1935–40. Epub 2009/11/26.

28. Mythen MG, Webb AR. Perioperative plasma volume expansion reduces the incidence of gut mucosal hypoperfusion during cardiac surgery. *Arch Surg.* 1995; 130[4]: 423–9. Epub 1995/04/01.

29. McKendry M, McGloin H, Saberi D, *et al.* Randomised controlled trial assessing the impact of a nurse delivered, flow monitored protocol for optimisation of circulatory status after cardiac surgery.[Erratum appears in *BMJ.* 2004 Aug 21;329[7463]:438]. *BMJ.* 2004; 329[7460]: 258.

30. Sinclair S, James S, Singer M. Intraoperative intravascular volume optimisation and length of hospital stay after repair of proximal femoral fracture: randomised controlled trial. *BMJ.* 1997; 315[7113]: 909–12.

31. Venn R, Steele A, Richardson P, *et al.* Randomized controlled trial to investigate influence of the fluid challenge on duration of hospital stay and

perioperative morbidity in patients with hip fractures. *Br J Anaesth.* 2002; 88[1]: 65–71.

32. Lassen K, Soop M, Nygren J, *et al.* Consensus review of optimal perioperative care in colorectal surgery: Enhanced Recovery After Surgery [ERAS] Group recommendations. *Arch Surg.* 2009; 144[10]: 961–9. Epub 2009/10/21.

33. Esophageal Doppler ultrasound-based cardiac output monitoring for real-time therapeutic management of hospitalized patients: a review. Database of Abstracts of Reviews of Effects (DARE). Rochville: Agency for Healthcare Research and Quality, Department of Health & Human Services, 2007.

34. Mowatt G, Houston G, Hernandex R. Evidence review: Oesophageal Doppler monitoring in patients undergoing high-risk surgery and in critically ill patients. NHS Purchasing and Supply Agency, 2008; http://www.deltexmedical.com/downloads/CEPreport .pdf.

35. Marik PE, Cavallazzi R, Vasu T, *et al.* Dynamic changes in arterial waveform derived variables and fluid responsiveness in mechanically ventilated patients: a systematic review of the literature. *Crit Care Med.* 2009; 37[9]: 2642–7. Epub 2009/07/16.

36. Berkenstadt H, Margalit N, Hadani M, *et al.* Stroke volume variation as a predictor of fluid responsiveness in patients undergoing brain surgery. *Anesth Analg.* 2001; 92[4]: 984–9.

37. Michard F. Long live dynamic parameters! *Crit Care.* 2014; 18[1]: 413.

38. Renner J, Gruenewald M, Quaden R, *et al.* Influence of increased intra-abdominal pressure on fluid responsiveness predicted by pulse pressure variation and stroke volume variation in a porcine model. *Crit Care Med.* 2009; 37[2]: 650–8. Epub 2008/12/31.

39. Tavernier B, Robin E. Assessment of fluid responsiveness during increased intra-abdominal pressure: keep the indices, but change the thresholds. *Crit Care.* 2011; 15[2]: 134.

40. Guinot PG, de Broca B, Bernard E, *et al.* Respiratory stroke volume variation assessed by oesophageal Doppler monitoring predicts fluid responsiveness during laparoscopy. *Br J Anaesth.* 2014; 112[4]: 660–4.

41. Squara P, Denjean D, Estagnasie P, *et al.* Noninvasive cardiac output monitoring [NICOM]: a clinical validation. *Intensive Care Med.* 2007; 33[7]: 1191–4. Epub 2007/04/27.

42. Raval NY, Squara P, Cleman M, *et al.* Multicenter evaluation of noninvasive cardiac output measurement by bioreactance technique. *J Clin Monit Comput.* 2008; 22[2]: 113–19.

43. Waldron NH, Miller TE, Thacker JK, *et al.* A prospective comparison of a noninvasive cardiac output monitor versus esophageal Doppler monitor for goal-directed fluid therapy in colorectal surgery patients. *Anesth Analg.* 2014; 118[5]: 966–75.

44. Eeftinck Schattenkerk DW, van Lieshout JJ, van den Meiracker AH, *et al.* Nexfin noninvasive continuous blood pressure validated against Riva-Rocci/Korotkoff. *Am J Hypertens.* 2009; 22[4]: 378–83.

45. Broch O, Renner J, Gruenewald M, *et al.* A comparison of the Nexfin[R] and transcardiopulmonary thermodilution to estimate cardiac output during coronary artery surgery. *Anaesthesia.* 2012; 67[4]: 377–83.

46. Forget P, Lois F, de Kock M. Goal-directed fluid management based on the pulse oximeter-derived pleth variability index reduces lactate levels and improves fluid management. *Anesth Analg.* 2010; 111[4]: 910–14.

47. Spiess BD, Patel MA, Soltow LO, *et al.* Comparison of bioimpedance versus thermodilution cardiac output during cardiac surgery: evaluation of a second-generation bioimpedance device. *J Cardiothorac Vasc Anesth.* 2001; 15[5]: 567–73. Epub 2001/11/01.

48. Suttner S, Schollhorn T, Boldt J, *et al.* Noninvasive assessment of cardiac output using thoracic electrical bioimpedance in hemodynamically stable and unstable patients after cardiac surgery: a comparison with pulmonary artery thermodilution. *Intensive Care Med.* 2006; 32[12]: 2053–8. Epub 2006/10/14.

49. Miller TE, Scott MJ. Enhanced recovery and the changing landscape of major abdominal surgery. *Anesthesiol Clinics.* 2015; 33[1]: xv–xvi.

50. Greco M, Capretti G, Beretta L, *et al.* Enhanced recovery program in colorectal surgery: a meta-analysis of randomized controlled trials. *World J Surg.* 2014; 38[6]: 1531–41.

51. Brandstrup B, Svendsen PE, Rasmussen M, *et al.* Which goal for fluid therapy during colorectal surgery is followed by the best outcome: near-maximal stroke volume or zero fluid balance? *Br J Anaesth.* 2012; 109[2]: 191–9. Epub 2012/06/20.

52. Srinivasa S, Taylor MH, Singh PP, *et al.* Randomized clinical trial of goal-directed fluid therapy within an enhanced recovery protocol for elective colectomy. *Br J Surg.* 2013; 100[1]: 66–74. Epub 2012/11/08.

53. Pestana D, Espinosa E, Eden A, *et al.* Perioperative goal-directed hemodynamic optimization using noninvasive cardiac output monitoring in major abdominal surgery: a prospective, randomized, multicenter, pragmatic trial: POEMAS Study [PeriOperative goal-directed thErapy in Major Abdominal Surgery]. *Anesth Analg.* 2014; 119[3]: 579–87.

54. Pearse RM, Harrison DA, MacDonald N, *et al.* Effect of a perioperative, cardiac output-guided hemodynamic therapy algorithm on outcomes following major gastrointestinal surgery: a randomized clinical trial and systematic review. *JAMA.* 2014; 311[21]: 2181–90.

55. Minto G, Struthers R. Stroke volume optimisation: is the fairy tale over? *Anaesthesia.* 2014; 69[4]: 291–6. Epub 2014/03/20.

56. Grocott MP, Dushianthan A, Hamilton MA, *et al.* Perioperative increase in global blood flow to explicit defined goals and outcomes after surgery: a Cochrane Systematic Review. *Br J Anaesth.* 2013; 111[4]: 535–48. Epub 2013/05/11.

57. Roger C, Muller L, Deras P, *et al.* Does the type of fluid affect rapidity of shock reversal in an anaesthetized-piglet model of near-fatal controlled haemorrhage? A randomized study. *Br J Anaesth.* 2014; 112[6]: 1015–23. Epub 2013/12/03.

58. Perel P, Roberts I, Ker K. Colloids versus crystalloids for fluid resuscitation in critically ill patients. *Cochrane Database Syst Rev.* 2013; 2: CD000567.

59. Yates DR, Davies SJ, Milner HE, *et al.* Crystalloid or colloid for goal-directed fluid therapy in colorectal surgery. *Br J Anaesth.* 2014; 112[2]: 281–9. Epub 2013/09/24.

60. Brienza N, Giglio MT, Marucci M, *et al.* Does perioperative hemodynamic optimization protect renal function in surgical patients? A meta-analytic study. *Crit Care Med.* 2009; 37[6]: 2079–90.

61. Giglio MT, Marucci M, Testini M, *et al.* Goal-directed haemodynamic therapy and gastrointestinal complications in major surgery: a meta-analysis of randomized controlled trials. *Br J Anaesth.* 2009; 103[5]: 637–46.

Chapter

16

Non-invasive guidance of fluid therapy

Maxime Cannesson

Summary

Optimization of oxygen delivery to the tissues during surgery cannot be conducted by monitoring arterial pressure alone. Therefore, apart from cardiac output monitoring, functional hemodynamic parameters have been developed. These parameters indicate "preload dependence," which is defined as the ability of the heart to increase stroke volume in response to an increase in preload. The Frank–Starling relationship links preload to stroke volume and presents two distinct parts: a steep portion and a plateau. If the patient is on the steep portion of the Frank–Starling relationship, then an increase in preload (induced by volume expansion) is going to induce an important increase in stroke volume. If the patient is on the plateau of this relationship, then increasing preload will have no effect on stroke volume. The functional hemodynamic parameters rely on cardiopulmonary interactions in patients under general anesthesia and mechanical ventilation and can be obtained invasively from the arterial pressure waveform or non-invasively from the plethysmographic waveform. Here, the effects of positive-pressure ventilation on preload and stroke volume are used to detect fluid responsiveness. If mechanical ventilation induces important respiratory variations in stroke volume (SVV) or in pulse pressure (PPV) it is more likely that the patient is preload-dependent. These dynamic parameters, including passive leg raising, have consistently been shown to be superior to static parameters, such as central venous pressure, for the prediction of fluid responsiveness.*

It is estimated that about 240 million anesthesia procedures are performed each year around the world.[1] Among them, 24 million (∼10%) are conducted in high-risk patients. If this is a small percentage of the whole population, one has to remember that this sample accounts for more than 80% of the overall mortality related to surgery.[2]

Moderate-risk surgery represents approximately 40% of the whole population (i.e. 96 million patients a year). Thankfully, most of these patients present with uncomplicated postoperative course. However, it is estimated that approximately 30% of them (i.e. ∼29 million patients a year) present with "minor" postoperative complications mainly related to gut injury inducing delayed enteral feeding, abdominal distension, nausea, vomiting, or wound complications such as wound dehiscence or pus from the operation wound.[3] Even if these complications are said to be "minor," they induce an increased postoperative medication, increased length of stay in hospital, and finally an increase in the cost of the medicosurgical management. In most of these patients, postoperative complications are related to tissue hypoperfusion and inadequate perioperative resuscitation.[3,4]

The function of the circulation system is to service the needs of the body tissues, to transport nutrients to the body tissues, to transport waste products away, to conduct hormones from one part of the body to another, and, in general, to maintain an appropriate environment in all the tissue fluids of the body for optimal survival and function of the cells.

---

* Summary compiled by the Editor.

Clinical Fluid Therapy in the Perioperative Setting, Second Edition, ed. Robert G. Hahn. Published by Cambridge University Press. © Cambridge University Press 2016.

To be achieved, this goal requires two physiological objectives: adequate perfusion pressure in order to force blood into the capillaries of all organs, and adequate cardiac output to deliver oxygen and substrates, and to remove carbon dioxide and other metabolic products.[5,6] This is so true that several studies have demonstrated that cardiac output maximization during high-risk surgery has the ability to improve postoperative patients' outcome and to decrease the cost of surgery.[7–10]

It is obvious that optimization of oxygen delivery to the tissues during surgery cannot be conducted by monitoring arterial pressure alone. Because arterial pressure and cardiac output are both dependent on systemic vascular resistances, a normal or even supra-normal arterial pressure does not guarantee that cardiac output is not low. However, flow measurement is technologically not as straightforward as pressure measurements.

Therefore, apart from cardiac output monitoring, new parameters (called *functional hemodynamic parameters*) have recently been developed. These parameters rely on cardiopulmonary interactions in patients under general anesthesia and mechanical ventilation, and can be obtained invasively from the arterial pressure waveform (pulse pressure variation or PPV [11,12]) or non-invasively from the plethysmographic waveform (ΔPOP, the amplitude of the pulse oximetric plethysmographic waveform,[13] or PVI, for pleth variability index [14]).[15,16]

In this chapter we describe the rationale and the potential applications of these non-invasive hemodynamic monitoring parameters during surgery and how they can improve patients' outcome by optimizing cardiac output and oxygen delivery during surgery.

Preload dependence

Hypovolemia induces hypotension, oliguria, and tachycardia. That's a fact. But one has to be very careful: these signs are not related to hypovolemia, but they are related to severe hypovolemia.[17] Moreover, they are not specific and can be present even in the absence of hypovolemia. Consequently, they are neither sensitive nor specific and cannot be used for assessing a patient's fluid status with accuracy.

Central venous pressure (CVP) or pulmonary capillary wedge pressure (PCWP) have been used for years for monitoring patients' volemia. However, this assumption has been made because CVP and PCWP

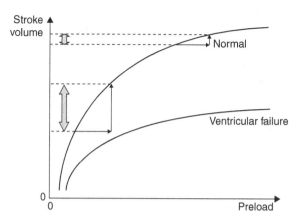

Figure 16.1 Frank–Starling relationship between ventricular preload and ventricular stroke volume. The first portion of this relationship is called the *steep portion* and the second portion is called the *plateau*. If the heart is working on the steep portion (low preload), then an increase in preload (induced by volume expansion) will induce a significant increase in stroke volume (here the heart is said to be preload-dependent). If the heart is working on the plateau (elevated preload), then an increase in preload (induced by volume expansion) will not induce any significant increase in stroke volume (here the heart is said to be preload-independent). The Frank–Starling relationship does not only depend on preload and stroke volume but also depends on ventricular function, and the Frank–Starling curve is flattened when ventricular function is impaired. Consequently, for a given preload value, it is not possible to predict the effects of an increase in preload on stroke volume.

were supposed to reflect ventricular preload or preload dependence, which is actually wrong. And almost all the studies focusing on the ability of CVP and PCWP to predict fluid responsiveness have failed to demonstrate any accuracy of these parameters for predicting the effects of volume expansion on cardiac output.[18]

The main question that anesthesiologists and/or intensivists have to answer before they perform volume expansion is: "Will my patient increase cardiac output in response to volume expansion?" What he or she wants to know is: "Is my patient preload-dependent or not?"

Preload dependence is defined as the ability of the heart to increase stroke volume in response to an increase in preload. To understand this concept, one has to be reminded of the Frank–Starling relationship. This relationship links preload to stroke volume and presents two distinct parts: a steep portion and a plateau (Figure 16.1). If the patient is on the steep portion of the Frank–Starling relationship, then an increase in preload (induced by volume expansion) is going to induce an important increase in stroke volume. If the patient is on the plateau of this relationship, then increasing preload will have no effect on stroke volume.

The Frank–Starling relationship does not only depend on preload and stroke volume, but also depends on cardiac function. When cardiac function is impaired, the Frank–Starling relationship is flattened and for the same level of preload the effects of volume expansion on stroke volume are going to be less important, explaining why preload parameters such as CVP or PCWP are not accurate predictors of fluid responsiveness (Figure 16.1). Instead of monitoring a given parameter, functional hemodynamic monitoring assesses the effects of a stress on this given parameter.[19]

Functional hemodynamic parameters

For the assessment of preload dependence, the stress is a "fluid challenge," and the parameter is stroke volume or one of its surrogates (pulse pressure or plethysmographic waveform amplitude for instance). In mechanically ventilated patients under general anesthesia, the effects of positive-pressure ventilation on preload and stroke volume are used to detect fluid responsiveness. If mechanical ventilation induces important respiratory variations in stroke volume (SVV) or in PPV, it is more likely that the patient is preload-dependent (Figure 16.2).[15]

These dynamic parameters – SVV, PPV, and passive leg raising (PLR) – have consistently been shown to be superior to static parameters (CVP, PCWP) for the prediction of fluid responsiveness. Today CVP and PCWP, as well as oliguria, hypotension, and tachycardia, should no longer be used for predicting the effects of volume expansion on cardiac output.[18,20]

Theoretically, the main interest of these dynamic parameters is that they can be used as a surrogate for cardiac output monitoring. As a matter of fact, if one considers that knowing whether the patient is preload-dependent (i.e. whether cardiac output can be improved using volume expansion) is more important than knowing the absolute cardiac output value, then monitoring these parameters could replace cardiac output monitoring itself (Figure 16.2).

However, dynamic parameters of fluid responsiveness based on cardiopulmonary interactions have several limitations that need to be clearly stated before they can be adequately used in the clinical setting.

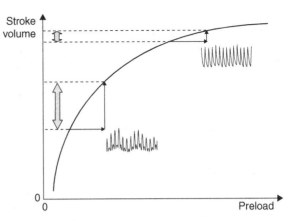

Figure 16.2 Frank–Starling relationship with associated respiratory variations in the arterial pressure waveform signal. Provided that respiratory variations in arterial pulse pressure are studied in adequate conditions, high respiratory variations reflect that the heart is working on the steep portion of the relationship (indicating a preload dependence), while low respiratory variations reflect that the heart is working on the plateau of the relationship (indicating a preload independence).

Firstly, these parameters have to be used in mechanically ventilated patients under general anesthesia. Up to now, studies conducted in spontaneously breathing patients have failed to demonstrate that PPV can predict fluid responsiveness in this setting.[21] Moreover, tidal volume has an impact on the predictive value of PPV and a tidal volume of 8 ml/kg of body weight is required.[22] Patients have to be in sinus rhythm, the chest must be closed (open chest as well as open pericardium strongly modifies cardiopulmonary interactions) and the intra-abdominal pressure has to be within the normal ranges.[23]

These dynamic indicators need to be further explored in children and in the setting of left ventricular failure and acute respiratory distress syndrome.

To summarize, the conditions of application of PPV for the purpose of fluid responsiveness are:

- patient under general anesthesia and mechanical ventilation;
- tidal volume >8 ml/kg of ideal body weight;
- sinus rhythm;
- no right ventricular failure;
- closed chest;
- normal intra-abdominal pressure.

Finally, PPV monitoring requires an arterial line and is more likely to be applied in high-risk surgery patients. In moderate-risk surgery patients, the pulse oximeter waveform can be used to assess preload dependence as described below.

Using the pulse oximeter to optimize fluid status

The pulse oximeter waveform is based on a signal proportional to light absorption between an emitter and a receptor, which are usually placed on the fingertip, on the forehead, or on the earlobe. Light absorption increases with the amount of hemoglobin present in the studied tissue.

The amplitude of the pulse oximeter plethysmographic waveform depends particularly on the vessel volume (venous, arterial, and microcirculation volume) and on the transmural pressure applied on the probe.[24] This waveform presents two components: the first component is said to be constant (DC, as direct current) and is due to light absorption by bone, tissue, pigments, non-pulsatile blood (venous), and skin. The second component is said to be pulsatile absorption (AC, as alternating current) and is mainly related to arterial pulse.

Venous blood is responsible for a slight pulsatile absorption on the plethysmographic waveform recorded at the forehead when the pulse oximetry sensor is not pressed by an elastic tensioning headband (i.e. when the transmural pressure is low).[25,26] Without the headband, venous saturation can induce false low-saturation readings. At the finger, the pulsatile component is due primarily to arterialized blood and the venous pulse is less frequently seen. Low-frequency oscillations due to changes in capillary density (sympathetic tone) have also been reported [27] and can alter the waveform quality.

Shamir *et al.* were the first to describe the respiratory variations in the plethysmographic waveform (SPVpleth) and in its Δdownpleth component (by analogy with the arterial Δdown) in patients presenting with various degrees of hypovolemia.[28] Then, in 2005 our team showed the relationship between the respiratory variations in the ΔPOP and in the PPV in mechanically ventilated patients under general anesthesia in the intensive care unit.[29] In this study, we showed that both indices were strongly related and that ΔPOP was easily measurable at the bedside. Using the PPV formula rather than the variations in the peak of the waveform for quantifying the respiratory variations in the plethysmographic waveform allowed us

to get rid of the fact that this waveform has no unit. By dividing the difference in amplitude by the mean of these amplitudes we observe a mathematical simplification for the unit, and then ΔPOP is expressed as a percentage.

Pulse oximeter waveform amplitude was then tested in clinical settings and was shown to be sensitive to venous return in mechanically ventilated patients [30] and to be an accurate predictor of fluid responsiveness in various settings,[13] including in the intensive care unit [31] and in the postoperative period following cardiac surgery.[32] In the operating room, a ΔPOP greater than 13% before volume expansion allowed discrimination between responders and non-responders with 80% sensitivity and 90% specificity.[30]

In the intensive care unit, in a septic hypotensive cohort, Feissel *et al.* showed that a ΔPOP value of 14% before volume expansion allowed discrimination between responders and non-responders with 94% and 80% specificity, respectively.[31] It is interesting to underline that patients were all under vasoactive drugs in this last study and that it did not seem to impact the ability of this index to predict fluid responsiveness.

We now have numerous evidence showing that ΔPOP has the ability to predict fluid responsiveness in mechanically ventilated patients under general anesthesia despite some limitations related to vasomotor tone.[27] The most recently published study comes from Pizov *et al.* and shows that respiratory variations in the plethysmographic waveform are early detectors of hypovolemia, and that this parameter increases before arterial pressure decreases and heart rate increases in patients in whom occult bleeding occurs.[33]

Pleth variability index

Most pulse oximeter waveforms displayed by conventional monitor screens are smoothed and filtered because it is impossible to accurately eyeball the respiratory variations in this waveform and to draw any reliable information regarding patients' fluid status from these screens.[34]

Recently, a new parameter extracted from this waveform allows clinicians to continuously and automatically monitor these respiratory variations. The PVI is continuously displayed as a percentage on Radical 7 Masimo Monitors (Masimo Corp., Irvine, CA).

Pleth variability index is an automatic measure of the dynamic change in perfusion index (PI) that occurs during a complete respiratory cycle.

For the measurement of SpO_2 via pulse oximetry, red and infrared lights are used. A constant amount of light (DC) from the pulse oximeter is absorbed by skin, other tissues, and non-pulsatile blood, while a variable amount of light is absorbed by the pulsatile arterial inflow (AC). For PI calculation, the infrared pulsatile signal is indexed against the non-pulsatile infrared signal and expressed as a percentage (PI = [AC/DC] × 100) reflecting the amplitude of the pulse oximeter waveform. Then PVI calculation is accomplished by measuring changes in PI over a time interval sufficient to include one or more complete respiratory cycles as $PVI = [(PI_{max} - PI_{min})/PI_{max}] \times 100$.

Several studies have now validated the ability of PVI to predict fluid responsiveness in mechanically ventilated patients undergoing general anesthesia.[14,35,36] A PVI higher than 10–15% is suggestive of preload dependence and indicates that volume expansion is more likely to increase cardiac output.

Functional hemodynamic monitoring and clinical outcome

In 2007, the literature regarding the influence of goal-directed therapy based on cardiac output maximization on postoperative outcome was reviewed.[37] The authors concluded that individualized goal-directed therapy in the perioperative period improves gut function and reduces postoperative nausea and vomiting, morbidity, and hospital length of stay.

More recently, a 15-year follow-up study of high-risk surgical patients even found that short-term goal-directed therapy based on cardiac output monitoring in the perioperative period may improve long-term outcomes, in part owing to the ability of such therapy to reduce the number of perioperative complications.[38]

Growing evidence indicates that goal-directed therapy using appropriate fluid monitoring methods, such as PPV and PVI, is effective in optimizing patient outcomes.[15] For example, in a randomized controlled trial published in 2007, monitoring and minimizing PPV by volume loading during high-risk surgery improved postoperative outcome and decreased hospital length of stay.[39] The median duration of postoperative hospital stay was lower in the intervention group than the control group (7 vs.

17 days, $p < 0.01$), as were the number of postoperative complications per patient (1.4 ± 2.1 vs. 3.9 ± 2.8, $p < 0.05$), and the median duration of mechanical ventilation (1 vs. 5 days, $p < 0.05$) and stay in the intensive care unit (3 vs. 9 days, $p < 0.01$).

Similarly, in a randomized controlled trial in 60 high-risk patients undergoing major abdominal surgery, a goal-directed hemodynamic optimization protocol using the FloTrac/Vigileo device was associated with a shorter median length of stay: 15 days for the goal-directed group vs. 19 days for the control group receiving a standard management protocol ($p = 0.006$).[10] The goal-directed group also had a reduced incidence of perioperative complications (20%) relative to the control group (50%) ($p = 0.03$). In another study, high-risk patients undergoing major abdominal surgery whose fluid management was guided by SVV had fewer complications than those receiving routine intraoperative care ($p = 0.0066$).[40]

PVI may also play a role in optimizing hemodynamic status in patients undergoing major abdominal surgery.[41] In a recently published randomized controlled trial, patients scheduled for major abdominal surgery ($n = 82$) were randomized into two groups: a PVI group monitored for PVI and a control group receiving standard care. In the PVI group, authors aimed at maintaining PVI under 13% by iterative volume expansion. The primary outcome measure, the perioperative serum lactate level, was significantly lower in the PVI group, and peri- and postoperative volume infused were lower in the PVI group. It was concluded that PVI improved perioperative fluid management in abdominal surgery. Other studies focusing on the ability of non-invasive technologies to be used in goal-directed therapy protocols are now ongoing and should be published in the near future.

Conclusion

"From flying blind to flying right?" [42]

Hemodynamic optimization is of major importance during surgery. This concept requires arterial pressure monitoring and optimization, and also cardiac output monitoring and optimization. High-risk surgery has been shown to benefit from cardiac output maximization using semi-invasive technologies. Patients undergoing moderate-risk surgery may also

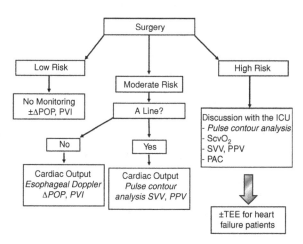

Figure 16.3 Proposed algorithm for hemodynamic monitoring during anesthesia depending on the type of surgery. ICU, intensive care unit; PAC, pulmonary artery catheter; Δ POP, respiratory variations in pulse oximeter waveform amplitude; PPV, pulse pressure variation; PVI, pleth variability index; ScvO$_2$, mixed venous oxygen saturation; SVV, stroke volume variation; TEE, transesophageal echocardiography.

benefit from this approach using non-invasive technologies. It is more likely that in the future, goal-directed therapy using more sophisticated and less invasive monitoring will help clinicians to optimize their patients' hemodynamic status during surgery (Figure 16.3).

References

1. Weiser TG, Regenbogen SE, Thompson KD, *et al.* An estimation of the global volume of surgery: a modelling strategy based on available data. *Lancet* 2008; 372: 139–44.

2. Pearse RM, Harrison DA, James P, *et al.* Identification and characterisation of the high-risk surgical population in the United Kingdom. *Crit Care* 2006; 10: R81.

3. Bennett-Guerrero E, Welsby I, Dunn TJ, *et al.* The use of a postoperative morbidity survey to evaluate patients with prolonged hospitalization after routine, moderate-risk, elective surgery. *Anesth Analg* 1999; 89: 514–19.

4. Gan TJ, Mythen MG. Does peroperative gut-mucosa hypoperfusion cause postoperative nausea and vomiting? *Lancet* 1995; 345: 1123–4.

5. Guyton AH, Hall JE. Heart muscle; the heart as a pump and function of the heart valves. In: *Textbook of Medical Physiology*, 11th edn. Philadelphia: Elsevier, Inc., 2006, pp.103–15.

6. Guyton AH, Hall JE. Overview of the circulation: medical physics of pressure, flow, and resistance. In:

7. *Textbook of Medical Physiology*, 11th edn. Philadelphia: Elsevier, Inc., 2006, pp. 161–70.

7. Gan TJ, Soppitt A, Maroof M, *et al.* Goal-directed intraoperative fluid administration reduces length of hospital stay after major surgery. *Anesthesiology* 2002; 97: 820–6.

8. Pearse R, Dawson D, Fawcett J, *et al.* Early goal-directed therapy after major surgery reduces complications and duration of hospital stay. A randomised, controlled trial. *Crit Care* 2005; 9: R687–93.

9. Wakeling HG, McFall MR, Jenkins CS, *et al.* Intraoperative oesophageal Doppler guided fluid management shortens postoperative hospital stay after major bowel surgery. *Br J Anaesth* 2005; 95: 634–42.

10. Mayer J, Boldt J, Mengistu AM, Rohm KD, Suttner S. Goal-directed intraoperative therapy based on autocalibrated arterial pressure waveform analysis reduces hospital stay in high-risk surgical patients: a randomized, controlled trial. *Crit Care* 2010; 14: R18.

11. Michard F, Boussat S, Chemla D, *et al.* Relation between respiratory changes in arterial pulse pressure and fluid responsiveness in septic patients with acute circulatory failure. *Am J Respir Crit Care Med* 2000; 162: 134–8.

12. Cannesson M, Slieker J, Desebbe O, *et al.* The ability of a novel algorithm for automatic estimation of the respiratory variations in arterial pulse pressure to monitor fluid responsiveness in the operating room. *Anesth Analg* 2008; 106: 1195–2000.

13. Cannesson M, Attof Y, Rosamel P, *et al.* Respiratory variations in pulse oximetry plethysmographic waveform amplitude to predict fluid responsiveness in the operating room. *Anesthesiology* 2007; 106: 1105–11.

14. Cannesson M, Desebbe O, Rosamel P, *et al.* Pleth variability index to monitor the respiratory variations in the pulse oximeter plethysmographic waveform amplitude and predict fluid responsiveness in the operating theatre. *Br J Anaesth* 2008; 101: 200–6.

15. Cannesson M. Arterial pressure variation and goal-directed fluid therapy. *J Cardiothorac Vasc Anesth* 2010; 24: 487–97.

16. Michard F. Changes in arterial pressure during mechanical ventilation. *Anesthesiology* 2005; 103: 419–28.

17. Perel A, Pizov R, Cotev S. Systolic blood pressure variation is a sensitive indicator of hypovolemia in ventilated dogs subjected to graded hemorrhage. *Anesthesiology* 1987; 67: 498–502.

18. Marik PE, Baram M, Vahid B. Does central venous pressure predict fluid responsiveness? A systematic

review of the literature and the tale of seven mares. *Chest* 2008; 134: 172–8.

19. Pinsky MR, Payen D. Functional hemodynamic monitoring. *Crit Care* 2005; 9: 566–72.

20. Marik PE, Cavallazzi R, Vasu T, Hirani A. Dynamic changes in arterial waveform derived variables and fluid responsiveness in mechanically ventilated patients: a systematic review of the literature. *Crit Care Med* 2009; 37: 2642–7.

21. De Backer D, Pinsky MR. Can one predict fluid responsiveness in spontaneously breathing patients? *Intensive Care Med* 2007; 33: 1111–13.

22. De Backer D, Heenen S, Piagnerelli M, Koch M, Vincent JL. Pulse pressure variations to predict fluid responsiveness: influence of tidal volume. *Intensive Care Med* 2005; 31: 517–23.

23. Duperret S, Lhuillier F, Piriou V, *et al.* Increased intra-abdominal pressure affects respiratory variations in arterial pressure in normovolaemic and hypovolaemic mechanically ventilated pigs. *Intensive Care Med* 2007; 33: 163–71.

24. Reisner A, Shaltis PA, McCombie D, Asada HH. Utility of the photoplethysmogram in circulatory monitoring. *Anesthesiology* 2008; 108: 950–8.

25. Shelley KH, Dickstein M, Shulman SM. The detection of peripheral venous pulsation using the pulse oximeter as a plethysmograph. *J Clin Monit* 1993; 9: 283–7.

26. Agashe GS, Coakley J, Mannheimer PD. Forehead pulse oximetry: headband use helps alleviate false low readings likely related to venous pulsation artifact. *Anesthesiology* 2006; 105: 1111–16.

27. Landsverk SA, Hoiseth LO, Kvandal P, *et al.* Poor agreement between respiratory variations in pulse oximetry photoplethysmographic waveform amplitude and pulse pressure in intensive care unit patients. *Anesthesiology* 2008; 109: 849–55.

28. Shamir M, Eidelman LA, Floman Y, Kaplan L, Pizov R. Pulse oximetry plethysmographic waveform during changes in blood volume. *Br J Anaesth* 1999; 82: 178–81.

29. Cannesson M, Besnard C, Durand PG, Bohe J, Jacques D. Relation between respiratory variations in pulse oximetry plethysmographic waveform amplitude and arterial pulse pressure in ventilated patients. *Crit Care* 2005; 9: R562–8.

30. Cannesson M, Desebbe O, Hachemi M, *et al.* Respiratory variations in pulse oximeter waveform amplitude are influenced by venous return in mechanically ventilated patients under general anaesthesia. *Eur J Anaesthesiol* 2007; 24: 245–51.

31. Feissel M, Teboul JL, Merlani P, *et al.* Plethysmographic dynamic indices predict fluid responsiveness in septic ventilated patients. *Intensive Care Med* 2007; 33: 993–9.

32. Wyffels PA, Durnez PJ, Helderweirt J, Stockman WM, De Kegel D. Ventilation-induced plethysmographic variations predict fluid responsiveness in ventilated postoperative cardiac surgery patients. *Anesth Analg* 2007; 105: 448–52.

33. Pizov R, Eden A, Bystritski D, *et al.* Arterial and plethysmographic waveform analysis in anesthetized patients with hypovolemia. *Anesthesiology* 2010; 113: 83–91.

34. Feldman JM. Can clinical monitors be used as scientific instruments? *Anesth Analg* 2006; 103: 1071–2.

35. Cannesson M, Delannoy B, Morand A, *et al.* Does the pleth variability index indicate the respiratory induced variation in the plethysmogram and arterial pressure waveforms? *Anesth Analg* 2008; 106: 1189–94.

36. Zimmermann M, Feibicke T, Keyl C, *et al.* Accuracy of stroke volume variation compared with pleth variability index to predict fluid responsiveness in mechanically ventilated patients undergoing major surgery. *Eur J Anaesthesiol* 2009; 27: 555–61.

37. Bundgaard-Nielsen M, Holte K, Secher NH, Kehlet H. Monitoring of perioperative fluid administration by individualized goal-directed therapy. *Acta Anaesthesiol Scand* 2007; 51: 331–40.

38. Rhodes A, Cecconi M, Hamilton M, *et al.* Goal-directed therapy in high-risk surgical patients: a 15-year follow-up study. *Intensive Care Med* 2010: 36: 1327–32.

39. Lopes MR, Oliveira MA, Pereira VO, *et al.* Goal-directed fluid management based on pulse pressure variation monitoring during high-risk surgery: a pilot randomized controlled trial. *Crit Care* 2007; 11: R100.

40. Benes J, Chytra I, Altmann P, *et al.* Intraoperative fluid optimization using stroke volume variation in high risk surgical patients: results of prospective randomized study. *Crit Care* 2010; 14: R118.

41. Forget P, Lois F, de Kock M. Goal-directed fluid management based on the pulse oximeter-derived pleth variability index reduces lactate levels and improves fluid management. *Anesth Analg* 2010; 111: 910–14.

42. Cannesson M, Vallet B, Michard F. Pulse pressure variation and stroke volume variation: from flying blind to flying right? *Br J Anaesth* 2009; 103: 896–7; author reply 7–9.

Chapter

17

Hemodilution

Philippe van der Linden

Summary

Acute normovolemic hemodilution entails the removal of blood either immediately before or shortly after the induction of anesthesia and its simultaneous replacement by an appropriate volume of crystalloids and/or colloids to maintain "isovolemic" conditions. As a result, blood subsequently lost during surgery will contain proportionally fewer red blood cells, thus reducing the loss of autologous erythrocytes. Although still frequently used in some surgical procedures, the real efficacy of acute normovolemic hemodilution in reducing allogeneic blood transfusion remains discussed. The aim of this article is to describe the physiology, limits, and efficacy of acute normovolemic hemodilution.

Acute normovolemic hemodilution (ANH) was introduced into clinical practice in the 1970s to reduce requirements for allogeneic blood products.[1] Acute normovolemic hemodilution entails the removal of blood either immediately before or shortly after the induction of anesthesia and its simultaneous replacement by an appropriate volume of crystalloids and/or colloids to maintain "isovolemic conditions.[2] As a result, blood subsequently lost during surgery will contain proportionally fewer red blood cells (RBCs), thus reducing the loss of autologous erythrocytes.

Acute normovolemic hemodilution therefore presents all the advantages associated with a reduction in allogeneic blood exposure, including a reduction of transfusion reactions from exposure to donor's blood antigens and a decreased exposure to blood-borne pathogens, but also offers several advantages in comparison to other blood conservation techniques. It is quite inexpensive and easily available, it improves tissue oxygenation through its microcirculatory effects, and it provides fresh autologous blood units for later transfusion after the achievement of surgical hemostasis. However, the real efficacy of ANH in reducing allogeneic blood transfusion remains discussed. The aim of this article is to describe the physiology, limits, and efficacy of ANH.

Physiological compensatory mechanisms

The acute reduction in RBC concentration induced by hemodilution elicits intrinsic compensatory mechanisms, allowing the maintenance of adequate tissue oxygenation.[3,4] The development of these mechanisms is closely related to the improvement of whole blood fluidity achieved by the hemodilution process, providing the maintenance of "isovolemic" conditions. Basic determinants of blood fluidity are the red cell concentration, the plasma viscosity, the cell-to-cell interactions, and the prevailing shear rate (i.e. the mean linear flow velocity). The lower the shear rate, the more pronounced is the improvement in blood fluidity based on changes in hematocrit.[5] The sympathetic nervous system also plays an important role in the maintenance of optimal oxygen delivery during ANH.[6] Elicited compensatory mechanisms mainly involve an increase in cardiac output and an increase in tissue oxygen extraction.

Increase in cardiac output

At the systemic level, improvement in blood fluidity results in an increase of venous return and a reduction of left ventricular afterload. Enhancement of shear rate with subsequent release of nitric oxide may also contribute to systemic vasodilation, while hemodilution-induced stimulation of aortic chemoreceptors increases the sympathetic activity of the heart, resulting in improved myocardial performance.[7] These entire phenomena are responsible for the increase in cardiac output, mainly through a rise in stroke volume, but also to some extent through an increase in heart rate.

Increase in tissue oxygen extraction

The second compensatory mechanism aims at a better matching of oxygen delivery to oxygen demand at the tissue level. This mechanism entails physiological alterations at both the systemic and the microcirculatory level. At the systemic level, a redistribution of blood flow to areas of high metabolic demand from areas where demand is low has been repeatedly demonstrated during isovolemic ANH.[8] Experimental models of extreme hemodilution have recently demonstrated that tolerance to anemia is organ-specific, the brain and the heart being more tolerant than organs from the splanchnic area, and more specifically the kidneys.[9,10] This regional redistribution of blood flow is partly due to alpha-adrenergic stimulation, but seems unaltered in the presence of beta-adrenergic blockade.

At the microcirculatory level, several physiological alterations develop to provide a more efficient utilization of the remaining blood oxygen content. Increased RBC velocity appears the most important one, resulting from increased arteriolar pressure, which, alone, stimulates arterial vasomotion.[11] Increased RBC velocity and arterial vasomotion provide a better spatial and temporal spread of RBCs within the capillary network, and result in improved tissue oxygen extraction capacity.[12] Lastly, a right shift of the oxygen dissociation curve may reduce the affinity of hemoglobin for oxygen and therefore improve oxygen availability. This shift, related to a rise in the RBC's 2,3-diphosphoglycerate level, takes some hours to occur and has been demonstrated only in chronic anemia.[13]

Effects of anesthesia

Anesthesia can alter the physiological adjustments to isovolemic hemodilution at several levels (Table 17.1). The most striking effect of anesthesia appears to be a decreased cardiac output response, mainly related

Table 17.1 Effects of anesthesia on the physiological response to hemodilution

1. Effects on the cardiac output response
   Alteration in cardiac preload and afterload conditions
   Negative inotropic effect
   Depressed autonomic nervous system activity
2. Effects on the O_2 extraction response
   Vasodilation
   Depressed sympathetic nervous system activity
3. Effects on gas exchange
   Decreased functional residual capacity
4. Effects on tissue oxygen demand
   Relief of pain, stress, anxiety
   Decreased muscular activity
   Decreased myocardial O_2 demand (negative chronotropic and inotropic effect)

to a complete blunting of the increase in heart rate [14,15] (Figure 17.1). This reduced cardiac output response resulted in a decreased oxygen delivery, but oxygen consumption remained unchanged as the oxygen extraction ratio increased (Figure 17.2).

Interestingly, ANH appears to be associated with increased oxygen consumption in awake patients, which could be related at least in part to an increase in myocardial oxygen demand. In the Ickx et al. study,[15] when the patients undergoing ANH while awake were anesthetized, all the measured parameters returned to values similar to those obtained in patients undergoing hemodilution while anesthetized. Therefore, performing ANH before or after induction of anesthesia did not result in a significant different physiological response at the time of surgery.

Limits of hemodilution

As described above, maintenance of tissue oxygenation during ANH results from an increase in cardiac output and oxygen extraction. Several experimental and clinical studies have demonstrated the involvement of both mechanisms even in the early stage of ANH.[16] The relative contribution of these mechanisms will depend on the ability of the organism to recruit them. They allow the maintenance of adequate tissue oxygenation until the hemoglobin concentration falls to about 3 to 4 g/dl (hematocrit 10–12%). Below this "critical" value, oxygen delivery can no longer match tissue oxygen demand, and cellular hypoxia will develop, as demonstrated in several experimental studies.[17–20] Van Woerkens et al., who studied a Jehovah's Witness patient who died from extreme hemodilution, reported a critical hemoglobin concentration of 4 g/dl.[21]

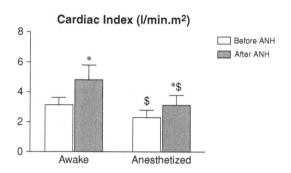

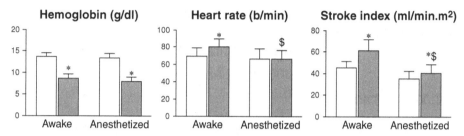

Figure 17.1 Effects of anesthesia on the physiological response to acute normovolemic hemodilution (ANH).
∗ $p < 0.05$ after ANH versus before ANH.
$ $p < 0.05$ anesthetized versus awake.
Adapted from Ref. [15].

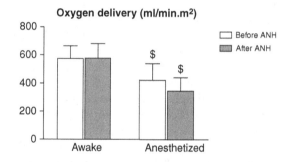

Figure 17.2 Effects of anesthesia on oxygen delivery, oxygen consumption, and oxygen extraction during acute normovolemic hemodilution (ANH).
∗ $p < 0.05$ after ANH versus before ANH.
$ $p < 0.05$ anesthetized versus awake.
Adapted from Ref. [15].

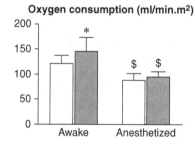

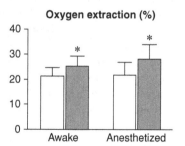

The efficacy of the mechanisms maintaining tissue oxygen delivery when the oxygen-carrying capacity of the blood is reduced depends primarily on the maintenance of an adequate circulating blood volume. Indeed, hypovolemia blunts the effects of decreased blood viscosity on venous return.[22] Although "normovolemic" conditions are difficult to define, replacement of the blood and fluid losses with at least a volume of substitute having the same expanding effect on the intravascular volume is required. Only a few studies have compared the effects of different plasma substitutes on the hemodynamic response to ANH: colloids appeared superior to crystalloids.[23,24] On the one hand, compared with colloids, crystalloids have a very low volume-expanding effect in the context of ANH.[25] On the other hand, colloids and in particular tetrastarches appeared to have potential beneficial effects on renal tissue [26] and modulation of inflammation.[27]

Tolerance to acute isovolemic hemodilution not only depends on the integrity of the compensatory mechanisms described above, but also on the level of tissue oxygen demand. For a given cardiac output and oxygen extraction response, any increase in tissue oxygen demand will require a higher hemoglobin concentration.

Acute normovolemic hemodilution and the cardiac patient

Maintenance of myocardial oxygen delivery during ANH depends essentially on the increase in the coronary blood flow as oxygen extraction is already nearly maximal at the level of the heart under resting conditions.[8] This is achieved by a reduction in coronary vascular resistance related to the decreased blood viscosity and to specific coronary vasodilation. Heart rate and possibly myocardial contractility have been shown to increase during hemodilution,[28] which results in an augmentation of myocardial oxygen demand. When the hematocrit is reduced to about 10%, myocardial oxygen consumption more than doubles and coronary vasodilation is nearly maximal. Below such a hematocrit, coronary blood flow can no longer match myocardial oxygen demand and ischemia develops, ultimately resulting in cardiac failure.

The dependency of myocardial oxygen supply to the coronary blood flow highlights the vulnerability of the heart during ANH, especially in patients with coronary artery disease (CAD) in whom coronary blood flow cannot increase. The lowest tolerable hemoglobin concentration in CAD patients remains unknown.[29] A recent pilot study addressing specifically the problem remained inconclusive.[30] It probably depends on several factors, including the severity of the disease.[31] There is, however, increased evidence that tolerance of CAD patients to isovolemic anemia closely depends on the level of myocardial oxygen demand.

In anesthetized patients scheduled for coronary surgery, several studies demonstrated that moderate ANH (target hematocrit value 27–33%) is well tolerated, and may be even cardioprotective if associated with a decreased myocardial oxygen demand.[32] Myocardial oxygen balance is profoundly influenced by the level of heart rate, and recent clinical data confirm that tolerance of CAD patients to moderate anemia is closely related to the level of heart rate.[33] The anesthetic technique also may play a role.[34] The early postoperative period is certainly critical in hemodiluted CAD patients, because they have to face an increased tissue metabolic demand.[35]

Acute normovolemic hemodilution and hemostasis

Hemodilution could affect hemostasis in different ways. Firstly, it will dilute not only plasmatic factors, but also cellular coagulation factors, such as platelets and, of course, RBCs. Red blood cells have been shown to interfere with hemostasis through a mechanical effect but also through biological effects related to the release of intracellular adenosine diphosphate and to the generation of thrombin.[36] The clinical consequences (i.e. importance of perioperative bleeding) of these interactions between RBCs and hemostasis remain to be determined.

Hemodilution could also affect hemostasis through the direct effects of plasma substitution fluids on the platelets and the coagulation mechanisms.[37] These effects are more marked with colloids than with crystalloids. Among colloids, they are more marked with dextrans than with gelatins and albumin. For hydroxyethyl starches, these effects seem to be closely related to the intrinsic properties of the different solutions, such as a high *in vitro* molecular weight and a high degree of hydroxyethyl substitution.[38] Several *in vitro* studies have confirmed these effects in the context of ANH.[39,40] In addition, patients with Type O blood may demonstrate more coagulation compromise than those with non-O blood when undergoing hemodilution with low molecular weight hydroxyethyl starch.[41]

Storage of whole blood during ANH might be associated with disturbances in platelet aggregation,[42] although the clinical relevance of this observation remains unknown. Agitation during storage of ANH blood does not seem to have any effect on platelet function.[43]

Despite the fact that ANH may directly interfere with normal hemostasis, there is no evidence from the literature that ANH is associated with increased perioperative bleeding,[44,45] although it may affect standard coagulation tests.[46]

Efficacy

Theoretical aspects

The basic concept behind ANH is that patients undergoing such procedure will lose fewer erythrocytes per milliliter of lost blood during surgery and after transfusion of the collected autologous blood in the immediate postoperative period.[5]

Several equations have been developed to calculate the efficacy of ANH as a function of surgical blood loss, initial hematocrit, target post-ANH hematocrit, and hematocrit used as the transfusion trigger. Presuming a "usual" surgical patient without preoperative anemia, and a transfusion decision based exclusively on a trigger hemoglobin concentration of 6–7 g/dl, Weiskopf [47] calculated that 55 to 77% of patient's total blood volume must be lost during surgery in order to achieve savings of about 180 ml of RBCs, which represents one standard blood unit. However, the usefulness of the different published equations in clinical practice remains limited, as several factors have not been always taken into account in the proposed formulae.[2]

Results from the literature

Although efficacy of ANH as a blood conservation technique remains highly debated,[44,45,48,49] this technique is still currently used in many adult and pediatric centers.[50,51] Most of the studies reviewed were performed in the setting of cardiac or orthopedic surgery. Adequate evaluation of the published results was hampered by the relative poor quality of the studies and the marked heterogeneity observed between trials, partly explained by study factors (patient populations, target hematocrit values, transfusion triggers, ANH technique, etc.). Efficacy of ANH was found to be relatively modest in terms of likelihood of exposure to allogeneic blood and units transfused. It closely depends on the use or not of protocols to guide transfusion practice. There was no obvious increase in adverse events with ANH, but the incidence of complications was poorly reported.

Studies that demonstrated a clear efficacy of ANH in reducing the likelihood of patient's exposure to allogeneic blood in the perioperative period have been performed in major liver resection [52,53] or major abdominal surgery.[54] In all of them, a high volume of blood was collected. Surgery was associated with significant blood loss, and a low hemoglobin concentration (7–8 g/dl) was used as the transfusion trigger. Adequate selection of patients may also play a role.[55] All these observations indicate that efficient ANH requires significant expertise in the field from the care-giving team.

Conclusions

Acute normovolemic hemodilution entails the removal of blood from a patient shortly after the beginning of the surgical procedure, and its replacement with crystalloids or colloids to maintain the circulating blood volume. It is a relatively simple, cheap, and effective tool to avoid or reduce allogeneic blood transfusion. Factors that influence the efficacy of the technique have been clearly identified. This reduces the field of application of ANH to patients undergoing surgery with high bleeding risk in whom a great volume of blood can be collected.

Knowledge of the physiological compensatory mechanisms that occur during normovolemic hemodilution and their limits is essential for the safe use of the technique. In addition, the anesthesiologist must be familiar with its practical aspects. Although ANH has a place in different types of surgery, it must be regarded as an integral part of a blood conservation strategy tailored to the individual patient's needs and adapted to specific surgical procedures.

References

1. W.P. Klövekorn, H. Laks, R.N. Pilon, *et al*. Effects of acute hemodilution in man. *Eur Surg Res* 1973; 5(Suppl 2): 27–8.

2. M. Jamnicki, R. Kocian, P. van der Linden, M. Zaugg, D.R. Spahn. Acute normovolemic hemodilution: physiology, limitations, and clinical use. *J Cardiothorac Vasc Anesth* 2003; 17: 747–54.

3. P. Van der Linden. The physiology of acute isovolaemic anaemia. *Acta Anaesthesiol Belg* 2002; 53: 97–103.

4. P.C. Hébert, P. Van der Linden, G.P. Biro, L. Qun. Physiologic aspects of anemia. *Crit Care Clin* 2004; 20: 187–212.

5. U. Kreimeier, K. Messmer. Perioperative hemodilution. *Transfus Apher Sci* 2002; 27: 59–72.

6. A.K. Tsui, N.D. Dattani, P.A. Marsden, *et al.* Reassessing the risk of hemodilutional anemia: Some new pieces to an old puzzle. *Can J Anaesth* 2010; 57: 779–91.

7. C.K. Chapler, C.M. Cain. The physiologic reserve in oxygen carrying capacity: studies in experimental hemodilution. *Can J Physiol Pharmacol* 1986, 64: 7–12.

8. F.C. Fan, R.Y.Z. Chen, G.B. Schuessler, S. Chien. Effects of hematocrit variations on regional hemodynamics and and oxygen transport in the dog. *Am J Physiol* 1980; 238: H545–52.

9. P. Lauscher, H. Kertscho, O. Schmidt, *et al.* Determination of organ-specific anemia tolerance. *Crit Care Med* 2013; 41: 1037–45.

10. G.J. Crystal. Regional tolerance to acute normovolemic hemodilution: evidence that the kidney may be at greatest risk. *J Cardiothorac Vasc Anesth* 2015; 29: 320–7.

11. K. Messmer, G. Gutierrez, J.L. Vincent. Blood rheology factors and capillary blood flow. In: *Tissue Oxygen Utilization*. Berlin, Heidelberg, New-York: Springer-Verlag; 1991: 103–13.

12. P. Van der Linden, E. Gilbart, P. Paques, C. Simon, J.L. Vincent. Influence of hematocrit on tissue O_2 extraction capabilities during acute hemorrhage. *Am J Physiol* 1993; 264: H1942–7.

13. T. Rodman, H.P. Close, M.K. Purcell. The oxyhemoglobin dissociation curve in anemia. *Ann Intern Med* 1960; 52: 295–301.

14. G. Kungys, D.D. Rose, N.W. Fleming. Stroke volume variation during acute normovolemic hemodilution. *Anesth Analg* 2009; 109: 1823–30.

15. B. Ickx, M. Rigolet, P. Van der Linden. Cardiovascular and metabolic response to acute normovolemic anemia: effects of anesthesia. *Anesthesiology* 2000; 93: 1011–16.

16. D.R. Spahn, B.J. Leone, J.G. Reves, T. Pasch. Cardiovascular and coronary physiology of acute isovolemic hemodilution: a review of nonoxygen-carrying and oxygen-carrying solutions. *Anesth Analg* 1994; 78: 1000–21.

17. J. Räsänen. Supply-dependent oxygen consumption and mixed venous oxyhemoglobin saturation during isovolemic hemodilution in pigs. *Chest* 1992; 101: 1121–4.

18. P. Van der Linden, F. De Groote, N. Mathieu, *et al.* Critical haemoglobin concentration in anaesthetized dogs: comparison of two plasma substitutes. *Br J Anaesth* 1998; 81: 556–62.

19. P. Van der Linden, S. De Hert, N. Mathieu, *et al.* Tolerance to acute isovolemic hemodilution: effect of anesthetic depth. *Anesthesiology* 2003; 99: 97–104.

20. A. Pape, S. Kutschker, H. Kertscho, *et al.* The choice of the intravenous fluid influences the tolerance of acute normovolemic anemia in anesthetized domestic pigs. *Crit Care* 2012; 16: R69.

21. E.C.S.M. van Woerkens, A. Trouwborst, J.J.B. Van Lanschot. Profound hemodilution: what is the critical level of hemodilution at which oxygen delivery-dependent oxygen consumption starts in an anesthetized human? *Anesth Analg* 1992; 75: 818–21.

22. T.Q. Richardson, A.C. Guyton. Effects of polycythemia and anemia on cardiac output and other circulatory factors. *Am J Physiol* 1959; 197: 1167–70.

23. D.A. Otsuki, D.T. Fantoni, C.B. Margarido, *et al.* Hydroxyethyl starch is superior to lactated Ringer as a replacement fluid in a pig model of acute normovolaemic haemodilution. *Br J Anaesth* 2007; 98: 29–37.

24. V.K. Arya, N.G. Nagdeve, A. Kumar, S.K. Thingnam, R.S. Dhaliwal. Comparison of hemodynamic changes after acute normovolemic hemodilution using Ringer's lactate versus 5% albumin in patients on beta-blockers undergoing coronary artery bypass surgery. *J Cardiothorac Vasc Anesth* 2006; 20: 812–18.

25. M. Jacob, D. Chappell. Reappraising Starling: the physiology of the microcirculation. *Curr Opin Crit Care* 2013; 19: 282–9.

26. F.M. Konrad, E.G. Mik, S.I. Bodmer, *et al.* Acute normovolemic hemodilution in the pig is associated with renal tissue edema, impaired renal microvascular oxygenation, and functional loss. *Anesthesiology* 2013; 119: 256–69.

27. M. Kahvegian, D. Aya Otsuki, C. Holms, *et al.* Modulation of inflammation during acute normovolemic anemia with different fluid replacement. *Minerva Anestesiol* 2013; 79: 1113–25.

28. R.B. Weiskopf, J. Feiner, H. Hopf, *et al.* Heart rate increases linearly in response to acute isovolemic anemia. *Transfusion* 2003; 43: 235–40.

29. J.L. Carson, P.A. Carless, P.C. Hebert. Transfusion thresholds and other strategies for guiding allogeneic red blood cell transfusion. *Cochrane Database Syst Rev* 2012; 4: CD002042.

30. J.L. Carson, M.M. Brooks, J. Abbott, *et al.* Liberal versus restrictive transfusion thresholds for patients with symptomatic coronary artery disease. *Am Heart J* 2013; 165: 964–71.

31. R. Tircoveanu, P. Van der Linden. Hemodilution and anemia in patients with cardiac disease: what is the safe limit? *Curr Opin Anaesthesiol* 2008; 21: 66–70.

32. M. Licker, C. Ellenberger, J. Sierra, *et al.* Cardioprotective effects of acute normovolemic hemodilution in patients undergoing coronary artery bypass surgery. *Chest* 2005; 128: 838–47.

33. S. Cromheecke, S. Lorsomradee, P.J. Van der Linden, S.G. De Hert. Moderate acute isovolemic hemodilution alters myocardial function in patients with coronary artery disease. *Anesth Analg* 2008; 107: 1145–52.

34. S.G. De Hert, S. Cromheecke, S. Lorsomradee, P.J. Van der Linden. Effects of moderate acute isovolaemic haemodilution on myocardial function in patients undergoing coronary surgery under volatile inhalational anaesthesia. *Anaesthesia* 2009; 64: 239–45.

35. C.W. Hogue, L.T. Goodnough, T. Monk. Perioperative myocardial ischemic episodes are related to hematocrit level in patients undergoing radical prostatectomy. *Transfusion* 1998; 38: 1070–7.

36. B. Ouakine-Orlando, C.M. Samama, P. de Moerloose, *et al.* Hématocrite et hémostase. In: *Hémorragies et thromboses périopératoires: approche pratique.* Paris: Masson; 2000: 113–19.

37. P. Van der Linden, B.E. Ickx. The effects of colloid solutions on hemostasis. *Can J Anaesth* 2006; 53(Suppl): S30–9.

38. M. Westphal, M.F. James, S. Kozek-Langenecker, *et al.* Hydroxyethyl starches: different products–different effects. *Anesthesiology* 2009; 111: 187–202.

39. S.B. Jones, C.W. Whitten, G.J. Despotis, T.G. Monk. The influence of crystalloid and colloid replacement solutions in acute normovolemic hemodilution: a preliminary survey of hemostatic markers. *Anesth Analg* 2003; 96: 363–8, table of contents.

40. C. Thyes, C. Madjdpour, P. Frascarolo, *et al.* Effect of high- and low-molecular-weight low-substituted hydroxyethyl starch on blood coagulation during acute normovolemic hemodilution in pigs. *Anesthesiology* 2006; 105: 1228–37.

41. J.G. Kangg, H.J. Ahn, G.S. Kim, *et al.* The hemostatic profiles of patients with Type O and non-O blood after acute normovolemic hemodilution with 6% hydroxyethyl starch (130/0.4). *Anesth Analg* 2006; 103: 1543–8.

42. C. Reyher, T.M. Bingold, S. Menzel, *et al.* Impact of acute normovolemic hemodilution on primary hemostasis. *Anaesthesist* 2014; 63: 496–502.

43. S.Y. Lu, G. Konig, M.H. Yazer, *et al.* Stationary versus agitated storage of whole blood during acute normovolemic hemodilution. *Anesth Analg* 2014; 118: 264–8.

44. G.L. Bryson, A. Laupacis, G.A. Wells. Does acute normovolemic hemodilution reduce perioperative allogeneic transfusion? A meta-analysis. *Anesth Analg* 1998; 86: 9–15.

45. J.B. Segal, E. Blasco-Colmenares, E.J. Norris, E. Guallar. Preoperative acute normovolemic hemodilution: a meta-analysis. *Transfusion* 2004; 44: 632–44.

46. J.R. Guo, X.J. Jin, J. Yu, *et al.* Acute normovolemic hemodilution effects on perioperative coagulation in elderly patients undergoing hepatic carcinectomy. *Asian Pacif J Cancer Prevent* 2013; 14: 4529–32.

47. R.B. Weiskopf. Efficacy of acute normovolemic hemodilution assessed as a function of fraction of blood volume lost. *Anesthesiology* 2001; 94: 439–46.

48. P. Carless, A. Moxey, D. O'Connell, D. Henry. Autologous transfusion techniques: a systematic review of their efficacy. *Transfus Med* 2004; 14: 123–44.

49. G. Singbartl, A.L. Held, K. Singbartl. Ranking the effectiveness of autologous blood conservation measures through validated modeling of independent clinical data. *Transfusion* 2013; 53: 3060–79.

50. N. White, S. Bayliss, D. Moore. Systematic review of interventions for minimizing perioperative blood transfusion for surgery for craniosynostosis. *J Craniofac Surg* 2015; 26: 26–36.

51. V.M. Voorn, P.J. Marang-van de Mheen, M.M. Wentink, *et al.* Frequent use of blood-saving measures in elective orthopaedic surgery: a 2012 Dutch blood management survey. *BMC Musculoskel Dis* 2013; 14: 230.

52. I. Matot, O. Scheinin, O. Jurim, A. Eid. Effectiveness of acute normovolemic hemodilution to minimize allogeneic blood transfusion in major liver resections. *Anesthesiology* 2002; 97: 794–800.

53. W.R. Jarnagin, M. Gonen, S.K. Maithel, *et al.* A prospective randomized trial of acute normovolemic hemodilution compared to standard intraoperative management in patients undergoing major hepatic resection. *Ann Surg* 2008; 248: 360–9.

54. D.R. Spahn, K.F. Waschke, T. Standl, *et al.* Use of perflubron emulsion to decrease allogeneic blood transfusion in high-blood-loss non-cardiac surgery: results of a European phase 3 study. *Anesthesiology* 2002; 97: 1338–49.

55. T.L. Frankel, M. Fischer, F. Grant, *et al.* Selecting patients for acute normovolemic hemodilution during hepatic resection: a prospective randomized evaluation of nomogram-based allocation. *J Am Coll Surg* 2013; 217: 210–20.

The ERAS concept

18

Katie E. Rollins and Dileep N. Lobo

Summary

Optimum perioperative fluid administration as part of an Enhanced Recovery After Surgery (ERAS) program is dependent on a range of factors which are becoming increasingly well documented. Following previous ambiguous terms and definitions for fluid management strategies, appreciation of the importance of "zero balance" (where amount infused equals the amount lost from the body) of both water and salt is increasing, with both over- and underhydration resulting in significantly worse clinical outcomes (in a U-shaped distribution). Excessive fluid loads have a significant negative impact upon outcome. Electrolyte balance, from pre- to post-operative stages, is also now understood to play a key role.

Enhanced Recovery After Surgery (ERAS) programs employ a multimodal approach to perioperative care including fluid management, with key aims including rapid restoration of physiological function, reduction of the metabolic and physiological stress response, and reduced length of hospital stay, as well as decreased morbidity and mortality. Consensus guidelines for the ERAS programs, including perioperative fluid management, have been published in recent years in the fields of gastric,[1] colorectal,[2,3] bladder,[4] and pancreatic surgery.[5] These guidelines with respect to perioperative fluid management have placed particular emphasis upon optimizing near-zero fluid balance by targeting cardiac output, avoiding overhydration, preferential use of balanced crystalloids over 0.9% saline, and judicious use of vasopressors for arterial hypotension. Historical terms used to describe fluid management in the perioperative period include "restrictive," "liberal," and "standard"; however, these have been replaced largely in this setting by the concept of "balanced" versus "unbalanced" fluid regimens.

A meta-analysis of nine randomized controlled trials (including 801 patients undergoing elective abdominal surgery) examining the impact of these fluid regimes [6] found no significant difference in outcome when comparing "restricted" (<1.75 liter/day) and "standard or liberal" (>2.75 liter/day) fluid strategies. However, when these were reclassified as "fluid balance" versus "fluid imbalance," the balanced group had a significantly lower rate of overall complications (risk ratio 0.59 [95% CI 0.44 to 0.81], $p = 0.0008$) as well as hospital length of stay (weighted mean difference -3.44 days [95% CI -6.33 to -0.54 days], $p = 0.02$). The occurrence of one or more complications following surgery is associated with adverse effects not only on short- and long-term survival but also increasing healthcare costs.[7,8] "Near-zero balance" fluid administration has now become a key principle of fluid management in the perioperative period,[9] with patients incurring minimal or no weight gain, although the range for safe fluid therapy is a narrow one.

Optimal perioperative fluid management requires careful intervention in the pre-, intra- and postoperative stages, with imbalance during any of these stages potentially compromising clinical outcomes. Patient body weight can be used as a surrogate of hydration status during the perioperative period, with patient weight gain of just 2.5 kg (excessive fluid administration of 2.5 liters) being associated with a detrimental effect upon outcome.[10]

Preoperative fluid management

The aim of preoperative fluid management as part of an ERAS pathway is for the patient to arrive in the anesthetic room in a euvolemic state. Patients are kept in a starved state prior to elective anesthesia to reduce the risk of aspiration, but should not undergo prolonged periods of starvation which result in preoperative dehydration and increased insulin resistance.[11] Current National and European guidelines recommending a 2-hour preoperative starvation period for clear non-carbonated fluids and 6 hours for solids.[12,13] However, in practice starvation times may exceed those recommended, owing to changes in operative scheduling, and fluid status must be carefully monitored during these delays. Mechanical bowel preparation is another potential source of preoperative salt and water depletion, particularly in the elderly, and following recent meta-analyses [14,15] demonstrating no benefit in terms of overall complications, anastomotic leak rate, requirement for re-operation, and mortality, this is no longer recommended preoperatively as part of ERAS programs for colonic surgery. Conversely, the administration of large volumes of fluid, particularly salt-containing fluid, in the preoperative period is known to affect clinical outcomes adversely. If bowel preparation is deemed necessary preoperatively (e.g. in rectal surgery) then fluid administered should be titrated to hydration status, gastrointestinal losses, and patient body weight.

Oral carbohydrate drink administration containing a defined concentration (12%) of complex carbohydrates up to 2 hours preoperatively facilitates the patient's being in a "metabolically fed" state, which has been seen to reduce insulin resistance by approximately 50% [16] without the increased risk of aspiration as well as significantly reducing anxiety, hunger, thirst, and overall hospital length of stay.[17] The administration of a carbohydrate drink in the immediate preoperative period is now recommended as part of ERAS programs.

Combination of these preoperative fluid management strategies makes it less likely that patients will be fluid-responsive (i.e. underhydrated) in the anesthetic room than with traditional preoperative fluid strategies. Patients in a fluid-depleted state preoperatively often require preoperative fluid boluses to avoid the hypotensive effects associated with induction of anesthesia caused by decreased sympathetic tone.

Intraoperative fluid management

Evidence in the field of perioperative fluid management has shown a significant benefit conveyed by aiming for "near-zero balance" of both fluid and electrolyte in the reduction of postoperative complications.[6] However, the clinical assessment of "zero balance" can be problematic in an operative setting, with fluid deficits often not becoming apparent until they exceed 10% of patient body weight. This may be further impaired by the induction of a CO_2 pneumoperitoneum and Trendelenburg positioning, with laparoscopy a frequently employed technique in ERAS programs. Perioperative tissue oxygenation is in part dictated by cardiac output, which in turn relies on fluid status. Inadequate intravascular volume can be seen following a loss of circulating blood volume of just 10–15% and this may result in splanchnic hypoperfusion as well as hypoperfusion of other key organs, microcirculatory compromise, and altered coagulation, and this frequently outlasts the period of hypovolemia.[18] The combination of hypoperfusion and hypoxia is associated with an increased release of reactive oxygen species, and with mitochondrial and endothelial dysfunction, which all act to increase perioperative morbidity. This resultant hypoperfusion can precipitate a range of complications related to impaired gastrointestinal function, including prolonged ileus and a tendency towards anastomotic dehiscence. On the other hand, excessive fluid administration can similarly result in bowel edema, ileus, and increased surgical complications in the perioperative period.[19] This occurs through an increase in the intravascular hydrostatic pressure. Evidence suggests that a cumulative fluid load exceeding 10.5 liters in the first 72 hours following surgery is associated with an increased risk of anastomotic breakdown.[20] Postoperative morbidity is associated in a U-shaped manner with intraoperative fluid volumes;[21] thus it is important to aim for sufficient but not excessive fluid infusion.

Goal-directed therapy (GDT) was developed to guide intravenous fluid and vasopressor/inotrope administration using measurements of cardiac output and other hemodynamic parameters to optimize stroke volume and cardiac index. Several techniques have been developed to facilitate GDT, including trans-esophageal Doppler (TED), lithium dilution, thoracic electric bioimpedance, and trans-pulmonary thermodilution techniques. Algorithms used for GDT frequently involve the assessment of stroke volume

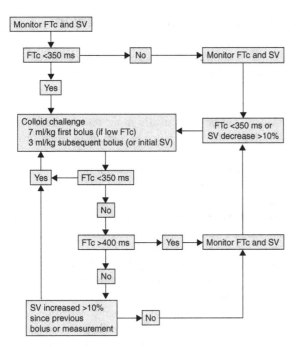

Figure 18.1 Algorithm for intraoperative goal-directed fluid administration. FTc – descending aortic corrected flow time; SV – stroke volume. From Ref. [24], with permission.

and stroke volume corrected flow time (FTc) in the descending aorta prior to and after an infusion of 200–250 ml fluid over a 5–10-min period (Figure 18.1). A change in stroke volume exceeding 10% or an FTc of less than 0.35 seconds following bolus administration indicates a hypovolemic patient and thus the requirement for a further fluid bolus. If, however, the stroke volume changes by less than 10% or the FTc exceeds 0.4 seconds, this suggests the patient is adequately filled, and there is no current requirement for a further fluid bolus in addition to background fluid infusion. These hemodynamic parameters should be continuously monitored throughout the operation and a further bolus administered if a fall below these parameters occurs. Perioperatively, maintenance fluid infusion should be limited to 2 ml/kg per hour, including any drug infusions, to limit the risk of fluid overload and resultant adverse clinical effects. This volume is guided by a combination of both any preoperative fluid deficits as well as any sensible and insensible intraoperative fluid losses. Currently, the use of GDT is recommended from commencement of the surgical procedure in:

- Major surgery with a 30-day mortality rate of >1%
- Major surgery with an anticipated blood loss of >500 ml
- Major intra-abdominal surgery
- Intermediate surgery (30-day mortality >0.5%) in high-risk patients (age >80 years, history of cardiovascular disease or peripheral arterial disease)
- Unexpected blood loss and/or fluid loss requiring >2 liters of fluid replacement
- Patients with ongoing evidence of hypovolemia and/or tissue hypoperfusion (e.g. persistent lactic acidosis).

Randomized controlled trials published in the early twenty-first century suggested that GDT was associated with a significant reduction in perioperative morbidity as well as hospital length of stay.[22–24] This evidence led to a recommendation by the UK National Institute of Health and Clinical Excellence (NICE) that intraoperative GDT be used as a standard of care. In addition, the British Consensus Guidelines on Intravenous Fluid Therapy for Adult Surgical Patients (GIFTASUP) further supported the use of this technique for the reduction of postoperative complications.

Despite this, in more recent studies when GDT was administered in combination with ERAS programs which controlled more accurately for postoperative salt and water overload than in conventional fluid administration, there was no longer a clinical benefit conveyed by this technique.[25] This is further evidenced by several recent systematic reviews and meta-analyses [26,27] which show a significantly attenuated clinical benefit when the two techniques are used in combination. A recent meta-analysis of 23 randomized controlled trials [28] including 2,099 patients demonstrated that although GDT was associated with a significant reduction in morbidity and hospital length of stay when patients were managed in a traditional care pathway, when managed in an ERAS setting the only benefit seen was to length of stay in intensive care.

Salt balance has become considered an increasingly important aspect of perioperative fluid management, with excess administration of 0.9% saline resulting in hyperchloremic acidosis, and as such, balanced crystalloids have become an increasingly important aspect of perioperative fluid management.

Postoperative fluid management

Increasing importance is now being placed upon the maintenance of normovolemia as well as electrolyte balance in the postoperative phase, as this is associated with a reduction in complication rates and hospital length of stay.[29,30] However, despite this recommendation it is not uncommon for patients in the postoperative period to receive 5–10 liters of fluid with large sodium loads in the first 24 hours following surgery. This is often related to errors in prescribing, with studies suggesting this to occur in up to 20% of patients. Excess fluid administration in the postoperative period is further compounded by the metabolic response to trauma precipitated by surgery which causes the retention of salt and water in order to maintain intravascular volumes. This excess water and sodium load can take several weeks to be offloaded in the postoperative period. Excessive fluid administration in the intra- and postoperative period can have multisystem complications following surgery, including respiratory (increased pneumonia), gastrointestinal (decreased mesenteric blood flow, prolonged ileus, increased anastomotic leak rates, and splanchnic edema), mobility (increased peripheral edema), and general patient status (increased nausea, impaired wound healing, and impaired cognitive abilities). In contrast, underhydration in the postoperative period is known to have significant hemodynamic effects including decreased venous return and preload, increased blood viscosity, and decreased tissue perfusion.

Once oral intake is reestablished postoperatively, intravenous fluid administration should be tailored to intake requirements, with cessation at the earliest opportunity, encouraging early postoperative mobility. Intravenous fluids should only be recommenced if clinically indicated. ERAS guidelines advocate rapid treatment of postoperative nausea and vomiting (PONV) in order to encourage early oral intake, with prophylaxis indicated in specific circumstances. ERAS guidelines recommend the avoidance of nasogastric tubes following evidence suggesting that their placement increases the incidence of pneumonia and time to passage of flatus but makes no difference to length of hospital stay.[31,32] Recommencement of normal diet as early as possible following surgery should be a major target of any ERAS protocol, with evidence that delay in commencement of feeding is associated with increased hospital length of stay and infectious complications.[33]

A frequently employed technique in ERAS protocols is the use of thoracic epidural analgesia (TEA), particularly following open surgery, owing to superior analgesic quantities in the first 72 hours following surgery.[34] This technique, however, often results in a degree of sympathetic blockade, reducing venous tone and capacitance, and resulting in fluid-resistant hypotension. It is key that when managing epidural-induced hypotension (EIH), a combination of judicious intravenous fluid administration as well as vasopressor use is adopted to prevent significant fluid overload (Figure 18.2) which is associated with worsening of clinical outcomes.[35]

The vast majority of the evidence for ERAS programs originates from the speciality of colorectal surgery, and thus its extrapolation to other fields of surgery is not without limitations.

Choice of fluid

A vast amount of research has been conducted into the potential risks and benefits associated with the type of fluid infused (colloid versus crystalloid; balanced versus unbalanced).

"Normal" 0.9% saline has historically been used as a maintenance fluid method and has previously been the most commonly prescribed crystalloid in the UK and USA, using 10 and 200 million liters annually. However, excessive administration of "normal saline," owing to its extra-physiological content of both sodium and chloride (10% and 50% higher than the content in extracellular fluid, respectively), is now understood to result in a significant hyperchloremic acidosis which may result in reduced renal cortical perfusion. This acidosis has been found to be associated with a significant reduction in mean renal artery flow velocity and perfusion [36] as well as increased postoperative morbidity and mortality [37,38] when compared with a balanced crystalloid, even in healthy volunteers. Bolus administration of 0.9% saline versus balanced crystalloid solutions in healthy human volunteers is associated with slower fluid excretion but equivalent blood volume expansion,[36,39] therefore increasing the likelihood of prolonged fluid retention and resultant edema. In addition, human studies have shown that sodium balance remains

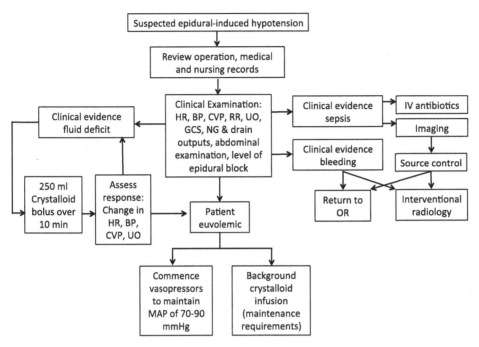

Figure 18.2 Postoperative algorithm for the management of epidural-induced hypotension (EIH). BP, blood pressure; CVP, central venous pressure; GCS, Glasgow coma scale; HR, heart rate; MAP, mean arterial pressure; NG, nasogastric; OR, operating room; RR, respiratory rate; UO, urine output. With permission from Ref. [45].

abnormal for up to 2 days following infusion of 0.9% saline, as the mechanisms for sodium excretion are dependent upon prolonged suppression of the renin–angiotensin–aldosterone system. No clinical studies have found 0.9% saline to be superior to balanced crystalloids, and two randomized controlled trials [40,41] have shown saline to be associated with an increased side-effect profile versus Ringer's lactate. ERAS guidelines [1–5] now place much emphasis upon the administration of balanced crystalloid as the maintenance fluid of choice, reinforced by GIFTASuP, which recommend the use of balanced crystalloids in the majority of clinical settings. The main exceptions to this are patients with high output from the upper gastrointestinal tract (vomiting, high volume nasogastric drainage) which may result in hypochloremic alkalosis, and neurosurgical patients in whom hypo-osmolar fluid administration may be harmful.

The administration of colloid versus crystalloid fluids remains a much debated topic. Colloid fluids are of an increased molecular size; as such, they are retained in the intravascular compartment more readily and therefore provide increased expansion of this space. This is particularly useful in the hypovolemic patient, in whom colloid administration

results in a greater ability to expand intravascular volume, although excessive administration results in damage to the endothelial glycocalyx. Much research into GDT has utilized hydroxyethyl starch (HES) for bolus fluid infusion, but owing to concerns raised about HES from level I evidence regarding the risk of increased mortality [42,43] as well as acute kidney injury rates,[44] this fluid is no longer in use in Europe. Recent evidence has suggested that balanced crystalloid (Hartmann's solution) and colloid (6% HES) as the bolus agent in GDT result in equivalent rates of morbidity and coagulopathy, suggesting this may become increasingly utilized in a GDT strategy.

Summary

Optimal fluid management in the setting of an ERAS program is a careful balance of pre-, intra-, and postoperative factors, all aiming for "zero balance" of both water and salt. The range of balanced fluid administration is fairly narrow, with both under- and overhydration having significant harmful effects on the surgical patient. ERAS guidelines have recommended the preferential use of balanced crystalloids as the fluid of choice in this setting rather than 0.9% saline, excessive administration of which is associated with detrimental effects.

References

1. Mortensen K, Nilsson M, Slim K, *et al.* Consensus guidelines for enhanced recovery after gastrectomy: Enhanced Recovery After Surgery (ERAS(R)) Society recommendations. *Br J Surg* 2014; 101: 1209–29.

2. Gustafsson UO, Scott MJ, Schwenk W, *et al.* Guidelines for perioperative care in elective colonic surgery: Enhanced Recovery After Surgery (ERAS(R)) Society recommendations. *World J Surg* 2013; 37: 259–84.

3. Nygren J, Thacker J, Carli F, *et al.* Guidelines for perioperative care in elective rectal/pelvic surgery: Enhanced Recovery After Surgery (ERAS(R)) Society recommendations. *Clin Nutr* 2012; 31: 801–16.

4. Cerantola Y, Valerio M, Persson B, *et al.* Guidelines for perioperative care after radical cystectomy for bladder cancer: Enhanced Recovery After Surgery (ERAS(R)) Society recommendations. *Clin Nutr* 2013; 32: 879–87.

5. Lassen K, Coolsen MM, Slim K, *et al.* Guidelines for perioperative care for pancreaticoduodenectomy: Enhanced Recovery After Surgery (ERAS(R)) Society recommendations. *Clin Nutr* 2012; 31: 817–30.

6. Varadhan KK, Lobo DN. A meta-analysis of randomised controlled trials of intravenous fluid therapy in major elective open abdominal surgery: getting the balance right. *Proc Nutr Soc* 2010; 69: 488–98.

7. Khuri SF, Henderson WG, DePalma RG, *et al.* Determinants of long-term survival after major surgery and the adverse effect of postoperative complications. *Ann Surg* 2005; 242: 326–41; discussion 341–3.

8. Dimick JB, Chen SL, Taheri PA, *et al.* Hospital costs associated with surgical complications: a report from the private-sector National Surgical Quality Improvement Program. *J Am Coll Surg* 2004; 199: 531–7.

9. Doherty M, Buggy DJ. Intraoperative fluids: how much is too much? *Br J Anaesth* 2012; 109: 69–79.

10. Lobo DN. Fluid overload and surgical outcome: another piece in the jigsaw. *Ann Surg* 2009; 249: 186–8.

11. Faria MS, de Aguilar-Nascimento JE, Pimenta OS, *et al.* Preoperative fasting of 2 hours minimizes insulin resistance and organic response to trauma after video-cholecystectomy: a randomized, controlled, clinical trial. *World J Surg* 2009; 33: 1158–64.

12. Smith I, Kranke P, Murat I, *et al.* Perioperative fasting in adults and children: guidelines from the European Society of Anaesthesiology. *Eur J Anaesthesiol* 2011; 28: 556–69.

13. Practice guidelines for preoperative fasting and the use of pharmacologic agents to reduce the risk of pulmonary aspiration: application to healthy patients undergoing elective procedures: an updated report by the American Society of Anesthesiologists Committee on Standards and Practice Parameters. *Anesthesiology* 2011; 114: 495–511.

14. Cao F, Li J, Li F. Mechanical bowel preparation for elective colorectal surgery: updated systematic review and meta-analysis. *Int J Colorectal Dis* 2012; 27: 803–10.

15. Guenaga KF, Matos D, Wille-Jorgensen P. Mechanical bowel preparation for elective colorectal surgery. *Cochrane Database Syst Rev* 2011: CD001544.

16. Nygren J. The metabolic effects of fasting and surgery. *Best Pract Res Clin Anaesthesiol* 2006; 20: 429–38.

17. Awad S, Varadhan KK, Ljungqvist O, *et al.* A meta-analysis of randomised controlled trials on preoperative oral carbohydrate treatment in elective surgery. *Clin Nutr* 2013; 32: 34–44.

18. Giglio MT, Marucci M, Testini M, *et al.* Goal-directed haemodynamic therapy and gastrointestinal complications in major surgery: a meta-analysis of randomized controlled trials. *Br J Anaesth* 2009; 103: 637–46.

19. Bundgaard-Nielsen M, Secher NH, Kehlet H. 'Liberal' vs. 'restrictive' perioperative fluid therapy–a critical assessment of the evidence. *Acta Anaesthesiol Scand* 2009; 53: 843–51.

20. Schnuriger B, Inaba K, Wu T, *et al.* Crystalloids after primary colon resection and anastomosis at initial trauma laparotomy: excessive volumes are associated with anastomotic leakage. *J Trauma* 2011; 70: 603–10.

21. Bellamy MC. Wet, dry or something else? *Br J Anaesth* 2006; 97:755–7.

22. Pearse R, Dawson D, Fawcett J, *et al.* Early goal-directed therapy after major surgery reduces complications and duration of hospital stay. A randomised, controlled trial [ISRCTN38797445]. *Crit Care* 2005; 9: R687–93.

23. Gan TJ, Soppitt A, Maroof M, *et al.* Goal-directed intraoperative fluid administration reduces length of hospital stay after major surgery. *Anesthesiology* 2002; 97: 820–6.

24. Noblett SE, Snowden CP, Shenton BK, *et al.* Randomized clinical trial assessing the effect of Doppler-optimized fluid management on outcome after elective colorectal resection. *Br J Surg* 2006; 93: 1069–76.

25. Phan TD, D'Souza B, Rattray MJ, *et al*. A randomised controlled trial of fluid restriction compared to oesophageal Doppler-guided goal-directed fluid therapy in elective major colorectal surgery within an Enhanced Recovery After Surgery program. *Anaesth Intensive Care* 2014; 42: 752–60.

26. Srinivasa S, Taylor MH, Sammour T, *et al*. Oesophageal Doppler-guided fluid administration in colorectal surgery: critical appraisal of published clinical trials. *Acta Anaesthesiol Scand* 2011; 55: 4–13.

27. Srinivasa S, Lemanu DP, Singh PP, *et al*. Systematic review and meta-analysis of oesophageal Doppler-guided fluid management in colorectal surgery. *Br J Surg* 2013; 100: 1701–8.

28. Rollins KE, Lobo DN. Intraoperative goal-directed fluid therapy in elective major abdominal surgery: A meta-analysis of randomized controlled trials. *Ann Surg* 2015; 263: 465–76.

29. Lobo DN, Bostock KA, Neal KR, *et al*. Effect of salt and water balance on recovery of gastrointestinal function after elective colonic resection: a randomised controlled trial. *Lancet* 2002; 359: 1812–18.

30. Brandstrup B, Tonnesen H, Beier-Holgersen R, *et al*. Effects of intravenous fluid restriction on postoperative complications: comparison of two perioperative fluid regimens: a randomized assessor-blinded multicenter trial. *Ann Surg* 2003; 238: 641–8.

31. Cheatham ML, Chapman WC, Key SP, *et al*. A meta-analysis of selective versus routine nasogastric decompression after elective laparotomy. *Ann Surg* 1995; 221: 469–76.

32. Nelson R, Edwards S, Tse B. Prophylactic nasogastric decompression after abdominal surgery. *Cochrane Database Syst Rev* 2007: CD004929.

33. Lewis SJ, Andersen HK, Thomas S. Early enteral nutrition within 24 h of intestinal surgery versus later commencement of feeding: a systematic review and meta-analysis. *J Gastrointest Surg* 2009; 13: 569–75.

34. Block BM, Liu SS, Rowlingson AJ, *et al*. Efficacy of postoperative epidural analgesia: a meta-analysis. *JAMA* 2003; 290: 2455–63.

35. Holte K, Foss NB, Svensen C, *et al*. Epidural anesthesia, hypotension, and changes in intravascular volume. *Anesthesiology* 2004; 100: 281–6.

36. Chowdhury AH, Cox EF, Francis ST, *et al*. A randomized, controlled, double-blind crossover study on the effects of 2-L infusions of 0.9% saline and Plasma-Lyte(R) 148 on renal blood flow velocity and renal cortical tissue perfusion in healthy volunteers. *Ann Surg* 2012; 256: 18–24.

37. McCluskey SA, Karkouti K, Wijeysundera D, *et al*. Hyperchloremia after noncardiac surgery is independently associated with increased morbidity and mortality: a propensity-matched cohort study. *Anesth Analg* 2013; 117: 412–21.

38. Krajewski ML, Raghunathan K, Paluszkiewicz SM, *et al*. Meta-analysis of high- versus low-chloride content in perioperative and critical care fluid resuscitation. *Br J Surg* 2015; 102: 24–36.

39. Lobo DN, Stanga Z, Simpson JA, *et al*. Dilution and redistribution effects of rapid 2-litre infusions of 0.9% (w/v) saline and 5% (w/v) dextrose on haematological parameters and serum biochemistry in normal subjects: a double-blind crossover study. *Clin Sci (Lond)* 2001; 101: 173–9.

40. O'Malley CM, Frumento RJ, Hardy MA, *et al*. A randomized, double-blind comparison of lactated Ringer's solution and 0.9% NaCl during renal transplantation. *Anesth Analg* 2005; 100: 1518–24.

41. Waters JH, Gottlieb A, Schoenwald P, *et al*. Normal saline versus lactated Ringer's solution for intraoperative fluid management in patients undergoing abdominal aortic aneurysm repair: an outcome study. *Anesth Analg* 2001; 93: 817–22.

42. Brunkhorst FM, Engel C, Bloos F, *et al*. Intensive insulin therapy and pentastarch resuscitation in severe sepsis. *N Engl J Med* 2008; 358: 125–39.

43. Perner A, Haase N, Guttormsen AB, *et al*. Hydroxyethyl starch 130/0.42 versus Ringer's acetate in severe sepsis. *N Engl J Med* 2012; 367: 124–34.

44. Myburgh JA, Finfer S, Bellomo R, *et al*. Hydroxyethyl starch or saline for fluid resuscitation in intensive care. *N Engl J Med* 2012; 367: 1901–11.

45. Awad S, Lobo DN. Fluid management. In: Feldman LS, Delaney CP, Ljungqvist O, Carli F, eds. *The SAGES/ERAS Manual of Enhanced Recovery Programs for Gastrointestinal Surgery*. Switzerland, Springer International. 2015; 119–132.

Chapter

19

Spinal anesthesia

Michael F. M. James and Robert A. Dyer

Summary

Fluid therapy is widely used in conjunction with spinal anesthesia to minimize hypotensive events. The use of crystalloids for this purpose seems to be only minimally effective, particularly when given prior to the administration of the spinal anesthetic. To be effective, substantial fluid boluses must be administered – of the order of 20 ml/kg – and then preferably as a rapid coload simultaneously with the induction of spinal anesthesia. Several studies and meta-analyses suggest that colloids, either as preload or coload, are more effective than crystalloids and may result in a smaller volume of fluid loading being required. However, fluids alone, whether crystalloid or colloid, are generally inadequate to prevent or treat significant hypotension associated with spinal anesthesia, and the concomitant use of a vasopressor will frequently be necessary, particularly in obstetrics. The best that can be achieved with optimal fluid therapy is an overall reduction in the total dose of vasopressor required. The best available management of spinal hypotension would appear to be optimal fluid therapy combined with carefully graded administration of the appropriate vasopressor. It is possible that goal-directed fluid therapy, using an appropriate analysis of cardiac performance to assess the response dynamic indices to a fluid challenge, may improve fluid therapy in the future, but, at present, the evidence for this is insufficient to make a firm recommendation.

Introduction

Spinal anesthesia is inevitably associated with some degree of hypotension. Estimates of the incidence of clinically relevant hypotension vary from 25% to over 80%, depending on the criteria used to identify clinically relevant decreases in blood pressure, and on the population group studied.

Two groups of patients have been extensively studied. The first patient population of concern comprises elderly patients undergoing a variety of surgical procedures for which spinal anesthesia is appropriate, including bladder and prostate procedures and lower limb surgery, particularly joint replacements. The second important group is the obstetric population, in whom hypotension has implications for the fetus (reduction in placental perfusion) and for the mother (cardiovascular collapse and unpleasant side effects of nausea and vomiting).

A variety of causative factors have been suggested to explain the hypotension following spinal anesthesia. These include diminished cardiac output as a result of inadequate compensation for arteriolar- and venodilatation in elderly patients with impaired ventricular function, and an only partial compensatory increase in cardiac output in obstetrics patients with normal ventricular function. There may also be paralysis of the sympathetic nerve supply to the heart and adrenal glands resulting in reduced catecholamine responsiveness and unmasking of hypovolemia. In the pregnant patient these may be complicated by aorto-caval compression. Pre-existing hypertension may increase the risk of spinal anesthesia-associated hypotension in older patients,[1] but pre-eclampsia is associated with less spinal hypotension than in healthy parturients, since the usual cardiovascular status is one of increased inotropy together with elevated systemic vascular resistance.[2]

Older texts refer to the value of electrolyte solutions in minimizing the hypotensive response and suggest that volumes of 2 liters may be adequate. These assumptions have been challenged by a substantial body of research over the past 20 years.

Non-obstetric spinal anesthesia

In a study conducted in elderly patients aged 60 years or over, the overall incidence of arterial hypotension during spinal anesthesia was 27%, rising to 60% when temperature sensation was blocked to T7. If the block reached T4, all patients required vasopressor therapy. Patients were divided into three groups receiving 16 ml/kg, 8 ml/kg, or zero acetated Ringer's lactate solution (RL) as a preload; crystalloid preloading had no effect on the incidence of hypotension.[3] However, a relatively small preload (7 ml/kg) of 3% hypertonic saline was significantly better than 0.9% saline at reducing the requirement for vasopressor support in patients undergoing prostatectomy.[4] RL was shown to sustain, but not increase cardiac output in healthy patients undergoing lower extremity surgery.[5]

Fluid kinetics modeling has shown that crystalloids rapidly redistribute away from the central compartment, and tend to enhance the second compartment. The redistribution time constants of crystalloid are quite rapid,[6] and these kinetics may contribute to the relative lack of efficacy of crystalloid solutions in preventing spinal anesthesia-associated hypotension. Volunteer studies have shown that an infusion rate of 50 ml/min is required to yield an increase in blood volume of approximately 10%, and that this would need be maintained for at least 40 min to produce the required volume expansion; this volume load rapidly dissipates.[7] In a review of spinal anesthesia in elderly patients, Critchley concluded that an adequate venous preload was necessary, but any fluid loading should be ideally administered as the block is developing (subsequently termed *coload* in an obstetric anesthesia study [8]), rather than as a preload.[9] In an early study of volume kinetics during epidural anesthesia, it was shown that a crystalloid coload of 15 ml/kg was better retained within the circulation in those patients who showed a substantial decrease in systolic pressure. Nevertheless, despite volume loading, there was a relative hypovolemia, as evidenced by hemodilution, in all patients throughout the development of hypotension.[10] A recent study using either crystalloid (1,000 ml) or colloid (500 ml) coload in older patients showed that both forms of fluid therapy sustained cardiac output above baseline values for 30 min, but the effect of crystalloids waned after 20 min.[11]

Goal-directed fluid therapy

Levy and colleagues recommended the use of goal-directed fluid therapy with colloids together with spinal (but not epidural) anesthesia to optimize patient outcomes after laparoscopic surgery.[12] In a subsequent study, patients undergoing laparoscopic colorectal surgery were randomized to receive spinal or epidural analgesia or intravenous morphine. All patients were treated with volume optimization against esophageal Doppler measurements. Patients who failed to achieve an indexed oxygen delivery of >400 ml/min/m² had a higher rate of anastomotic leak than those achieving this level, but the fluid therapy itself and the mode of analgesia were not individual predictors.[13] A recent study examined the effects of goal-directed fluid therapy using the LiDCO® device in patients undergoing hip surgery and found no evidence of improved outcome relative to a standard care group, and no evidence of benefit. These authors concluded that there was insufficient evidence either to support or discount routine use of goal-directed fluid administration in these patients.[14] In a clinical study of isobaric spinal anesthesia in patients undergoing transurethral bladder tumor resection, patients receiving crystalloid (15 ml/kg) showed a significantly longer mean time to reach the peak sensory block and a lower median sensory block at 15 and 20 min than those receiving colloid (5 ml/kg). In the crystalloid group, cerebrospinal fluid (CSF) flow in the cranial direction decreased significantly and attenuated pulsatile movement of CSF at the L2–3 intervertebral intrathecal space. However, this was not observed with colloid.[15]

Obstetric spinal anesthesia

The management of spinal hypotension in obstetrics is crucial for the safety and comfort of the mother, and the well-being of her baby.

An early obstetrics study showed that the administration of a 20 ml/kg crystalloid preload failed to prevent significant hypotension whether the load was given rapidly over 10 min or more slowly over 20 min. However, in the rapid preload group, three patients were found to have a marked rise in central venous pressure. The authors queried the role of isotonic crystalloid preload in the management of spinal anesthesia for elective Cesarean section,[16] and the same group recommended that if time was scarce the spinal anesthesia should not be delayed by awaiting administration of the crystalloid preload.[17] Jackson and colleagues evaluated the use of a preload of 1,000 ml prior to spinal anesthesia for Cesarean section and were unable to demonstrate any advantage over a preload of 200 ml. They also concluded that crystalloid preload was not of value.[18]

A study in pre-eclamptic patients has also failed to demonstrate significant benefit from a preload of 1,000 ml crystalloid, although the authors commented that changes in uterine artery velocity waveforms were minimal and there was no adverse effect on the neonate.[19] There have been a number of concerns regarding the possible adverse consequences of saline-based solutions given in large volumes in terms of generating hyperchloremic metabolic acidosis, but this does not seem to be of particular consequence to either mother or child when saline solution is compared with lactated Ringer's for preload,[20] and this has since been confirmed in a study of starch in a balanced salt solution compared with a similar starch in saline.[21]

Crystalloid coload

The relative lack of efficacy of crystalloid loading prior to spinal anesthesia can be explained by a number of factors including the physiological responses of patients with normal fluid balance status to a rapid fluid load, and the volume kinetics of crystalloid solutions. Pouta and colleagues demonstrated a significant increase in the release of atrial natriuretic peptide, and a lesser effect on endothelin-1, following crystalloid loading of 2,000 ml lactated Ringer's solution in healthy parturients. They concluded that this could offset the effects of volume load on blood pressure during Cesarean delivery.[22] This release of hormone was correlated significantly with the increase in atrial stretch as indicated by an increase in central venous pressure. Pre-eclamptic patients showed a

greater response, possibly in line with reduced diastolic function in these patients.[23]

A dose-defining study of 90 parturients looked at the effect of three fluid volume groups receiving 10, 15, or 20 ml/kg of RL respectively within 15 min before the spinal block. Spinal anesthesia was followed immediately by an infusion of ephedrine of 3 mg/min in all groups. The incidence of hypotension was 60%, 36.7%, and 13.4% in groups 10RL, 15RL, and 20RL, respectively ($p < 0.05$). Additional ephedrine dosage was lowest in group 20RL compared with the other groups ($p < 0.05$). The incidence of nausea and vomiting in group 20RL was significantly less than in group 10RL ($p = 0.02$). It was concluded that preloading with 20 ml/kg of RL prior to spinal anesthesia followed by an ephedrine infusion reduced the incidence of hypotension and of nausea and vomiting, and decreased the total dose of ephedrine.[24]

Since the administration of crystalloids to healthy, volume-replete subjects is likely to trigger physiological responses such as secretion of atrial natriuretic peptide and increased renal excretion of the fluid, and volume kinetics suggest very rapid redistribution of fluid loads in the absence of a hypovolemic state, the administration of fluids as a coload at the time of onset of spinal anesthesia might be more efficacious than administering a preload. Initial studies using 20 ml/kg of crystalloid as a rapid bolus at the time of the performance of spinal anesthesia suggested that a significant reduction in ephedrine requirements could be achieved by this method.[8]

A meta-analysis of preload vs. coload failed to confirm the advantage of coload, although the authors commented that the only study in which coload was effective was the one that used the highest infusion volume, i.e. 20 ml/kg.[25] Fluid kinetic studies have shown that the distribution of crystalloids from the plasma to the interstitium is markedly delayed during the onset of spinal, epidural, and general anesthesia,[26] and this lends support to the concept that coload with crystalloids may be more effective than preload, but definitive data are lacking. There is also no evidence that colloid coload is more effective than colloid preload.[27]

Colloids

The final issue to be resolved is whether the use of colloid solutions would be advantageous by virtue of their retention in the circulating blood volume for a longer period than crystalloids.

Studies on the effects of spinal anesthesia on cardiac output suggested that volume preloading had to be sufficient to produce a significant increase in cardiac output if hypotension was to be minimized.[28] These authors showed that colloid preload was more effective than crystalloid in enhancing cardiac output and, consequently, in reducing spinal hypotension during elective Cesarean section.

Whilst logic would suggest that colloid preloading would be advantageous compared with crystalloid loading, the data on this topic are inconsistent. Riley and colleagues suggested that a preload of 500 ml hydroxyethyl starch (HES) together with 1 liter RL was superior to 2 liters of RL in terms of reductions in the incidence of hypotension and requirements for ephedrine in obstetrics patients.[29] However, a study found that 500 ml of gelatin colloid preload was not superior to a similar volume of crystalloid or no preload at all in parturients.[30] The same group also failed to show a benefit of a combination of 500 ml each of HES and crystalloid in elderly patients receiving spinal anesthesia.[31]

Obstetrics studies using 1 liter colloid showed significantly less hypotension than no preload,[32] or preloading with either 1.5 liters lactated Ringer's or 500 ml HES.[28] A systematic review at this time concluded that crystalloid preload was inconsistent in preventing hypotension, whereas colloid was generally effective in minimizing hypotension, but neither was effective in minimizing maternal nausea, and there were few differences in neonatal outcomes.[33] Dahlgren and colleagues confirmed that 1 liter of colloid was more effective than an equivalent volume of crystalloid for the prevention of hypotension [34] and subsequently demonstrated that supine stress testing could accurately predict those patients in whom a colloid preload would likely be beneficial.[35] Davies and French demonstrated that 10 ml/kg of colloid was more effective than 5 ml/kg at minimizing obstetric spinal hypotension.[36]

A comparison between combinations of 1 liter each of RL combined with gelatin or HES-based colloids demonstrated that the HES-RL was superior to either the gelatin combination or 1 liter HES alone.[37] A recent Cochrane review concluded that crystalloids were more effective than no fluids (relative risk [RR] 0.78, 95% confidence interval [CI] 0.60–1.00; one trial, 140 women, sequential analysis) and colloids were more effective than crystalloids (RR 0.68, 95% CI 0.52–0.89; 11 trials, 698 women) in preventing hypotension following spinal anesthesia at Cesarean section.[38] Although no differences were detected for different doses, rates, or methods of administering colloids or crystalloids, the literature review presented above suggests that at least 1 liter of colloid is required to produce a significant reduction in the incidence of hypotension in healthy patients.

In terms of cardiac output, a study using Doppler monitoring during 1 liter coload with crystalloid or colloid found similar cardiac outputs between the groups, with no differences in secondary outcomes of vasopressor use or hemodynamic stability.[39] However, a subsequent meta-analysis involving 10 trials with 853 parturients (and including the previous study) concluded that, when colloid was used, there were significantly fewer hypotensive events (odds ration (OR) 3.21, 95% CI 2.15–4.53, number needed to treat = 4), less demand for vasopressors (standard mean difference SMD 0.77, 95% CI 0.34–1.21) and improved cardiac output (SMD −1.08, 95% CI −2.00 to −0.17).[40]

A study has recently been published comparing 500 ml of 6% HES (130/0.4) + 500 ml of RL (HES group) or 1,000 ml of RL (RL group) i.v. before spinal anesthesia. The incidence of both hypotension and symptomatic hypotension was significantly lower in the HES group than in the RL group. There was no detectable placental transfer of HES in six umbilical cord blood samples analyzed in the HES group, and neonatal outcomes were comparable.[41]

In reviewing the current trends, Mitra *et al.* concluded that intravenous crystalloid pre-hydration is not very efficient and that the focus has changed toward co-hydration and use of colloids.[42]

Fluids and vasopressors

It is well established that fluids alone are inadequate for the prophylaxis or management of obstetric spinal hypotension.[43] In elective cases in which left lateral tilt is correctly practiced, spinal hypotension is predominantly due to a decrease in systemic vascular resistance, and the pure alpha-agonist phenylephrine is the obvious antidote.[44]

Over the past 15 years, many studies by Ngan Kee and others have confirmed that phenylephrine is the vasopressor of choice for obstetric spinal hypotension. Close control of maternal blood pressure

Table 19.1 Suggested fluid options in spinal anesthesia. These volumes represent the best guidelines that can currently be obtained from the literature, but conclusive evidence for these suggestions is lacking

Patient	Fluid type	Volume (ml/kg)	Timing
Healthy obstetrics	Crystalloid	20	Coload
Healthy obstetrics	Colloid	15	Preload or coload
Pre-eclamptics	Colloid (?)	5–7	Preload or coload
Older patients block *below* T10	No fluid load	Replacement and maintenance fluids only	
Older patients block *above* T10	Colloid	5–7	Coload

employing coload, together with either early boluses or infusions of phenylephrine, provides the best hemodynamic stability and the lowest incidence of maternal symptoms.[45]

Conclusions

Current data suggest that crystalloids are only minimally effective at limiting hypotension and then only if given in doses of 20 ml/kg or greater, preferably as a rapid coload immediately after induction of spinal anesthesia. Such a large fluid bolus may be disadvantageous in elderly patients with limited cardiac reserve and in pre-eclamptic patients in whom diastolic dysfunction may predispose to the development of pulmonary edema.

Colloid fluid loading given as either a coload or preload appears to be more successful as a preventative strategy, and the weight of evidence appears to suggest that a volume of 15 ml/kg may be optimal in the healthy pregnant patient. Cost– and to some extent risk–benefit considerations have, however, resulted in the widespread adoption of crystalloid coloading.

A smaller volume load of colloid may be appropriate in older patients undergoing spinal anesthesia, and similar conditions may apply in pre-eclampsia, although firm data in this area are lacking. The height of the block required for surgery may also be important as most elderly patients require a much lower block than do Cesarean section patients and may thus require a smaller fluid load (Table 19.1).

The use of fluids to manage hypotension during spinal anesthesia is, at best, only moderately effective, and early intervention with vasopressors, particularly in obstetrics, will be required in many patients regardless of the fluid strategy adopted, if hypotension is to be minimized. The best that can be achieved with optimal fluid therapy is an overall reduction in the total dosage of vasopressor required. However, this endpoint is worth achieving since vasopressors may have adverse consequences in both obstetric and non-obstetric patients undergoing spinal anesthesia.

The best possible management of spinal hypotension would appear to be optimal fluid therapy combined with early, carefully graded management of subsequent hypotension with the appropriate vasopressor, dependent on cardiovascular status. Newer techniques involving analysis of cardiac performance, using the response of dynamic indices to a fluid challenge, may give better guidance in the individual case, for the administration of the appropriate volume of fluid in association with spinal anesthesia.

References

1. Critchley LA, Stuart JC, Short TG, Gin T. Haemodynamic effects of subarachnoid block in elderly patients. *Br J Anaesth* 1994; 73: 464–70.

2. Dennis AT. Transthoracic echocardiography in women with preeclampsia. *Curr Opin Anaesthesiol* 2015; 28: 254–60.

3. Coe AJ, Revanas B. Is crystalloid preloading useful in spinal anaesthesia in the elderly? *Anaesthesia* 1990; 45: 241–3.

4. Baraka A, Taha S, Ghabach M, *et al.* Hypertonic saline prehydration in patients undergoing transurethral resection of the prostate under spinal anaesthesia. *Br J Anaesth* 1994; 72: 227–8.

5. Kamenik M, Paver-Erzen V. The effects of lactated Ringer's solution infusion on cardiac output changes after spinal anesthesia. *Anesth Analg* 2001; 92: 710–14.

6. Svensen CH, Rodhe PM, Prough DS. Pharmacokinetic aspects of fluid therapy. *Best Pract Res Clin Anaesthesiol* 2009; 23: 213–24.

7. Hahn RG, Svensen C. Plasma dilution and the rate of infusion of Ringer's solution. *Br J Anaesth* 1997; 79: 64–7.

8. Dyer RA, Farina Z, Joubert IA, *et al*. Crystalloid preload versus rapid crystalloid administration after induction of spinal anaesthesia (coload) for elective caesarean section. *Anaesth Intensive Care* 2004; 32: 351–7.

9. Critchley LA. Hypotension, subarachnoid block and the elderly patient. *Anaesthesia* 1996; 51: 1139–43.

10. Drobin D, Hahn RG. Time course of increased haemodilution in hypotension induced by extradural anaesthesia. *Br J Anaesth* 1996; 77: 223–6.

11. Zorko N, Kamenik M, Starc V. The effect of Trendelenburg position, lactated Ringer's solution and 6% hydroxyethyl starch solution on cardiac output after spinal anesthesia. *Anesth Analg* 2009; 108: 655–9.

12. Levy BF, Scott MJ, Fawcett WJ, Day A, Rockall TA. Optimizing patient outcomes in laparoscopic surgery. *Colorectal Dis* 2011; 13(Suppl 7) : 8–11.

13. Levy BF, Fawcett WJ, Scott MJ, Rockall TA. Intra-operative oxygen delivery in infusion volume-optimized patients undergoing laparoscopic colorectal surgery within an enhanced recovery program: the effect of different analgesic modalities. *Colorectal Dis* 2012; 14: 887–92.

14. Moppett IK, Rowlands M, Mannings A, *et al*. LiDCO-based fluid management in patients undergoing hip fracture surgery under spinal anaesthesia: a randomized trial and systematic review. *Br J Anaesth* 2015; 114: 444–59.

15. Shin BS, Kim CS, Sim WS, *et al*. A comparison of the effects of preanesthetic administration of crystalloid versus colloid on intrathecal spread of isobaric spinal anesthetics and cerebrospinal fluid movement. *Anesth Analg* 2011; 112: 924–30.

16. Rout CC, Akoojee SS, Rocke DA, Gouws E. Rapid administration of crystalloid preload does not decrease the incidence of hypotension after spinal anaesthesia for elective caesarean section. *Br J Anaesth* 1992; 68: 394–7.

17. Rout CC, Rocke DA, Levin J, Gouws E, Reddy D. A reevaluation of the role of crystalloid preload in the prevention of hypotension associated with spinal anesthesia for elective cesarean section. *Anesthesiology* 1993; 79: 262–9.

18. Jackson R, Reid JA, Thorburn J. Volume preloading is not essential to prevent spinal-induced hypotension at caesarean section. *Br J Anaesth* 1995; 75: 262–5.

19. Karinen J, Rasanen J, Alahuhta S, Jouppila R, Jouppila P. Maternal and uteroplacental haemodynamic state in pre-eclamptic patients during spinal anaesthesia for Caesarean section. *Br J Anaesth* 1996; 76: 616–20.

20. Chanimov M, Gershfeld S, Cohen ML, Sherman D, Bahar M. Fluid preload before spinal anaesthesia in Caesarean section: the effect on neonatal acid–base status. *Eur J Anaesthesiol* 2006; 23: 676–9.

21. Marciniak A, Wujtewicz M, Owczuk R. The impact of colloid infusion prior to spinal anaesthesia for caesarean section on the condition of a newborn – a comparison of balanced and unbalanced hydroxyethyl starch 130/0.4. *Anaesthesiol Intensive Ther* 2013; 45: 14–19.

22. Pouta AM, Karinen J, Vuolteenaho OJ, Laatikainen TJ. Effect of intravenous fluid preload on vasoactive peptide secretion during Caesarean section under spinal anaesthesia. *Anaesthesia* 1996; 51: 128–32.

23. Pouta A, Karinen J, Vuolteenaho O, Laatikainen T. Pre-eclampsia: the effect of intravenous fluid preload on atrial natriuretic peptide secretion during caesarean section under spinal anaesthesia. *Acta Anaesthesiol Scand* 1996; 40: 1203–9.

24. Faydaci F, Gunaydin B. Different preloading protocols with constant ephedrine infusion in the prevention of hypotension for elective cesarean section under spinal anesthesia. *Acta Anaesthesiol Belg* 2011; 62: 5–10.

25. Banerjee A, Stocche RM, Angle P, Halpern SH. Preload or coload for spinal anesthesia for elective Cesarean delivery: a meta-analysis. *Can J Anaesth* 2010; 57: 24–31.

26. Hahn RG. Volume kinetics for infusion fluids. *Anesthesiology* 2010; 113: 470–81.

27. Siddik-Sayyid SM, Nasr VG, Taha SK, *et al*. A randomized trial comparing colloid preload to coload during spinal anesthesia for elective cesarean delivery. *Anesth Analg* 2009; 109: 1219–24.

28. Ueyama H, He YL, Tanigami H, Mashimo T, Yoshiya I. Effects of crystalloid and colloid preload on blood volume in the parturient undergoing spinal anesthesia for elective Cesarean section [see comments]. *Anesthesiology* 1999; 91: 1571–6.

29. Riley ET, Cohen SE, Rubenstein AJ, Flanagan B. Prevention of hypotension after spinal anesthesia for cesarean section: six percent hetastarch versus lactated Ringer's solution. *Anesth Analg* 1995; 81: 838–42.

30. Buggy D, Higgins P, Moran C, *et al*. Prevention of spinal anesthesia-induced hypotension in the elderly: comparison between preanesthetic administration of crystalloids, colloids, and no prehydration. *Anesth Analg* 1997; 84: 106–10.

31. Buggy D, Fitzpatrick G. Intravascular volume optimisation during repair of proximal femoral fracture. Regional anaesthesia is usually technique of choice. *BMJ* 1998; 316: 1090.

32. Ngan Kee WD, Khaw KS, Lee BB, Ng FF, Wong MM. Randomized controlled study of colloid preload before spinal anaesthesia for caesarean section. *Br J Anaesth* 2001; 87: 772–4.

33. Morgan PJ, Halpern SH, Tarshis J. The effects of an increase of central blood volume before spinal anesthesia for cesarean delivery: a qualitative systematic review. *Anesth Analg* 2001; 92: 997–1005.

34. Dahlgren G, Granath F, Pregner K, *et al.* Colloid vs. crystalloid preloading to prevent maternal hypotension during spinal anesthesia for elective cesarean section. *Acta Anaesthesiol Scand* 2005; 49: 1200–6.

35. Dahlgren G, Granath F, Wessel H, Irestedt L. Prediction of hypotension during spinal anesthesia for Cesarean section and its relation to the effect of crystalloid or colloid preload. *Int J Obstet Anesth* 2007; 16: 128–34.

36. Davies P, French GW. A randomised trial comparing 5 mL/kg and 10 mL/kg of pentastarch as a volume preload before spinal anaesthesia for elective Caesarean section. *Int J Obstet Anesth* 2006; 15: 279–83.

37. Vercauteren MP, Hoffmann V, Coppejans HC, Van Steenberge AL, Adriaensen HA. Hydroxyethylstarch compared with modified gelatin as volume preload before spinal anaesthesia for Caesarean section. *Br J Anaesth* 1996; 76: 731–3.

38. Cyna AM, Andrew M, Emmett RS, Middleton P, Simmons SW. Techniques for preventing hypotension during spinal anaesthesia for Caesarean section. *Cochrane Database Syst Rev* 2006: CD002251.

39. McDonald S, Fernando R, Ashpole K, Columb M. Maternal cardiac output changes after crystalloid or colloid coload following spinal anesthesia for elective Cesarean delivery: a randomized controlled trial. *Anesth Analg* 2011; 113: 803–10.

40. Li L, Zhang Y, Tan Y, Xu S. Colloid or crystalloid solution on maternal and neonatal hemodynamics for Cesarean section: a meta-analysis of randomized controlled trials. *J Obstet Gynaecol Res* 2013; 39: 932–41.

41. Mercier FJ, Diemunsch P, Ducloy-Bouthors AS, *et al.* 6% Hydroxyethyl starch (130/0.4) vs. Ringer's lactate preloading before spinal anaesthesia for Caesarean delivery: the randomized, double-blind, multicentre CAESAR trial. *Br J Anaesth* 2014; 113: 459–67.

42. Mitra JK, Roy J, Bhattacharyya P, Yunus M, Lyngdoh NM. Changing trends in the management of hypotension following spinal anesthesia in Cesarean section. *J Postgrad Med* 2013; 59: 121–6.

43. Sharwood-Smith G, Drummond GB. Hypotension in obstetric spinal anaesthesia: a lesson from pre-eclampsia. *Br J Anaesth* 2009; 102: 291–4.

44. Dyer RA, Reed AR, van Dyk D, *et al.* Hemodynamic effects of ephedrine, phenylephrine, and the coadministration of phenylephrine with oxytocin during spinal anesthesia for elective Cesarean delivery. *Anesthesiology* 2009; 111: 753–65.

45. Ngan Kee WD. Phenylephrine infusions for maintaining blood pressure during spinal anesthesia for Cesarean delivery: finding the shoe that fits. *Anesth Analg* 2014; 118: 496–8.

Chapter

20

Day surgery

Jan Jakobsson

Summary

Rapid recovery and a minimum of residual effects are factors of utmost importance when handling the day-case patient. Prolonged preoperative fasting should be avoided. Many countries have adopted revised fasting guidelines that allow patients without risk factors to eat a light meal up to 6 hours and to ingest clear fluids up to 2 hours prior to the induction of anesthesia. Postoperative fatigue can be reduced by fluid intake up to 2–3 hours prior to surgery.

Perioperative intravenous fluid therapy should be instituted on the basis of the case profile. In general, fluid infused during minor surgery may not exert a major effect, but during intermediate surgery, such as laparoscopic cholecystectomy, a liberal fluid program has been shown to improve recovery and reduce postoperative fatigue. Administration of about 1 liter isotonic electrolyte solution to compensate for the fasting, and a further 1 liter during surgery, improves the postoperative course. Liberal fluid administration also reduces the risk for postoperative nausea and the risk vs. benefit seems to be in favor for its routine use in ASA 1–2 patients. The potential benefit in adding dextrose to the intravenous fluid during the early postoperative phase has been assessed, but the benefit seems to be very minor.

Resumption of oral intake, drinking, and eating are traditional variables for the assessment of eligibility for discharge and thus an essential part

of day surgery. However, there is no need for patients to drink before discharge; intake of fluid and food should be recommended but not pushed.*

Day surgery is expanding. More patients and procedures are transferred from traditional in-hospital care to day-case or short-stay logistics. This trend – to shorten the hospital stay – affects the preparation and planning of patient care. The concept of fast tracking has become well established in a variety of surgical settings and is a most fundamental part of day surgery.[1] Rapid recovery and a minimum of residual effects are factors of utmost importance for the handling of the day-case patient. Resumption of oral intake, drinking, and eating are traditional variables for the assessment of eligibility for discharge and thus an essential part of day surgery.

Most surgical specialities are today performing day-case surgery, and the proportion of traditional in-hospital vs. day surgery is, in many disciplines, much in favor of the day cases. However, the proportion of day-case surgery for one and the same procedure varies considerably between countries and may also vary considerably within nations between different institutions. Explanations for these differences include tradition and economical factors.

Day surgery calls for vigilant assessment and preparation. The patient, the procedure, institutional resources, anesthesia, and a structured and quality-assured plan are needs to be considered. A structured anesthesia and analgesia protocol is fundamental. Multimodal analgesia should include a combination of local anesthesia and non-opioid analgesics (paracetamol and non-steroidal anti-inflammatory drugs, NSAIDs), then add on a weak opioid, and, as further

---

* Summary compiled by the Editor.

Clinical Fluid Therapy in the Perioperative Setting, Second Edition, ed. Robert G. Hahn. Published by Cambridge University Press. © Cambridge University Press 2016.

rescue, oral strong opioids in an escalating fashion. These factors are cornerstones in the widely accepted standard of care.[1]

The adoption of day surgery must not jeopardize safety. However, the experience of day surgery as of today is reassuring. The outcomes at 30 days in large cohorts of patients show very low mortality and incidences of major morbidity. Classical follow-up studies, such as the ones by Warner *et al.* [2], and Mezei and Chung,[3] and the 60-day follow up of day surgery in Copenhagen,[4] have all documented most reassuring safety. On the other hand, the increasing numbers of more complex procedures and acceptance of patients with more extensive medical history for day-case surgery must be acknowledged, and surveillance of outcome is of great importance in order to evaluate the maintenance of safe practice.

More elderly patients

The number of elderly patients undergoing day surgery increases. A positive result of this trend is that avoidance of hospitalization and change in environment reduces the risk of postoperative cognitive impairment. However, further effort to evaluate the outcome of day surgery in the growing elderly population is warranted. Alternatively, the experience from cataract surgery in office-based or day-surgery practice is most reassuring and has gained wide acceptance as a cost-effective approach with high patient satisfaction.

Elderly patients are also, in increasing numbers, scheduled for day surgery that requires general anesthesia. The elderly are prone to have somewhat more minor perioperative cardiovascular events, the most frequent being hypertension and dysrhythmias. Hypotension and hypovolemia are relatively less frequent in this patient group compared with patients of all ages; hypotension constitutes about one-tenth of all cardiovascular events seen.[5]

Preoperative fasting routines

One important part of patient care is proper preparation with regard to intake of food and fluid in order to minimize the risk of regurgitation and aspiration in conjunction with the anesthesia.

Many countries have adopted revised *fasting guidelines* that allow patients without risk factors to eat a light meal up to 6 hours and to ingest clear fluids up to 2 hours prior to the induction of anesthesia.[6] The safety of a more liberal fasting regime in patients without obvious risk factors for delayed gastric emptying receives support from a recent Cochrane systematic meta-analysis review.[7] The acceptable safety of intake of clear fluid up to 2 hours prior to surgery has also been shown in obese patients and in children.[8–10]

Avoiding prolonged fasting and fluid restriction has beneficial effects on patient satisfaction, and may also have positive effects on outcome, reduced fatigue, postoperative nausea and vomiting (PONV), and glucose intolerance.[11]

Adherence to the new more physiological fasting guidelines is not yet well adopted. For simplicity, it may be easier to inform a patient not to take food or fluids after midnight.

Elective day-case surgery should allow proper planning and timing and, thus, information about intake of clear fluids up to 2–3 hours prior to anesthesia should be promoted in patients without risk factors. Shortening the preoperative fasting and promoting intake of clear liquid for up to 2 hours prior to anesthesia is today considered to be well established and evidence-based.

The authors' conclusion in the Cochrane meta-analysis is clear; there was no evidence to suggest that a shortened fluid fast results in an increased risk of aspiration, regurgitation, or related morbidity compared with the standard "nil by mouth from midnight" fasting policy. Permitting patients to drink water preoperatively resulted in significantly smaller gastric volumes.

Clinicians should be encouraged to appraise this evidence for themselves and, when necessary, adjust any remaining standard fasting policies (nil-by-mouth from midnight) for patients who are not considered "at risk" during anesthesia.[7]

Preoperative nutrition: correction of deficits

Correction of malnutrition and specific nutritional or vitamin deficits should always be assessed before elective surgery and, as far as possible, substituted. The typical day-surgery patients are rarely those exhibiting a more extensive degree of malnourishment but, if present, it should be handled in accordance with general nutritional routines.

Preoperative testing of the clinically healthy patient has been questioned in recent years.[12] Patients showing signs or symptoms of being malnourished should be identified and possibly supported in order to restore proper nutritional status before surgery. Likewise, in patients with severe obesity, proper preoperative diet preparations have become standard care in most bariatric centers. Fluid deficits, low plasma/blood volume, and/or a low hematocrit should be evaluated and corrected whenever there are any signs, symptoms, or history raising suspicion about its occurrence.

Preoperative nutrition: "energy loading"

There are reports from studies evaluating the effects of preoperative nutritive fluid intake suggesting potential benefits without risk.[13] An increasing amount of evidence indicates that instead of being operated on in the traditional overnight fasted state, undergoing surgery in the carbohydrate-fed state has many clinical benefits. Many of these clinical effects can be related to the reduced postoperative insulin resistance by preoperative carbohydrate loading.

In many centers, preoperative carbohydrates have become established for use before major surgery. Those who advocate preoperative energy support suggest that carbohydrate loading should be considered for all patients who are scheduled for elective surgery and are allowed to drink clear fluid.[14] The value of such efforts in minor intermediate elective day surgery in ASA 1–2 patients may be debated.

Perioperative fluid therapy: anesthetic considerations

Perioperative fluid therapy in day surgery should be instituted on the basis of the case profile.

The benefit of fluid therapy can be questioned in minor surgical procedures of short duration (less than 15–20 min) and without any substantial fluid losses during the procedure.

Fluid therapy is more clearly beneficial in intermediate surgery, and administration of more liberal volumes probably leads to better recovery compared with lower volumes. Study design, fluid administered, and variables used for evaluation of effects vary between studies, and thus it is hard to provide clear, explicit guidelines (Table 20.1). The administered fluid has, in most studies, consisted of crystalloid fluid solutions such as lactated Ringer's solution.

Administration of about 1 liter of isotonic electrolyte solution to compensate for the fasting, and a

further 1 liter during surgery seems to improve the postoperative course of laparoscopic cholecystectomy. The group of Holte et al. has conducted several studies of the effects of perioperative fluid on outcome. They showed that administration of 30–40 ml/kg compared with 10–15 ml/kg lactated Ringer's solution for laparoscopic cholecystectomy improves recovery of organ functions and reduces hospital stay.[15] In contrast, a benefit from using a liberal fluid regime during thyroid surgery was not supported in a study of similar design.[16]

Administration of crystalloids i.v. has been shown to influence the occurrence of PONV. Apfel et al. found in a quantitative review that a more liberal use of crystalloid infusion reduced nausea and need for rescue antiemetics, supporting a liberal approach in day-case patients without history of cardiac disease.[17]

The effects of high volume (30–40 ml/kg) perioperatively should also be put into perspective. Infusion of 40 ml/kg of lactated Ringer's solution in volunteers with a mean age of 63 years decreased pulmonary function for 8 hours and also resulted in a significant weight gain that lasted for 24 hours [18]. Therefore, a more restricted fluid therapy should be adopted in the elderly. The risk of reduced lung function and edema must be acknowledged in the elderly, and fluid volume be adjusted accordingly.

Large volumes of crystalloid and colloid fluid have been compared in one study showing no difference in outcome with regard to the variables studied.[19]

The independent effect of adding glucose to the infused fluid has been studied by McCaul et al.[20] They could see no major benefit in adding glucose, which rather increased thirst and the incidence of pain besides elevating the blood glucose concentration.

The expansion of day-case surgery is moving rapidly, and there are reports of successful bariatric surgery performed on an ambulatory basis. Some institutions perform transurethral prostatectomy in day-case practice. The fluid management for these special procedures is addressed in other chapters. Procedure-specific fluid protocols should be used regardless of whether the patient is operated on in ambulatory practice or as an in-patient.

Postoperative fluids

The potential benefit in adding dextrose to the i.v. fluid during the early postoperative phase has been assessed, but the benefit, if any, seems minor.[21,22]

Table 20.1 Clinical trials of fluid therapy in intermediate-sized day surgery

Reference	Surgery	Active	Control	Fluid	No. of patients	Results
Yogendran et al. 1995 [29]	Ambulatory surgery	20 ml/kg	2 ml/kg	Isotonic electrolyte solution	2 × 100	Significant positive thirst, drowsiness, and dizziness
Elhakim et al. 1998 [30]	Termination of pregnancy	1,000 ml	0	Sodium lactate	2 × 50	Significant positive PONV
Bennett et al. 1999 [31]	Dental surgery	17 ml/kg	2 ml/kg	Isotonic solution	2 × 77	Significant positive feelings of well-being
McCaul et al. 2003 [20]	Gynecological laparoscopy	1.5 ml/kg ± glucose		Sodium lactate ± glucose	3 × 40	Glucose; higher blood glucose and more thirst
Ali et al. 2003 [32]	Laparoscopic cholecystectomy/ gynecological surgery	15 ml/kg	2 ml/kg	Hartmann's solution	2 × 40	Significant positive PONV
Holte et al. 2004 [15]	Laparoscopic cholecystectomy	40 ml/kg	15 ml/kg	Lactated Ringer's	2 × 24	Significant positive pulmonary function, dizziness, drowsiness, and fatigue
Magner et al. 2004 [33]	Gynecological laparoscopy	30 ml/kg	10 ml/(kg h)	Sodium lactate	2 × 70	Significant positive PONV
Maharaj et al. 2005 [34]	Gynecological laparoscopy	2 ml/(kg h)	3 ml/kg	Sodium lactate	2 × 40	Significant positive PONV and pain
Chohedri et al. 2006 [35]	Ambulatory surgery	20 ml/kg	2 ml/kg	Isotonic electrolyte solution	2 × 100	Significant positive PONV and thirst
Goodarzi et al. 2006 [36]	Strabism	30 ml/(kg h)	10 ml/(kg h)	Lactated Ringer's	2 × 50	Significant positive PONV and thirst
Chaudhary et al. 2008 [19]	Open cholecystectomy	12 ml/kg	2 ml/kg	Lactated Ringer's hetastarch	2 × 30	Significant positive PONV, no diff. crystalloid vs. colloid
Dagher et al. 2009 [16]	Thyroid surgery	30 ml/kg	1 ml/kg	Sodium lactate	2 × 50	No effect
Lambert et al. 2009 [37]	Gynecological laparoscopy	1,000 ml	2 ml/kg		2 × 23	Significant positive PONV

PONV, postoperative nausea and vomiting.

Rapid recovery, which allows the patient to possibly bypass the conventional recovery room stay, is a common goal in minor day-case procedures. Rapid regain of vital function and thus capacity to drink is also part of the management of intermediate day cases. Traditional discharge criteria include drinking, although the necessity of oral intake has been questioned in later versions.[23]

Allowing and supporting patients to drink clear fluids up to 2 hours before induction of anesthesia and promoting early postoperative intake reduce the need for administration of intravenous fluids. Hence, intravenous fluids may be used only to maintain venous access, which is a prerequisite for the rapid administration of anesthetics and analgesics.

Adjunct medications with impact on fluid balance

Steroids have become increasingly popular as part of the anesthetic management for day-case surgery in order to reduce pain, emesis, and fatigue. However, the impact of 4–8 mg dexamethasone or betametasone on fluid balance is not well studied.

The potential effect of NSAIDs on renal function and subsequent risk of fluid retention should also be acknowledged. NSAIDs have become a key part of pain management in day-case surgery. Renal impairment has been described, associated to the use of ketorolac.

Outcome

Major morbidity is rarely seen in conjunction with day surgery. Several major follow-up studies have documented good safety associated to elective day surgery.[2–4] For example, a huge 60-day follow-up after day surgery study in Copenhagen revealed a very low incidence of adverse events. Wound-related complications, hematoma, and infection were the most commonly seen.[4] Minor perioperative cardiovascular events, dysrhythmia, and hypertensive episodes are not uncommon, but signs of hypovolemia are rare.[5]

Rapid return of vital functions is an important goal in day surgery. However, fatigue, dizziness, and nausea are often reported during the early postoperative period. The independent effects of preoperative and perioperative fluid administration on quality of recovery have been evaluated to some extent, while the effects of postoperative fluid therapy (parenteral or oral) are not well studied.

Fatigue can be reduced by supporting fluid intake up to 2–3 hours prior to surgery. Administration of intravenous fluid during minor surgery may not exert a major effect, but during intermediate surgery such as laparoscopic cholecystectomy a liberal fluid program has been shown to improve recovery and reduce postoperative fatigue.

Postoperative nausea and vomiting – the "little big problem" – is still a major concern in day-case anesthesia and surgery. There are beneficial effects of liberal fluid administration in reducing the risk for PONV, and the risk vs. benefit seems to be in favor of its routine use in ASA 1–2 patients.[19]

Efforts to minimize postoperative pain are of huge importance in day surgery, and all opioid-sparing techniques should be acknowledged. Some studies evaluating the effects of liberal fluid administration have shown positive effects, including a reduction of postoperative pain.

Adequate hydration is needed when NSAID analgesics are used, in order to minimize the risk of renal impairment.

The risk for postoperative urinary retention in day surgery must be acknowledged. Studies have reported incidences of about 10 percent after laparoscopic

hernia repair. In this group, age and history of prostate hyperplasia are shown to be risk factors, but length of surgery also contributes to its occurrence.[24,25] The risk related to fluid volume administered has not been assessed.

A more liberal fluid regime has been shown to facilitate recovery and discharge after laparoscopic bariatric surgery.[26] The data do not support a restrictive fluid strategy, but rather a liberal fluid strategy, in laparoscopic bariatric surgery among patients without history of myocardial disease. The low urinary output during surgery is, however, commonly seen also with more liberal fluid administration.[27]

Conclusions

Day surgery is growing in importance. More patients and procedures are being transferred from traditional in-hospital care to day surgery. A number of factors have contributed to the growth of day-case surgery; these include the development of minimally invasive techniques, and better understanding of the surgical trauma and how the surgical stress response can be reduced. Introduction of new anesthetics with rapid onset and offset of action after cessation of administration has also contributed. Better use of the multimodal approach to reduce pain and pain-associated distress is also of huge importance.

Day surgery includes minor and intermediate surgery and is not commonly associated with major perioperative fluid losses. The anesthetist should still strive to maintain normal physiology by avoiding fluid and energy depletion.

Ambulatory surgery and the enhanced recovery guidelines strongly support avoidance of prolonged preoperative fasting.[28]

Efforts to avoid fluid shifts and circulatory disturbances during the entire perioperative period improve the postoperative course. They promote rapid recovery and combat adverse effects such as fatigue, nausea, and vomiting, and may also have effects on pain, thus improving well-being and satisfaction.

References

1. Jakobsson J. *Day Case Anaesthesia*. Oxford, UK: Oxford Library Press, 2009.

2. Warner MA, Shields SE, Chute CG. Major morbidity and mortality within 1 month of ambulatory surgery and anesthesia. *JAMA* 1993; 270: 1437–41.

3. Mezei G, Chung F. Return hospital visits and hospital readmissions after ambulatory surgery. *Ann Surg* 1999; 230: 721–7.

4. Engbaek J, Bartholdy J, Hjortsø NC. Return hospital visits and morbidity within 60 days after day surgery: a retrospective study of 18,736 day surgical procedures. *Acta Anaesthesiol Scand* 2006; 50: 911–19.

5. Chung F, Mezei G, Tong D. Adverse events in ambulatory surgery. A comparison between elderly and younger patients. *Can J Anaesth* 1999; 46: 309–21.

6. Søreide E, Eriksson LI, Hirlekar G, *et al.* Pre-operative fasting guidelines: an update. *Acta Anaesthesiol Scand* 2005; 49: 1041–7.

7. Brady M, Kinn S, Stuart P. Preoperative fasting for adults to prevent perioperative complications. *Cochrane Database Syst Rev* 2003: CD004423.

8. Brady M, Kinn S, Ness V, *et al.* Preoperative fasting for preventing perioperative complications in children. *Cochrane Database Syst Rev* 2009: CD005285.

9. Maltby JR, Pytka S, Watson NC, Cowan RA, Fick GH. Drinking 300 mL of clear fluid two hours before surgery has no effect on gastric fluid volume and pH in fasting and non-fasting obese patients. *Can J Anaesth* 2004; 51: 111–15.

10. Cook-Sather SD, Gallagher PR, Kruge LE, *et al.* Overweight/obesity and gastric fluid characteristics in pediatric day surgery: implications for fasting guidelines and pulmonary aspiration risk. *Anesth Analg* 2009; 109: 727–36.

11. Meisner M, Ernhofer U, Schmidt J. Liberalisation of preoperative fasting guidelines: effects on patient comfort and clinical practicability during elective laparoscopic surgery of the lower abdomen. *Zentralbl Chir* 2008; 133: 479–85.

12. Chung F, Yuan H, Yin L, Vairavanathan S, Wong DT. Elimination of preoperative testing in ambulatory surgery. *Anesth Analg* 2009; 108: 467–75.

13. Nygren J, Soop M, Thorell A, Sree Nair K, Ljungqvist O. Preoperative oral carbohydrates and postoperative insulin resistance. *Clin Nutr* 1999; 18: 117–20.

14. Ljungqvist O. Modulating postoperative insulin resistance by preoperative carbohydrate loading. *Best Pract Res Clin Anaesthesiol* 2009; 23: 401–9.

15. Holte K, Klarskov B, Christensen DS, *et al.* Liberal versus restrictive fluid administration to improve recovery after laparoscopic cholecystectomy: a randomized, double-blind study. *Ann Surg* 2004; 240: 892–9.

16. Dagher CF, Abboud B, Richa F, *et al.* Effect of intravenous crystalloid infusion on postoperative nausea and vomiting after thyroidectomy: a prospective, randomized, controlled study. *Eur J Anaesthesiol* 2009; 26: 188–91.

17. Apfel CC, Meyer A, Orhan-Sungur M, *et al.* Supplemental intravenous crystalloids for the prevention of postoperative nausea and vomiting: quantitative review. *Br J Anaesth* 2012; 108: 893–902.

18. Holte K, Jensen P, Kehlet H. Physiologic effects of intravenous fluid administration in healthy volunteers. *Anesth Analg* 2003; 96: 1504–9.

19. Chaudhary S, Sethi AK, Motiani P, Adatia C. Pre-operative intravenous fluid therapy with crystalloids or colloids on postoperative nausea & vomiting. *Indian J Med Res* 2008; 127: 577–81.

20. McCaul C, Moran C, O'Cronin D, *et al.* Intravenous fluid loading with or without supplementary dextrose does not prevent nausea, vomiting and pain after laparoscopy. *Can J Anaesth* 2003; 50: 440–4.

21. Dabu-Bondoc S, Vadivelu N, Shimono C, *et al.* Intravenous dextrose administration reduces postoperative antiemetic rescue treatment requirements and postanesthesia care unit length of stay. *Anesth Analg* 2013; 117: 591–6.

22. Patel P, Meineke MN, Rasmussen T, *et al.* The relationship of intravenous dextrose administration during emergence from anesthesia to postoperative nausea and vomiting: a randomized controlled trial. *Anesth Analg* 2013; 117: 34–4.

23. Ead H. From Aldrete to PADSS: reviewing discharge criteria after ambulatory surgery. *J Perianesth Nurs* 2006; 21: 259–67.

24. Sivasankaran MV, Pam T, Divino CM. Incidence and risk factors for urinary retention following laparoscopic inguinal hernia repair. *Am J Surg* 2014; 207: 288–92.

25. Antonescu I, Baldini G, Watson D, *et al.* Impact of a bladder scan protocol on discharge efficiency within a care pathway for ambulatory inguinal herniorraphy. *Surg Endosc* 2013; 27: 4711–20.

26. Nossaman VE, Richardson WS 3rd, Wooldridge JB Jr, Nossaman BD. Role of intraoperative fluids on hospital length of stay in laparoscopic bariatric surgery: a retrospective study in 224 consecutive patients. *Surg Endosc* 2014; 29: 2960–9.

27. Matot I, Paskaleva R, Eid L, *et al.* Effect of the volume of fluids administered on intraoperative oliguria in laparoscopic bariatric surgery: a randomized controlled trial. *Arch Surg* 2012; 147: 228–34.

28. Nelson G, Kalogera E, Dowdy SC. Enhanced recovery pathways in gynecologic oncology. *Gynecol Oncol* 2014; 135: 586–94.

29. Yogendran S, Asokumar B, Cheng DC, Chung F. A prospective randomized double-blinded study of the effect of intravenous fluid therapy on adverse outcomes on outpatient surgery. *Anesth Analg* 1995; 80: 682–6.

30. Elhakim M, el-Sebiae S, Kaschef N, Essawi GH. Intravenous fluid and postoperative nausea and vomiting after day-case termination of pregnancy. *Acta Anaesthesiol Scand* 1998; 42: 216–19.

31. Bennett J, McDonald T, Lieblich S, Piecuch J. Perioperative rehydration in ambulatory anesthesia for dentoalveolar surgery. *Oral Surg Oral Med Oral Pathol Oral Radiol Endod* 1999; 88: 279–84.

32. Ali SZ, Taguchi A, Holtmann B, Kurz A. Effect of supplemental pre-operative fluid on postoperative nausea and vomiting. *Anaesthesia* 2003; 58: 780–4.

33. Magner JJ, McCaul C, Carton E, Gardiner J, Buggy D. Effect of intraoperative intravenous crystalloid infusion on postoperative nausea and vomiting after gynaecological laparoscopy: comparison of 30 and 10 ml/kg. *Br J Anaesth* 2004; 93: 381–5.

34. Maharaj CH, Kallam SR, Malik A, *et al.* Preoperative intravenous fluid therapy decreases postoperative nausea and pain in high risk patients. *Anesth Analg* 2005; 100: 675–82.

35. Chohedri AH, Matin M, Khosravi A. The impact of operative fluids on the prevention of postoperative anesthetic complications in ambulatory surgery – high dose vs. low dose. *Middle East J Anesthesiol* 2006; 18: 1147–56.

36. Goodarzi M, Matar MM, Shafa M, Townsend JE, Gonzalez I. A prospective randomized blinded study of the effect of intravenous fluid therapy on postoperative nausea and vomiting in children undergoing strabismus surgery. *Paediatr Anaesth* 2006; 16: 49–53.

37. Lambert KG, Wakim JH, Lambert NE. Preoperative fluid bolus and reduction of postoperative nausea and vomiting in patients undergoing laparoscopic gynecologic surgery. *AANA J* 2009; 77: 110–14.

Chapter 21

Abdominal surgery

Birgitte Brandstrup

Summary

Normal as well as pathological fluid losses should be replaced with a fluid resembling the loss in quantity and quality (electrolyte composition). Elective surgical patients can be allowed to eat until 6 hours and drink up to 2 hours before surgery without increasing the risk of fluid aspiration. Preoperative administration of sugar-containing fluids, intravenous or by mouth, improves postoperative well-being and muscle strength, and lessens the postoperative insulin resistance. It does not, however, reduce the number of patients with wound- or other complications, length of stay, or mortality. Surgery does not increase the normal fluid and electrolyte losses, but causes perspiration from the abdominal wound that approximately equals the decreased water loss from the lungs because of ventilation with moist air. It is not possible to treat a decrease in blood pressure caused by the use of epidural analgesia with fluid.

The goal of zero fluid balance (formerly called "restrictive") reduces postoperative complications and the risk of death in major abdominal surgery. The goal of zero balance in combination with a goal of near-maximum stroke volume provides equally good outcome. During outpatient surgical procedures the wellbeing of the patient is improved by giving approximately 1 liter of fluid. The role of glucose-containing fluid in this setting may be beneficial, but the evidence is sparse. "Postoperative restricted fluid therapy," allowing the patients to drink no more than 1,500 ml/day,

is not recommended. To measure the body weight is the best way to monitor the postoperative fluid balance. Fluid charts are insufficient.*

Hypovolemia may lead to postoperative complications, circulatory collapse, and death. However, fluid overload with i.v. fluid also leads to the formation of edema in all tissues but especially the tissue surrounding the anastomosis and the cardiopulmonary system, causing postoperative complications and increased risk of death.[1–10] For these reasons, it is important to give the right amount of fluid.[11]

Lately, the question in the literature has been what fluid to give and in how large an amount. The so-called "fixed volume regimens" have been questioned. Instead, fluid therapy guided by a goal has been praised, and enthusiasts have argued about which goal is the best. The different goals in mind may be hemodynamic (stroke volume or pulse pressure variation among others), biochemical (oxygen tension or lactate concentrations), or simple (zero fluid balance with no body weight increase). Most likely, however, the answer to the question is not one or the other, but rather to use a combination of them.

Perioperative intravenous fluid therapy therefore has several goals:

1. To correct preoperative fluid or electrolyte disturbances (hypovolemia, dehydration, anemia, hypokalemia, etc.);
2. To meet basal requirements;
3. To replace intraoperative and later postoperative fluid and blood losses;
4. To maintain physiological parameters within an acceptable normal range;

---

* Summary compiled by the Editor.

---

and to do it all with minimum risk for the patient in terms of side effects.

Basic fluid and electrolyte needs

Everybody has obligatory fluid and electrolyte losses (or fluid and electrolyte needs). Knowledge of these and their changes during surgery is mandatory for performing an adequate fluid therapy.

Insensible perspiration is the only loss of pure water, and is approximately 10 ml/kg per day, or 0.4 ml/kg per hour. About 2/3 of the volume comes from the skin, and 1/3 from the respiratory tract. Thus a patient on mechanical ventilation with moist air has a reduced fluid loss from the respiratory tract, and the insensible perspiration is reduced by 1/3 to 6.6 ml/kg per day or 0.275 ml/kg per hour. Increasing body temperature (fever) increases the respiratory frequency and thereby the insensible perspiration. The extra fluid lost with fever is, however, very small.

Sensible perspiration is visible sweat, consists of salt and water, and is increased by exercise and increasing environmental temperature. The loss is difficult to measure, but is small or zero for elective surgical patients. For patients with acute surgical conditions (sepsis, shock) and visible sweat it may be large.

Diuresis is approximately 1 liter per day for a healthy person with a normal body weight and normal food and fluid intake. For patients, a urinary output of 0.5–1.0 ml/kg per hour is therefore recommended. To evaluate the sufficiency of the diuresis for the individual patient, it is necessary to know the patient's osmotic load and the kidneys' ability to concentrate the urine. Healthy kidneys can concentrate the urine to maximum 900–1,200 milliosmol per liter of urine. The osmotic load consists primarily of ions and nitrogen compounds. Under maximal thirst, a healthy kidney can excrete sodium in an amount of approximately 300 mmol per liter urine. This means that if an 80 kg patient is administered 2 liters of saline 0.9% as the only fluid therapy, approximately 800 ml of the water will evaporate as insensible perspiration, leaving 1,200 ml to excrete the 308 mmol of sodium and the 308 mmol of chloride given with the infusion. This brings the kidneys very near the maximal concentration ability in a healthy person, but may exceed the kidneys' concentration ability during sickness. This is the reason that humans cannot survive by drinking sea water, and one of the reasons (together with

the surgical stress response) that intravenous infusion with normal saline causes edema formation and does not significantly increase the diuresis in surgical patients.

Edema formation in surgical patients should not be understood as overhydration (hydra = water) because something with osmotic capacity has to keep the water in the body, and that something is typically saline. Postoperative edema formation is better understood as over-salting, and giving water to help excrete the salt in combination with furosemide that promotes natriuresis will reduce the edema.

Lactated or acetated Ringer's solution has a lower chloride content, but the sodium content is 130 mmol per liter, and is not much different from that of normal saline. These fluids are still more easily excreted by the kidneys, which gives them a slightly smaller volume-expanding efficacy but also a shorter time of postoperative edema. Clinical trials have, however, so far not shown Ringer's solutions to be superior to saline in terms of clinical outcome. In addition, it is important to know that without a sufficient water intake, all colloids will form a gel in the tubuli of the kidneys and thereby impose a risk of kidney injury.

These normal fluid and electrolyte losses give the following fluid and electrolyte needs in a healthy person with a body weight of 70–80 kg:

- Potassium: 60–100 mmol.
- Sodium: 60–150 mmol (= 9 g) sodium (for the prevention of hypertension, new recommendations are as low as 33 mmol [= 2 g] sodium). It is possible to survive on a minimum of 10 mmol sodium per day.
- Glucose: 850 mmol (= 150 g) (for the basal metabolism of the brain).
- Water: 2–3 liters, or a normal fixed volume of approximately 1–1.5 ml/kg per hour.

Fluid therapy during preoperative fasting

Elective surgical patients are allowed to eat until 6 hours before surgery and to drink clear fluids until 2 hours before surgery without increasing the risk of aspiration to the lungs.[12] However, the volume of clear fluid allowed is inconsistent. In the European Society of Anaesthesiologists (ESA) guideline,[12] a maximal volume is not suggested at all, and practice varies from 500 ml to "no limit." To arrive well hydrated in the operating room, and lessen the need for intravenous fluid therapy, the patients should be encouraged to eat and drink before elective surgery.

Several trials have shown that sugar-containing fluid given preoperatively (orally or intravenously) increases well-being, reduces hunger and thirst, improves muscle strength, and decreases the postoperative insulin resistance in colorectal surgical patients.[13–15]

Intravenous glucose has been shown to reduce the postoperative insulin resistance,[14] and it is possible that ordinary lemonade or juice has the same effect. No evidence exists, however, that treatment with preoperative sugar-containing fluid has any effects on postoperative complications, length of stay, or mortality.

Intraoperative fluid therapy in major abdominal surgery

Zero-balance fluid therapy (also called restricted fluid therapy) has in several trials been shown to reduce postoperative morbidity and the risk of death following elective surgery.[1–4,6–10] However, the literature has been confusing, because some investigators have been testing "fixed volume regimens" without looking at the patient's individual fluid needs.[16]

Zero-balance fluid therapy is based on the principle that fluid lost should be replaced with a fluid that resembles the loss in quantity and quality. To ensure zero balance, it is necessary to know the patient's basal fluid and electrolyte needs, together with the magnitude of the pathological fluid losses and their electrolyte content.

Surgery does not increase the normal fluid and electrolyte losses, but results in an evaporative loss from the open abdomen, which approximately equals the reduced water loss from the lungs because the patient is ventilated with moist air (3.3 ml/kg per day or 0.14 ml/kg per hour). Moreover, the patient may have pathological blood losses or ascites.

The perspiration from the open abdomen is very small, and depends on the size of the incision and the exteriorization of the viscera.[17]

- A small incision without exteriorization of the viscera (for example open appendectomy): the evaporation is 2.1 ml/h.
- A medium incision and partial exposure of the viscera (for example open cholecystectomy): the evaporation is 8.0 ml/h.

- A large incision with totally exteriorized viscera: the evaporation is 32.2 ml/h.

This loss is reduced by 50% after 20 min,[17] and by keeping the viscera in a bowel bag of plastic the loss is reduced by approximately 87%[18].

The magnitude of the fluid loss during laparoscopic surgery is entirely unknown. It is often assumed to be small, but it may in fact be larger than the loss in open surgery because the insufflated air is dry, the entire visceral surface as well as the abdominal wall is exposed, and the air is replaced an unknown number of times during surgery.

The loss to third space

Previously it was believed that the surgical trauma resulted in a redistribution of the fluid in the body, so that a large volume of the extracellular fluid became unavailable for regeneration of lost plasma, and therefore had to be replaced with intravenous extracellular fluid. This was called a functional loss of extracellular fluid or a loss to third space. A critical review of the studies giving birth to this theory shows, however, that the concept depends on a flawed method, and that trials using newer and better methods are not finding this illogical loss.[19] The entire concept should therefore be abandoned.

Manipulation of the intestines and the surgical trauma does, however, result in cell damage that promotes the formation of minor edema. From studies of rabbits, we know that the formation of a small bowel anastomosis increases the water content in the tissue surrounding the anastomosis by 5–10%.[20] If the same occurs in humans and the tissue surrounding the anastomosis corresponds to the weight of the stoma removed by the reversal of the Hartmann's procedure (50 g [21]), the amount of fluid lost to the traumatized tissue is about 2.5–5 g, or 2.5–5 ml. If one imagines that the entire colon becomes edematous (and there is no evidence for that), the fluid lost would be approximately 150–200 ml. From these numbers it can be seen that any amount of fluid lost to traumatized tissue is very small.

However, replacing this loss with fluid increases the edema formation, which destabilizes the bowel anastomosis: if 15 ml/kg per hour is given, the water content more than doubles to 10–20%,[20] and the stability of the anastomosis decreases (the anastomosis bursts at lower pressure)[5] while the inflammation around the anastomosis increases.[3] This is supported by the findings of Rehm and co-workers,[22] who describe how fluid overload destroys the endothelial glycocalyx and causes inflammation and escape of fluid to the interstitial space.

The use of epidurals blocks the sensory as well as the sympathetic fibers in the affected area of the spinal cord, leading to a decrease in heart rate (for high blocks) and a dilatation of the vascular tree, and thus a decrease in arterial blood pressure.

Early trials showed that this drop in blood pressure could be counteracted by giving a fluid bolus of, for example, 500 ml of colloid or 1,000 ml of crystalloid. Randomized clinical trials have, however, not confirmed these results. On the contrary, they show that intravenous fluid is ineffective in the treatment of the blood pressure drop caused by epidural dilatation, and the cardiac output remains largely unchanged.[23–25]

Goal-directed fluid therapy (GDT) during anesthesia has been heavily argued for, and is recommended especially in Great Britain. Different goals have been used in these trials, and the goals that are accepted in order to call a trial "goal-directed" vary between the reviews published. The goal of "zero fluid balance" has been included in the family of goal-directed fluid therapies,[26] and is recommended for use in this chapter, but in most cases the accepted goals refer to central hemodynamic parameters. Trials testing the effect of GDT against a standard fluid regimen during abdominal surgical procedures are cited in Table 21.1.

An interesting feature is that the increase in stroke volume was achieved with a colloid solution while at the same time all the patients, regardless of the stroke volume measurements, received large amounts of crystalloid. This may have two interpretations: either the crystalloid is given as pure fluid overload and leaves the circulation almost immediately (as crystalloid fluid does when given to normovolemic persons), or crystalloid cannot raise stroke volume significantly.

Most of the trials have in common that the patient sample is small, and the trials are powered to show a difference in length of hospital stay, but also that the GDT intervention in most cases improved the outcome relative to standard fluid therapy. It is interesting that colloid including hydroxyethyl starch (Voluven) apparently has beneficial effects on outcome in elective bowel surgery, and not the side effects seen in a population of septic patients.[27] Recently the so-called

"restricted fluid therapy approach" (zero fluid balance) has been tested against GDT without the fluid overload with crystalloid (GDT on a zero balance basis) (Table 21.2).

The two regimens have shown an equally good outcome for the patients. However, all clinical randomized trials of fluid therapy in general have weaknesses. Firstly, it is very difficult to blind randomized clinical trials of fluid therapy. The fluids cause changes in the patient's body weight and in the urinary output, and if more than 20% of the extracellular fluid volume is given (≥3 liters for a 75 kg person), a visible subcutaneous edema is formed. The latter means that only trials with a fluid difference less than 3 liters between groups are possible to blind effectively.

Secondly, one has to be very careful in the choice of endpoints. Length of stay (LOS) has especial problems. The introduction of fast-track surgery has illustrated that the most important factor for LOS is expectations from patients as well as the doctors. They simply stay in hospital as long as everybody expects them to. Other important factors are traditions including the use of drains, the allowance of the patient to return to oral food, and the type of analgesia used postoperatively.

Thirdly, in all research concerning surgical patients, the many confounders are at best difficult-to-control. This is especially a problem for trials including a small number of patients. Large numbers of patients will equalize the confounders between the groups compared. For example, postoperative nausea and vomiting (PONV) is highly influenced by the fact that opiates have pronounced PONV side effects.

Intraoperative fluid therapy in outpatient surgery

The trials of different fluid volumes during outpatient and minor abdominal surgery are shown in Table 21.3.

These trials have shown that approximately 1 liter of fluid i.v. causes better postoperative well-being (less PONV) in patients undergoing outpatient surgery. This finding seems logical because patients undergoing outpatient surgery are told to fast from midnight before surgery, i.e. they have a fluid deficit of approximately 1 liter.[28]

A surprising finding was that by Holte *et al.* [29] who examined the effect of 3 liters versus 1 liter of fluid on PONV, postoperative ability to run on a treadmill, and pulmonary function measured by spirometry. The trial showed that patients receiving 3 liters had

Table 21.1 Trials of "goal-directed fluid therapy" (GDT) versus "standard therapy" in abdominal surgery

Author	Surgery	No. of patients	Blinding and intervention	Primary outcome	Intervention fluid	Preoperative fluid volume	Intraoperative fluid volume	Postoperative fluid volume	Results
Conway et al. 2002 [33]	Elective bowel surgery	57 in two groups	No blinding. Near maximal stroke volume EDM (CardiQ®)	LOS	HES 6%	Not given	Coll: 28 ml/kg (GDT) vs. 19 ml/kg Total 64 ml/kg (GDT) vs. 55 ml/kg	Not given	No differences for LOS or morbidity. Mortality: 0 (GDT) vs. 1
Gan et al. 2002 [34]	Elective general, urological or gynecological	100 in two groups	No blinding. Near maximal stroke volume, EDM (CardiQ®)	LOS	HES 6%	Not given	Coll: 847 (GDT) vs. 282 Cryst 4,405 (GDT) vs. 4375	Not given	GDT reduced LOS. No difference for morbidity. Mortality not reported
Wakeling et al. 2005 [35]	Elective colorectal resection	128 in two groups	Observer blinded. Near maximal stroke volume EDM (CardiQ®)	LOS	Haemaccel® or Gelofusine®	1,000–2,000 Hartmann's solution from midnight	Median coll: 2,000 (GDT) vs. 1,500. Cryst 3,000 both groups	Early oral intake, fluid volumes not given (i.v. or oral)	GDT reduced LOS and morbidity. Zero mortalities in 30 days, 1 (control) after 60 days
Noblett et al. 2006 [36]	Elective colorectal resection	108 in two groups	Observer blinded. Near maximal stroke volume EDM (CardiQ®)	LOS	Volplex®	Not given	Coll: 1,340 (GDT) vs. 1,209 Cryst 2,298 (GDT) vs. 2,625	Early oral intake, fluid volumes not given (i.v. or oral)	GDT reduced LOS and morbidity. Mortality: 0 (GDT) vs. 1 (control)
Lopes et al. 2007 [37]	Elective mixed GI and urological	33 in two groups	No blinding. Pulse pressure variation (PPV)	LOS	HES 6%	Not given	Coll: 2,247 (GDT) vs. 0 Cryst 2,176 (GDT) vs. 1,563	Patients transferred to ICU; fluid or other treatment not given	GDT reduced LOS and morbidity. Mortality: 2 (GDT) vs. 5 (followed until discharge)
Buettner et al. 2008 [38]	Elective general, urological or gynecological	80 in two groups	Not blinded. Stroke volume variation (PiCCOplus®)	ScvO$_2$ and serum lactate	HES 6% (Voluven®)	Not given	Coll: 1,500 (GDT) vs. 1,000. Cryst 4,500 (GDT) vs. 4,250	Not given	No difference in ScvO$_2$ or lactate Mortality: 1 patient in control group "after several weeks." "All others discharged from ICU alive"
Forget et al. 2010 [39]	Elective mixed GI surgery	82 in two groups	Observer blinded. Pleth variability index (PVI)	Whole blood lactate levels	HES 6% (Voluven®)	Not given	Coll: 890 (GDT) vs. 1,003 Cryst 1,363 (GDT) vs. 1,815	24 h postop. Col: 268 (GDT) vs. 358. Cryst: 3,107 (GDT) vs. 3,516	GDT reduced lactate levels. No difference in morbidity. Mortality: 2 (GDT) vs. 0

(cont.)

Table 21.1 (cont.)

Author	Surgery	No. of patients	Blinding and intervention	Primary outcome	Intervention fluid	Preoperative fluid volume	Intraoperative fluid volume	Postoperative fluid volume	Results
Mayer et al. 2010 [40]	Elective mixed GI surgery	60 in two groups	Observer blinded. Stroke volume variation (SVV) (FloTrac®)	LOS	Not given, just "colloid"	Not given	Coll: 1,180 (GDT) vs. 817 Cryst: 2,489 (GDT) vs. 3,153	Not given	GDT reduced LOS and morbidity. Mortality: 2 in each group
Benes et al. 2010 [41]	Elective mixed GI and vascular surgery	120 in two groups	Observer blinded. Stroke volume variation (SVV) (FloTrac®)	Postop complications	HES 6% (Voluven®)	Not given	Coll: 1,425 (GDT) vs. 1,000 Cryst: 2,321 (GDT) vs. 2,459	8 h postop: Col: 0 vs. 0 Cryst: 1,587 (GDT) vs. 1,528	GDT reduced morbidity and LOS. Mortality: 1 (GDT) vs. 2
Challand et al. 2012 [42]	Elective open or laparoscopic colorectal surgery	236 in four groups: fit vs. unfit and GDT vs. standard	Observer blinded. Near maximal stroke volume EDM (CardiQ®)	LOS	HES 6% (Voluven®)	1,273 (GDT) vs. 971 Hartmann's solution	Coll: 358 (GDT) vs. 336 Cryst: 3,479 (GDT) vs. 3,593	1. postop. day: 2,083 (GDT) vs. 2,011	GDT worsened LOS and morbidity for the fit. No difference for the unfit. Mortality 30 days: 2 vs. 2. 90 days: 5 (GDT) vs. 4
Salzwedel et al. 2013 [43]	Elective general, urological, or gynecological	160 in two groups	Patient blinded. Pulse pressure variation (PPV) and CI monitoring	Postop. complications	Not given	Not given	Coll: 774 (GDT) vs. 725 Cryst: 2,862 (GDT) vs. 2,680	24 h postop. Coll: 57 (GDT) vs. 147. Cryst: 3,204 (GDT) vs. 3,452	GDT reduced complications but not LOS. Mortality: not given

Fluid volumes are in ml.
LOS, length of stay; EDM, esophageal Doppler monitoring; CI, cardiac index; HES, hydroxyethyl starch; GI, gastrointestinal.
NOTE: One reference was excluded from the table because inclusion and exclusion criteria were unclear.[44]

Table 21.2 Trials of "goal-directed fluid therapy" (GDT) versus "restricted fluid therapy" in abdominal surgery

Author	Surgery	No. of patients	Blinding and intervention	Primary outcome	Intervention fluid	Preoperative fluid volume	Intraoperative fluid volume	Postoperative fluid volume	Results
Brandstrup et al. 2012 [45]	Elective laparoscopic or open colectomy	150 in two groups: GDT vs. "restricted"	Observer blinded. Near maximal stroke volume (EDM) (CardiQ®)	Patients with postop. complications	HES 6% (Voluven®)	2 h fasting for fluid. 500 ml saline if no fluid in 6 h	Coll: 810 (GDT) vs. 475 Total volume 1,877 (GDT) vs. 1,491 (restricted)	Oral fluid in an enhanced recovery protocol. i.v. fluid if oliguria, tachycardia, or hypotension	No difference in morbidity or LOS. Mortality: 1 in each group
Zhang et al. 2012 [46]	Elective open GI surgery	60 in three groups: 4 ml/(kg h) and GDT-Ringer's; 4 ml/(kg h) and GDT-HES; and 4 ml/(kg h) Ringer's	Observer blinded. Pulse pressure variation (PPV)	LOS	Ringer's lactate and HES 6%	Not given	Total volume: GDT-Ringer's: 2,109 vs. GDT-colloid: 1,742 vs. restricted Ringer's 1,260	1.5–2.0 ml/(kg h) crystalloid for 3 days. Oral intake not mentioned	LOS was shortest in GDT-colloid group, longest in the GDT-Ringer's group. Morbidity: no difference. Mortality: none
Srinivasa et al. 2013 [47]	Elective laparoscopic or open colectomy	85 in two groups GDT vs. "restricted"	Observer blinded. Near maximal stroke volume (EDM) (CardiQ®)	Surgical Recovery Score (SRS)	Succinylated gelatin colloid solution Gelofusine	13 patients with bowel preparation: 1,000 ml crystalloid	Coll: 591 (GDT) vs. 297 Total volume: 1,997 (GDT) vs. 1,614 (restricted)	Oral fluid in an enhanced recovery protocol. i.v. fluid if oliguria, tachycardia, or hypotension	No difference in SRS, LOS, or postoperative morbidity. Mortality: none
Phan et al. 2014 [48]	Elective colorectal surgery	100 in two groups GDT vs. "restricted"	Near maximal stroke volume (EDM) (CardiQ®)	LOS			Total volume 2,115 (GDT) vs. 1,500 (restricted)	Oral fluid in an enhanced recovery protocol	No difference in LOS or postoperative morbidity Mortality: none

LOS, length of stay; EDM, esophageal Doppler monitoring. Fluid volumes are in ml.

Table 21.3 Trials of outpatient abdominal surgery

Author	Surgery	No. of patients	Blinding	Duration of surgery	Intervention	Fast	Postop. oral fluid intake	Results
Keane & Murray 1986 [49]	Mixed outpatient surgery	212 in 2 groups	No	18 min	1,000 ml Hartmann's solution + 1,000 ml DW vs. No fluid	?	?	Fluid reduces thirst and drowsiness, and increases well-being. No effect on nausea
Spencer 1988 [50]	Minor gynecological surgery	100 in 2 groups	No	8 min	1,000 ml CSL vs. No fluid	?	?	Fluid reduces dizziness and nausea
Cook et al. 1990 [51]	Gynecological laparoscopy	75 in 3 groups	Yes	20 min	CSL 20 ml/kg vs. CSL + DW 20 ml/kg vs. No fluid	11–16 h	?	Fluid reduces dizziness and drowsiness. Hospital stay reduced in dextrose group
Yogendran et al. 1995 [52]	Mixed outpatient surgery	200 in 2 groups	Yes	28 min	Plasma-Lyte 20 ml/kg (1,215 ml) vs. Plasma-Lyte 2 ml/kg (164 ml)	8–13 h	?	Fluid reduces thirst, dizziness and drowsiness. No effect on nausea
McCaul et al. 2003 [53]	Gynecological laparoscopy	108 in 3 groups	Yes	22 min	CSL 1.5 ml/kg per fasting hour (1,115 ml) vs. CSL + DW 1.5 ml/kg per fasting hour (1,148 ml) vs. No fluid	11.5 h	?	No significant differences between the groups
Magner et al. 2004 [54]	Gynecological laparoscopy	141 in 2 groups	Yes	20 min	CSL 30 ml/kg vs. CSL 10 ml/kg	13 h	?	Fluid reduced nausea and vomiting. No effect on dizziness or thirst
Holte et al. 2004 [29]	Laparoscopic cholecystectomy	48 in 2 groups	Yes	68 min	LR 15 ml/kg (998 ml) vs. 40 ml/kg (2,928 ml)	2 h	Mean 600 ml	Fluid reduces thirst, nausea, dizziness, drowsiness; improves well-being and pulmonary function; and shortens hospital stay

DW, dextrose in water 5%; CSL, compound sodium lactose (Na:131, K:5, Ca:2, Cl:111, lactate:29 mmol/l); LR, lactated Ringer's solution.

less PONV and better exercise performance than the patients given 1 liter. This trial has, however, a problem with the doses of postoperative opiates, with smaller doses given to the patients in the group given most fluid.

Postoperative fluid therapy

Both fluid chart and body weight are needed to provide logical fluid and electrolyte therapy.[30] The fluid chart tells the type of fluid lost (the quality), and the body weight is needed for monitoring the quantity of fluid lost, i.e. the fluid balance. It is therefore necessary to measure the body weight of the patient in the morning before the operation, to ensure the recording of a fluid chart, and to continue to measure the body weight every morning postoperatively on one and the same scale.

Blood samples for control of electrolyte status (Na, K, Hb, creatinine) should be measured daily for as long as the patient does not eat a sufficient diet.

A drop in arterial pressure for any reason, including the use of epidurals or other drugs, decreases urinary output, because the glomerular filtration rate is pressure-dependent. In patients without a stenosis in the renal artery, a mean arterial pressure above 60 mmHg will be sufficient for the maintenance of glomerular filtration rate and thereby the urine production. Hypotension caused by epidurals is best treated with vasopressor substances. However, such drugs are not recommended for use in the surgical ward, and epidural hypotension is better treated with a reduction in the dose of epidural analgesia or interruption of habitual antihypertensive medication. If hypovolemia is suspected, a fluid bolus may be given and the effect observed.

A few trials have been performed to examine the effect of postoperative fluid restriction on colorectal surgical patients.[31,32] The results have not been consistent, probably in part because the trials have not been combined with zero-balance fluid therapy intraoperatively. It is not physiological to withhold water from thirsty patients, especially not if they have received large amounts of sodium and chloride during surgery.

It is recommended that patients are allowed to drink and eat freely postoperatively, and intravenous fluid therapy is indicated if the oral intake is insufficient, if the patient has paralytic ileus, or if a complication has occurred.

References

1. Brandstrup B, Tønnesen H, Beier-Holgersen R, *et al.* Effects of intravenous fluid restriction on postoperative complications: comparison of two perioperative fluid regimens. A randomized assessor blinded multicenter trial. *Ann Surg* 2003; 238: 641–8.

2. de Aguilar-Nascimento JE, Diniz BN, do Carmo AV, Silveira EA, Silva RM. Clinical benefits after the implementation of a protocol of restricted perioperative intravenous crystalloid fluids in major abdominal operations. *World J Surg* 2009; 33: 925–30.

3. Kulemann B, Timme S, Seifert G, *et al.* Intraoperative crystalloid overload leads to substantial inflammatory infiltration of intestinal anastomosis – a histomorphological analysis. *Surgery* 2013; 154: 596–603.

4. Lobo DN, Bostock KA, Neal KR, *et al.* Effect of salt and water balance on recovery of gastrointestinal function after elective colonic resection: a randomised controlled trial. *Lancet* 2002; 359: 1812–18.

5. Marjanovic G, Villain C, Juettner E, *et al.* Impact of different crystalloid volume fluid regimens on intestinal anastomotic stability. *Ann Surg* 2009; 249: 181–5.

6. McArdle GT, McAuley DF, McKinley A, *et al.* Preliminary results of a prospective randomized trial of restrictive versus standard fluid regime in elective open abdominal aortic aneurysm repair. *Ann Surg* 2009; 250: 28–34.

7. Neal JM, Wilcox RT, Allen HW, Low DE. Near-total esophagectomy: the influence of standardized multimodal management and intraoperative fluid restriction. *Reg Anesth Pain Med* 2003; 28: 328–334.

8. Nisanevich V, Felsenstein I, Almogy G, *et al.* Effect of intraoperative fluid management on outcome after intra-abdominal surgery. *Anesthesiology* 2005; 103: 25–32.

9. The National Heart, Lung, and Blood Institute Acute Respiratory Distress Syndrome (ARDS) Clinical Trials Network. Comparison of two fluid-management strategies in acute lung injury. *N Engl J Med* 2006; 354: 2564–75.

10. Wuethrich PY, Burchard FC, Thalmann GN, Stueber F, Studer UE. Restrictive deferred hydration combined with preemptive norepinephrine infusion during radical cystectomy reduces postoperative complications and hospitalization time: a randomized clinical trial. *Anesthesiology* 2014; 120: 365–77.

11. Varadhan KK, Lobo DN. A meta-analysis of randomised controlled trials of intravenous fluid therapy in major elective open abdominal surgery:

getting the balance right. *Proc Nutr Soc* 2010; 69: 488–98.

12. Preoperative faste for vokse of barn; retningslinie fra European Society of Anaesthesiology. www.dasaim.dk May 23, 2014.

13. Henriksen MG. Effects of preoperative oral carbohydrates and peptides on postoperative endocrine response, mobilization, nutrition and muscle function in abdominal surgery. *Acta Anaesthesiol Scand* 2003; 47: 191–9.

14. Ljungqvist O, Thorell A, Gutniak M, *et al.* Glucose infusion instead of preoperative fasting reduces postoperative insulin resistance. *J Am Coll Surg* 1994; 178: 329–36.

15. Nygren J, Soop M, Thorell A, Sree Nair K, Ljungqvist O. Preoperative oral carbohydrates and postoperative insulin resistance. *Clin Nutr* 1999; 18: 117–20.

16. Holte K, Foss NB, Andersen J, *et al.* Liberal versus restrictive fluid management in fast-track colonic surgery: a randomized, double-blind study. *Br J Anaesth* 2007; 99: 500–8.

17. Lamke LO, Nielsson GE, Reithner HL. Water loss by evaporation from the abdominal cavity during surgery. *Acta Chir Scand* 1977; 143: 279–84.

18. Roe CF. Effect of bowel exposure on body temperature during surgical operations. *Am J Surg* 1971; 122: 13–15.

19. Brandstrup B, Svendsen C, Engquist A. Hemorrhage and operation cause a contraction of the extracellular space needing replacement – evidence and implications? A systematic review. *Surgery* 2006; 139: 419–32.

20. Chan STF, Kapadia CR, Johnson AW, Radcliffe AG, Dudley HAF. Extracellular fluid volume expansion and third space sequestration at the site of small bowel anastomoses. *Br J Surg* 1983; 70: 36–9.

21. Brandstrup B. Restricted intravenous fluid therapy in colorectal surgery, results of a clinical randomised multi centre trial. 2003. Unpublished thesis/dissertation, University of Copenhagen.

22. Jacob M, Chappel D, Rehm M. The third space – fact or fiction? *Best Prac Res Clin Anaesthesiol* 2009; 23: 145–57.

23. Kinsella SM, Pirlet M, Mills MS, Tuckey JP, Thomas TA. Randomized study of intravenous fluid preload before epidural analgesia during labour. *Br J Anaesth* 2000; 85: 311–13.

24. Kubli M, Shennan AH, Seed PT, O'Sullivan G. A randomised controlled trial of fluid pre-loading before low dose epidural analgesia for labour. *Int J Obstet Anesth* 2003; 12: 256–60.

25. Nishimura N, Kajimoto Y, Kabe T, Sakamoto A. The effect of volume loading during epidural analgesia. *Resuscitation* 1985; 13: 31–9.

26. Navarro LH, Bloomstone JA, Auler JO Jr, *et al.* Perioperative fluid therapy: a statement from the international Fluid Optimization Group. *Perioper Med (Lond)* 2015; 4: 1–20.

27. Perner A, Haase N, Guttormsen AB, *et al.* Hydroxyethyl starch 130/0.42 versus Ringer's acetate in severe sepsis. *N Engl J Med* 2012; 367: 124–34.

28. Gan TJ, Mythen MG, Glass PS. Intraoperative gut hypoperfusion may be a risk factor for postoperative nausea and vomiting. *Br J Anaesth* 1997; 78: 476.

29. Holte K, Klarskov B, Christensen DS, *et al.* Liberal versus restrictive fluid administration to improve recovery after laparoscopic cholecystectomy. A randomized, double-blind study. *Ann Surg* 2004; 240: 892–9.

30. Tulstrup J, Brandstrup B. Clinical assessment of fluid balance is incomplete for colorectal surgical patients. *Scand J Surg* 2015; 104: 161–8.

31. Vermeulen H, Hofland J, Legemate DA, Ubbink DT. Intravenous fluid restriction after major abdominal surgery: a randomized blinded clinical trial. *Trials* 2009; 7: 10–50.

32. MacCay G, Fearon K, McConnachie A, *et al.* Randomized clinical trial of the effect of postoperative intravenous fluid restriction on recovery after elective colorectal surgery. *Br J Surg* 2006; 93: 1469–74.

33. Conway DH, Mayall R, Abdul-Latif MS, Gilligan S, Tackaberry C. Randomised controlled trial investigating the influence of intravenous fluid titration using oesophageal Doppler monitoring during bowel surgery. *Anaesthesia* 2002; 57: 845–9.

34. Gan TJ, Soppitt A, Maroof M, *et al.* Goal-directed intraoperative fluid administration reduces length of hospital stay after major surgery. *Anesthesiology* 2002; 97: 820–6.

35. Wakeling HG, McFall MR, Jenkins CS, *et al.* Intraoperative oesophageal Doppler guided fluid management shortens postoperative hospital stay after major bowel surgery. *Br J Anaesth* 2005; 95: 634–42.

36. Noblett SE, Snowden CP, Shenton BK, Horgan AF. Randomized clinical trial assessing the effect of Doppler-optimized fluid management on outcome after elective colorectal resection. *Br J Surg* 2006; 93: 1069–76.

37. Lopes MR, Oliveira MA, Pereira VO, *et al.* Goal-directed fluid management based on pulse pressure variation monitoring during high-risk

surgery: a pilot randomized controlled trial. *Crit Care* 2007; 11: R100.

38. Buettner M, Schummer W, Huettemann E, *et al.* Influence of systolic-pressure-variation-guided intraoperative fluid management on organ function and oxygen transport. *Br J Anaesth* 2008; 101: 194–9.

39. Forget P, Lois F, de Kock M. Goal-directed fluid management based on the pulse oximeter-derived pleth variability index reduces lactate levels and improves fluid management. *Anesth Analg* 2010; 111: 910–14.

40. Mayer J, Boldt J, Mengistu AM, Röhm KD, Suttner S. Goal-directed intraoperative therapy based on autocalibrated arterial pressure waveform analysis reduces hospital stay in high-risk surgical patients: a randomized, controlled trial. *Crit Care* 2010; 14: 1–9.

41. Benes J, Chytra I, Altmann P, *et al.* Intraoperative fluid optimization using stroke volume variation in high risk surgical patients: results of prospective randomized study. *Crit Care* 2010; 14: 1–15.

42. Challand C, Struthers R, Sneyd JR, *et al.* Randomized controlled trial of intraoperative goal-directed fluid therapy in aerobically fit and unfit patients having major colorectal surgery. *Br J Anaesth* 2012; 108: 53–62.

43. Salzwedel C, Puig J, Carstens A, *et al.* Perioperative goal-directed hemodynamic therapy based on radial arterial pulse pressure variation and continous cardiac index trending reduces postoperative complications: a multi-center, prospective, randomized study. *Crit Care* 2013; 17: 1–11.

44. Zheng H, Guo H, Ye J, Chen L, Ma H. Goal-directed fluid therapy in gastrointestinal surgery in older coronary heart disease patients: randomized trial. *World J Surg* 2013; 37: 2820–9.

45. Brandstrup B, Svendsen PE, Rasmussen M, *et al.* Which goal for fluid therapy during colorectal surgery is followed by the best outcome: near maximal stroke volume or zero fluid balance? A clinical randomized

double blinded multi centre trial. *Eur J Anaesth* 2010; 27: 4.

46. Zhang J, Qiao H, He Z, *et al.* Intraoperative fluid management in open gastrointestinal surgery: goal-directed versus restrictive. *Clinics* 2012; 67: 1149–55.

47. Srinivasa S, Taylor MH, Singh PP, *et al.* Randomized clinical trial of goal-directed fluid therapy within an enhanced recovery protocol for elective colectomy. *Br J Surg* 2013; 100: 66–74.

48. Phan TD, D'Sousa B, Rattray MJ, Johnston MJ, Cowie BS. A randomised controlled trial of fluid restriction compared to oesophageal Doppler-guided goal-directed fluid therapy in elective major colorectal surgery within an Enhanced Recovery After Surgery program. *Anaesth Intensive Care* 2014; 42: 752–60.

49. Keane PW, Murray PF. Intravenous fluids in minor surgery. Their effect on recovery from anaesthesia. *Anaesthesia* 1986; 41: 635–7.

50. Spencer EM. Intravenous fluids in minor gynaecological surgery. Their effect on postoperative morbidity. *Anaesthesia* 1988; 43: 1050–1.

51. Cook R, Anderson S, Riseborough M, Blogg CE. Intravenous fluid load and recovery. A double-blind comparison in gynaecological patients who had day-case laparoscopy. *Anaesthesia* 1990; 45: 826–30.

52. Yogendran S, Asokumar B, Cheng DC, Chung F. A prospective randomized double-blinded study of the effect of intravenous fluid therapy on adverse outcomes on outpatient surgery. *Anesth Analg* 1995; 80: 682–6.

53. McCaul C, Moran C, O'Cronin D, *et al.* Intravenous fluid loading with or without supplementary dextrose does not prevent nausea, vomiting and pain after laparoscopy. *Can J Anaesth* 2003; 5: 440–4.

54. Magner JJ, McCaul C, Carton E, Gardiner J, Buggy D. Effect of intraoperative intravenous crystalloid infusion on postoperative nausea and vomiting after gynaecological laparoscopy: comparison of 30 and 10 ml/kg. *Br J Anaesth* 2004; 93: 381–5.

Chapter 22

Cardiac surgery

Saqib H. Qureshi and Giovanni Mariscalco

Summary

Cardiac surgical patients have altered vascular and immunological factors that dictate short- and long-term clinical outcomes. So far, the evidence does not favor any single choice of fluid therapy. In fact, volume replacement is a determinant of "filling pressures" in isolation but requires a critical balance with other determinants of tissue-oxygen debt such as vasomotor tone, fluid responsiveness, and cardiac contractility. Lastly, none of the available fluid therapies have been assessed for their comparative endothelial homeostatic potential. This leaves a significant knowledge gap and an incentive for researchers, clinicians, and industry to design and test safer and more efficacious choices for clinical use.

Introduction

Cardiac surgical patients may receive fluid in excess of 10 liters of fluid therapy during the intraoperative and postoperative course. Such volume overload leads to peripheral edema, which is worsened by the alteration of capillary endothelial function that occurs during cardiopulmonary bypass (CPB).[1–5] This alteration might lead to depletion of intravascular volume and to organ dysfunction such as acute lung and acute kidney injury (AKI), thus increasing the length of stay in the intensive care unit (ICU) or hospital, with increased hospital healthcare costs. The choice of fluid therapy, the context in which it is indicated, and the target responses are often vague; hence the outcomes remain unpredictable in clinical practice.[1–5]

In this chapter we discuss why the debate is ongoing over whether colloids or crystalloids are superior, and how the evidence should be interpreted. We consider why we not only need novel fluids for intravascular resuscitation targeted for this population but also need better designed randomized controlled trials to assess the safety and efficacy of existing choices such as hydroxyethyl starch (HES), dextrans, and gelatin, and balanced or unbalanced crystalloids.

Cardiac surgery and vascular endothelial alterations

Perioperative factors – such as hypothermia, CPB-led cytokine storm, ischemia reperfusion and generation of reactive oxygen species, myocardial depression-led alterations in renin–angiotensin responses, or atrial natriuretic peptide (ANP) release from atrial tissue – can all affect vascular barrier function and in particular the integrity of the endothelial glycocalyx.[6–8] Surgical trauma has also been implicated in shedding of the glycocalyx in humans. Rehm *et al.* [8] showed an increase of the main components of the glycocalyx, syndecan-1 and heparan sulfate, in the plasma of vascular surgical patients with global or regional ischemia. The intraoperative damage was proportional to the duration of ischemia. Bruegger *et al.* [7] described increase levels of syndecan-1 and heparan sulfate in the arterial blood of patients undergoing coronary artery bypass surgery. In both investigations, shedding of the glycocalyx occurred concomitant with reperfusion.[7,8] It is important to realize that glycocalyx shedding has been demonstrated in patients undergoing both on-pump and off-pump coronary artery bypass grafting.[9] ANP, along with IL-8, IL-6, and IL-10, has been implicated.[10]

In addition, plasma-circulating enzymes play an important role in glycocalyx shedding. Human heparanase (HPSE-1) degrades heparan sulfate and glycosaminoglycans, and over-expression of HPSE-1 in transgenic mice leads to early proteinuria and renal failure.

Fluid therapy and effect on endothelial glycocalyx layer (EGL)

Rapid crystalloid infusion has been shown to cause a large increase in plasma hyaluronic acid, presumably by cleaving this essential polysaccharide from the endothelial glycocalyx.[11] Increased right atrial pressure resulting from large volume resuscitation as well as right atrial cannulation during cardiac surgery increases the release of natriuretic peptide.[12] Natriuretic peptides cleave off glycocalyx components (syndecan-1, hyaluronic acid, and heparan sulfate) into the circulation, compounding endothelial injury.[7] Owing to capillary leak, less than 5% of infused crystalloid remains intravascular within 3 hours after infusion.[13] The increased tissue edema compounds pre-existing myocardial dysfunction.[14]

Revised Starling equation and glycocalyx model paradigm: implications for fluid therapy

The traditional views of Ernest Starling's observations that capillaries were semipermeable membranes have essentially been re-written as our understanding of the role of the glycocalyx has increased.[15,16] The key objective behind infusion of colloids is to maintain and boost intravascular colloid osmotic pressure (COP) to prevent filtration and ensuing peripheral edema. However, the revised Starling equation and the glycocalyx model paradigm suggest that filtration in systemic capillaries is regulated not by COP difference between capillary and interstitial fluid, but rather by the COP difference between capillary and sub-glycocalyx space ($\pi c - \pi g$). The latter COP is zero, resulting in a much higher difference than for the original Starling hypothesis (Figure 22.1). Because of this, a "no-reabsorption rule" applies, suggesting that even with low mean capillary pressures, filtration of fluid to the interstitim will continue.[15] Resuscitation with colloids will oppose but will not reverse absorption. In addition, patients with sepsis lose their glycocalyx layer; hence the advantage affiliated with colloids of creating higher COP is lost, and with that, any superiority over crystalloids.

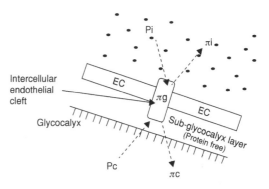

Classical Starling principle: Filtration Force = $(Pc - Pi) - \sigma(\pi p - \pi i)$
Revised Starling principle: Filtration Force = $(Pc - Pi) - \sigma(\pi p - \pi g)$

Figure 22.1 Two-dimensional glycocalyx–cleft model of capillary fluid exchange: the sub-glycocalyx space is protected and is protein free, forming the basis for the "no-reabsorption rule." The glycocalyx–cleft model identifies glycocalyx as a semipermeable layer. Its underside is subjected to the colloid osmotic pressure of fluid high inside the intercellular cleft rather than interstitial fluid (ISF), with important functional consequences. Pc, plasma capillary hydrostatic pressure; Pi, interstitial hydrostatic pressure; πc, oncotic pressure of plasma; πi, oncotic pressure of interstitial fluid; πg, oncotic pressure of intercellular endothelial cleft; EC, endothelial cell. Derived and modified from Ref. [16].

Types of resuscitation fluids

Colloids

Human albumin solutions

In healthy humans, albumin contributes 80% of the plasma oncotic pressure (25 mmHg) whereas in critically ill patients there is considerable reduction (to approx. 19 mmHg) and associated poor outcomes.[17] Albumin is involved in transport and metabolism of bile acids, eicosanoids, copper, zinc, folate and aquacobalamin, and drugs. Albumin imparts half of the normal anion gap, has significant antioxidant properties, and maintains vascular nitric oxide (NO) levels via stable S-nitrosothiol. Human albumin solutions (HAS) are produced by fractionation of blood and then heat treated to prevent transmission of viruses. The Saline versus Albumin Fluid Evaluation study (SAFE trial), on 6,997 patients randomized to either albumin or saline, concluded that albumin was not superior to saline when analyzed for 28-day mortality (relative risk, 0.99: 95% confidence interval, 0.91–1.09, $p = 0.870$).[18] Since then, follow-on trials such as FEAST study and ALBIOS have not shown any superiority of human albumin over crystalloids.[19,20]

Table 22.1 Pharmacological properties of different HES preparations. Molar substitution and the C2/C6 (i.e. quotient of the numbers of glucose residues hydroxyethylated at positions 2 and 6, respectively) dictate the kinetics of degradation: a higher C2/C6 substitution protects from hydrolysis, thus increasing plasma half-life and potential toxicity

Preparation[a]	Concentration	Trade name	MMW (kDa)	Specification range (kDa)	Top fraction[b] (kDa)	Bottom fraction[c] (kDa)	MS	C2/C6 ratio	In vitro COP (mmHg)	Initial volume effect	T½ alpha (h)	T½ beta (h)	Clearance (ml/min)
Hetastarch													
HES 450/0.7	6%	Plasmasteril, Hespan	450	150	2,170	19	0.7	4–5	26	100	n/a	300	n/a
HES 670/0.7	6%	Hextend	670	175	2,500	20	0.75	4	n/a	100	6.3	46.4	0.98
Hexastarch													
HES 200/0.62	6%	Elohes	200	25	900	15	0.62	9	25	110	5.08	69.7	1.23
Pentastarch													
HES 70/0.5	6%	Rheohes, Expafusin	70	10	180	7	0.5	3	30	90	n/a	n/a	n/a
HES 200/0.5	10%	HAES-steril, Hemohes	200	50	780	13	0.5	4–5	50–60	145	3.35	30.6	9.24
HES200/0.5	6%	HAES-steril, Hemohes	200	50	780	13	0.5	4–5	30–35	100	n/a	n/a	n/a
HES 200/0.5	3%	HAES-steril, Hemohes	200	50	780	13	0.5	4–5	15–18	60	n/a	n/a	n/a
Tetrastarch (waxy-maize-derived)													
HES 130/0.4	10%	Voluven	130	20	380	15	0.4	9	70–80	200	1.54	12.8	26
HES 130/0.4	6%	Voluven, Volulyte	130	20	380	15	0.4	9	36	100	1.39	12.1	31.4
Tetrastarch (potato-derived)													
HES 130/0.42	10%	Tetraspan	130	15	n/a	n/a	0.42	6	60	150	n/a	n/a	n/a
HES 130/0.42	6%	Venofundin, Tetraspan, VitaHES	130	15	n/a	n/a	0.42	6	36	100	n/a	12	19

Derived and modified from Ertmer et al. [24].

[a] Data extracted from manufacturer's product information.

[b] Bottom fraction: <10% of molecules are less than the molecular weight defined by bottom fraction.

[c] Top fraction: <10% of molecules exceed the molecular weight defined by bottom fraction.

COP, colloid osmotic pressure; MMW, molecular weight; MS, molar substitution; n/a, not applicable or not available; T½ alpha, distribution half-life; T½ beta, elimination half-life.

Semisynthetic colloids

Hydroxyethyl starches (HES)

The high cost of human albumin dictated the development of synthetic colloids. Currently HES are the most commonly used synthetic colloids (Table 22.1). HES are produced by hydroxyl substitution of amylopectin obtained from sorghum, maize, or potatoes. A high degree of substitution on glucose molecules protects against hydrolysis by non-specific amylases in the blood, but the action increases accumulation in liver and spleen macrophages, which constitute the reticuloendothelial system, probably because the reticuloendothelial system recognizes HES as a foreign substance and stores it (in the liver, spleen, and skin).[21] HES administration causes changes in coagulation and fibrinolysis.[22] The effect on fibrinolysis is driven by reduction in alpha2-antiplasmin/plasmin interactions with simultaneous reduction in all measures of coagulation such as clotting time, maximum clot firmness, and alpha-angle; these changes are driven by platelet dysfunction and loss of coagulation factors.[22,23] Growing evidence now questions the safety of traditional and modern HES owing to an increased incidence of mortality and renal failure observed in large randomized controlled trials (RCTs). However, these trials have only focused on critically ill septic patients, and have ignored trauma or cardiac surgical populations. Currently used HESs have a reduced concentration (6%) with a molecular weight (MW) of 130 kDa and a substitution of 0.38–0.45. HES is widely used for patients undergoing anesthesia for major surgery and in patients in ICU.

The raw material from which HES is synthesized is amylopectin (starch). HES is generated by nucleophilic substitution of amylopectin to ethylene oxide in the presence of an alkaline catalyst. Residual solvents are removed by repeated ultrafiltration. HES with a molar substitution of 0.5 or 0.6 is denoted as "pentastarch" or "hexastarch," respectively. In this regard, first-generation HESs consist of heta- and hexastarches, whereas pentastarch is allocated to the second generation. The latest, third-generation HESs consist of modern tetrastarches (HES 130/0.4 and HES 130/0.42).

Gelatins

These are prepared by hydrolysis of bovine collagen. Succinylated gelatin (Gelofusine™) is produced by enzymatic alterations of the basic gelatin peptide and is presented in isotonic saline. Urea-linked gelatin (Polygeline, Haemaccel™) is produced by thermal degradation of the raw material to small peptides (12,000–15,000 Da) followed by urea cross-linking to produce polymers of around 35,000 Da that are suspended in isotonic sodium chloride with 5.1 mmol/l potassium and 6.25 mmol/l calcium.[24] Concerns have been raised about association between the use of bovine-derived gelatin (but not pharmaceutically derived), bovine spongiform encephalitis, and Creutzfeld–Jakob disease.[24]

Dextrans

These are biosynthesized from sucrose by *Leuconostoc* bacteria using the enzyme dextran sucrase. This enzyme catalyzes the alpha-1,6-glycosidic linkage of glucose monomers. Dextrans are defined by their MW, with dextran 40 and 70 having MW 40,000 and 70,000 Da, respectively. Allergic reactions (<0.35%) have been associated with dextrans.[5] Injection of a hapten, dextran 1, before administering dextran solutions has significantly reduced the incidence to <0.0015%.[25] This involves a 20 ml injection of low-MW dextran 1 (1,000 Da MW) prior to infusion of a dextran volume expander, which leads to inactivation of anti-dextran IgGs in the recipient.

Crystalloids

The most commonly used crystalloid is normal (0.9%) saline (Na concentration = 154 mmol/l). The term "normal" was coined by Dutch physiologist Hartog Jacob Hamburger, who in 1882 suggested human blood salt to be 0.9% rather than 0.6%.

Concerns have been raised that normal saline (NS) induces hyperchloremic metabolic acidosis (NaCl + $H_2O \rightarrow$ HCl+ NaOH), but the clinical consequences of this are unclear.[26] In addition, owing to concerns regarding a fluid overload condition induced by large volumes, small-volume resuscitation with hypertonic saline (3%, 5%, or 7%) has been introduced.

Hypertonic saline

In 1980, de Felippe reported almost miraculous recovery from near-fatal hemorrhagic shock in 11 patients resuscitated with hypertonic saline (HS).[27] Various concentrations of HS have been used, and these are provided in Table 22.2. The plasma volume expansion is derived from increased fluid shift ability, secondary to the hyperosmotic and hyperoncotic abilities

Table 22.2 Physico-chemical properties of various HS solutions

Solution	Osmolarity (mosmol/l)	Sodium concentration (mosmol/l)
0.9% normal saline	308	154
Ringer's lactate	275	130
1.7% saline	291	582
3% saline	1,026	513
7.2% saline/6% HAES (200/0.6)	2,464	1,232
7.5% saline	2,566	1,283
7.5% saline/6% dextran 70	2,568	1,283
10% saline	3,424	1,712
23% saline	8,008	4,004
30% saline	10,000	5,000

Derived from Strandvik.[28]

of these solutions. The plasma volume expansion is approximately 750 ml for infusion of 1 liter of HS vs. 300 ml derived from 1 liter of crystalloid. Hypertonicity leads to vasodilatation by improving endothelial cell volume, improves cardiac output, and has also shown to reduce neutrophilic activation.[28] However, HS have not improved outcomes in patients with traumatic brain injury.[29]

Physiologically "balanced" and "unbalanced" fluids

Balanced or physiological fluids contain inorganic ions (calcium, potassium, magnesium), molecular glucose, and buffer components such as lactate or bicarbonate, and have a lower chloride component to prevent hyperchloremic metabolic acidosis. There is evidence

that patients randomized to these vs. unbalanced fluids had less impaired coagulation (less effect on thromboelastography and platelet aggregation).[30] Renal function may also be better preserved.

A typical example of balanced crystalloids is Hartmann's solution/Ringer's lactate. Balanced colloids are also available as 6% HES (Hextend®, Volulyte®). Table 22.3 summarizes the advantages and disadvantages of colloids and crystalloids, while Table 22.4 details compositions of commonly used colloids and crystalloids.

Controversies surrounding randomized clinical trials comparing efficacy of colloids with crystalloids

The clinical risks and benefits of crystalloids and colloids have remained controversial for decades. On the one hand, RCTs such as CHEST indicate that modern colloids such as hydroxyethyl starch (tetrastarch 130/0.4) may promote AKI in intensive care patients, and increased risk of mortality in septic patients.[31,32] On the other hand, trials such as FIRST, BaSES, and CRISTAL suggest that the outcomes for colloids and crystalloids are similar.[31–35] Within crystalloids, a growing body of evidence debates the safety of 0.9% saline when compared with balanced crystalloids.[36,37]

Unfortunately, much of the evidence is confounded by clinical, methodological, or statistical heterogeneity. Careful scrutiny of CHEST and 6S trials by adopting a standardized method shows lack of consistency in trial design, indications for colloid use, or maximum administered dose.[38] Such key limitations are highlighted in Table 22.5. Critics have used these and other observations such as lack of robust evidence of harm

Table 22.3 Comparative overview of generic advantages and disadvantages of colloids and crystalloids

Solution	Advantages	Disadvantages
Colloids	1. Smaller infused volumes 2. Prolong increase in plasma volumes 3. Less peripheral edema 4. Endothelial protection	1. Renal dysfunction (dextran>HES>albumin) 2. Coagulopathy (older HES>tetrastarch>albumin) 3. Pulmonary edema (capillary leak syndrome) 4. Pruritus (HES, dextran>albumin) 5. Anaphylaxis (dextran>HES>albumin) 6. Greater cost (albumin>other synthetic colloids)
Crystalloids	1. Lower cost 2. Higher glomerular filtration rate 3. Interstitial fluid replacement	1. Short-term increase in intravascular volume 2. Short-term hemodynamic improvement 3. Interstitial fluid accumulation

Table 22.4 Constituents of commonly used colloids and crystalloids

Variable	Human plasma	4% albumin	10% (200/0.5) HES	6% (450/0.7) HES	6% (130/0.4) HES		6% (130/0.42) HES		4% succinylated modified fluid gelatin	3.5% urealinked gelatin	0.9% saline	Compounded sodium lactate	Balanced salt solution
Trade name		Albumex	Hemohes	Hextend	Voluven	Voluyte	Venofundin	Tetraspan	Gelofusine	Haemaccel	Normal saline	Hartmann's or Ringer's lactate	Plasma-Lyte
Colloid source		Human donor	Potato starch	Maize starch	Maize starch	Maize starch	Potato starch	Potato starch	Bovine gelatin	Bovine gelatin			
Osmolarity (mosmol/l)	291	250	308	304	308	286	308	296	274	301	308	280.6	294
Sodium[a]	135–145	148	154	143	154	137	154	140	154	145	154	131	140
Potassium[a]	4.5–5.0	-	-	3.0	-	4	-	4	-	5.1	-	5.4	5
Calcium[a]	2.2–2.6	-	-	5	-	-	-	2.5	-	6.25	-	2	-
Magnesium[a]	0.8–1	-	-	0.9	-	1.5	-	1	-	-	-	-	3
Chloride[a]	94–111	128	154	124	154	110	154	118	120	145	154	111	98
Acetate[a]	-	-	-	-	-	34	-	24	-	-	-	-	27
Lactate[a]	1–2	-	-	28	-	-	-	-	-	-	-	29	-
Malate[a]	-	-	-	-	-	-	-	5	-	-	-	-	-
Gluconate[a]	-	-	-	-	-	-	-	-	-	-	-	-	23
Bicarbonate[a]	23–37	-	-	-	-	-	-	-	-	-	-	-	-
Octanoate[a]	-	6.4	-	-	-	-	-	-	-	-	-	-	-

Derived from Myburgh et al. [31].
[a] Units of measurement are mmol/l.

Table 22.5 Characteristics and relative risks of various outcomes in RCTs evaluating HES

Trial	VISEP	6S Trial	CHEST	CRYSTMAS	CRISTAL
Number of included patients	537	804	7,000	196	2,857
Disease condition	Severe sepsis	Severe sepsis	ICU admission requiring fluid administration	Severe sepsis	Sepsis, trauma, hypovolemic shock
Starch solution	10% 200/0.5	6% 130/0.42	6% 130/0.4	6% 130/0.4	Any colloid solution
Comparator	Ringer's lactate	Ringer's acetate	Saline	Saline	Isotonic or hypertonic saline, buffered solutions
Renal replacement therapy	1.66[a]	1.35[a]	1.21[a]	1.83	0.93
90-day mortality	1.21	1.17[a]	1.06, 95% CI 0.96, 1.18, $p = 0.26$	1.20	0.92[a]
Limitations	Considerable no. of patients received higher dose than manufacturer recommendation. Study used older HES. Considerable no. of patients in control group received HES	Randomization of 52% of patients after initial stabilization with colloids. Lack of valid resuscitation endpoints or resuscitation protocols. Failure to use pre-specified treatment algorithms. 36% of patients receiving HES had pre-existing renal impairment. No hemodynamic monitoring	Inclusion of patients after initial stabilization. Lack of valid resuscitation endpoints or resuscitation protocols. Failure to use pre-specified treatment algorithms	Not powered to assess renal safety. Publication and reporting bias. 68% of patients receiving HES had pre-existing renal impairment	Trial fluid not blinded. No stratified comparison according to subgroups

Derived and modified from Ghijselings and Rex [39].
[a] These relative risks differed from 1.00 with statistical significance at the 5% level.
CI, confidence interval.

with colloids in the non-critically ill/septic population as bases for their continued support.

An additional consideration is the increased cost of colloid solutions, which has been justified until now by the suggested clinical benefits conferred. In addition, publication of RCTs showing colloid harm have resulted in rapid regulatory steps to suspend marketing authorization of these colloids, but at the same time increased the downstream risk of blanket use of crystalloids even in patients with fragile microcirculation and fluid balance, a known risk factor for increased morbidity.[14,39,40]

Safety outcomes in cardiac surgery: an up-to-date review of randomized controlled trials

In a meta-analysis conducted by our group comparing safety outcomes in patients randomized to receive colloids or crystalloids (unpublished), we failed to observe any superiority of colloids over crystalloids. Interestingly, we did not receive any safety concerns such as renal morbidity attributed to HES in this subgroup of patients. We also undertook sensitivity analyses (not shown) by sensitizing against low-volume studies (fewer than 250 patients) and low-quality studies (high risk of selection or performance bias) to look at robustness of evidence. However, these by and large did not affect the summary estimates of effect.

- **Mortality.** Seven trials comparing colloids vs. crystalloids were included. Neither benefit nor harm was seen with either intervention (odds ratio (OR) 0.74, 95% CI 0.17 to 3.32; $p = 0.70$) (Figure 22.2).

- **Acute kidney injury.** This was analyzed in four studies showing neither benefit nor harm (OR

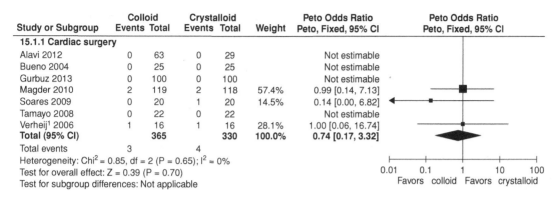

Figure 22.2 Comparison: colloid vs. crystalloid. Outcome: mortality. From Ref. [41].

Study or Subgroup	Colloid Events	Total	Crystalloid Events	Total	Weight	Peto Odds Ratio Peto, Fixed, 95% CI
15.2.1 Cardiac surgery						
Gurbuz 2013	9	100	6	100	29.5%	1.54 [0.54, 4.39]
Lee 2011	1	53	0	53	2.1%	7.39 [0.15, 372.38]
Magder 2010	19	119	18	118	66.3%	1.06 [0.52, 2.13]
Soares 2009	1	20	0	20	2.1%	7.39 [0.15, 372.38]
Total (95% CI)		**292**		**291**	**100.0%**	**1.28 [0.72, 2.26]**
Total events	30		24			

Heterogeneity: Chi^2 = 1.95, df = 3 (P = 0.58); I^2 = 0%
Test for overall effect: Z = 0.85 (P = 0.40)
Test for subgroup differences: Not applicable

Figure 22.3 Comparison: colloid vs. crystalloid. Outcome: acute kidney injury. From Ref. [41].

Study or Subgroup	Colloid Events	Total	Crystalloid Events	Total	Weight	Peto Odds Ratio Peto, Fixed, 95% CI
15.3.1 Cardiac surgery						
Lee 2011	1	53	0	53	33.4%	7.39 [0.15, 372.38]
Magder 2010	1	119	1	118	66.6%	0.99 [0.06, 15.95]
Total (95% CI)		**172**		**171**	**100.0%**	**1.94 [0.20, 18.71]**
Total events	2		1			

Heterogeneity: Chi^2 = 0.67, df = 1 (P = 0.41); I^2 = 0%
Test for overall effect: Z = 0.57 (P = 0.57)
Test for subgroup differences: Not applicable

Figure 22.4 Comparison: colloid vs. crystalloid. Outcome: renal replacement therapy. From Ref. [41].

1.28, 95% CI 0.72 to 2.26; $p = 0.40$) (Figure 22.3). No analyses could be performed after exclusion of low-volume studies owing to lack of studies remaining. Exclusion of low-quality studies had no effect on the outcome.

- **Renal replacement therapy.** This was analyzed in two studies showing neither benefit nor harm (OR 1.94, 95% CI 0.20 to 18.71; $p = 0.57$) (Figure 22.4). No analyses could be performed after exclusion of low-volume studies owing to lack of studies remaining. Exclusion of low-quality studies had no effect on the outcome.

- **Cerebrovascular accident.** An assessment on four studies was performed. No effect was observed in favor of colloids or crystalloids (OR 1.95, 95% CI 0.52 to 7.26; $p = 0.32$) (Figure 22.5).

- **ICU stay.** This was assessed in seven studies showing neither benefit nor harm (mean differences −0.04, 95% CI −0.16 to 0.08; $p = 0.54$) (Figure 22.6). No analyses could be performed after exclusion of low-volume studies owing to lack of studies remaining. Exclusion of low-quality studies had no effect on the outcome.

173

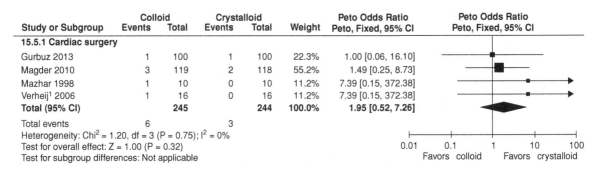

Figure 22.5 Comparison: colloid vs. crystalloid. Outcome: cerebrovascular accident. From Ref. [41].

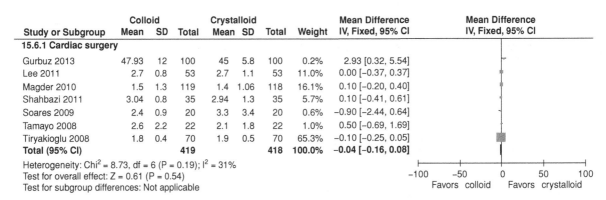

Figure 22.6 Comparison: colloid vs. crystalloid. Outcome: ICU length of stay (days). From Ref. [41].

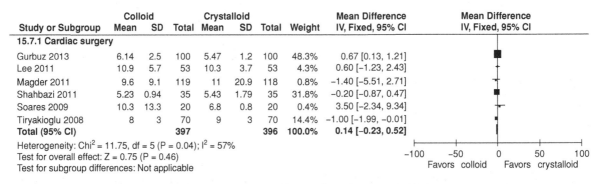

Figure 22.7 Comparison: colloid vs. crystalloid. Outcome: hospital length of stay (days). From Ref. [41].

- **Hospital stay.** This was assessed in six studies, showing non-significant effect estimate. (Mean differences 0.14, 95% CI −0.23 to 0.52; $p = 0.46$) (Figure 22.7). Significant heterogeneity was, however, observed. No analyses could be performed after exclusion of low-volume studies owing to lack of studies remaining. Exclusion of low-quality studies had no effect on the outcome.

References

1. Mariscalco G, Musumeci F. Fluid management in the cardiothoracic intensive care unit: diuresis–diuretics and hemofiltration. *Curr Opin Anaesthesiol* 2014; 27: 133–9.

2. Jakob SM, Ruokonen E, Takala J. Assessment of the adequacy of systemic and regional perfusion after cardiac surgery. *Br J Anaesth* 2000; 84: 571–7.

3. Habicher M, Perrino A, Spies CD, *et al.* Contemporary fluid management in cardiac anesthesia. *J Cardiothorac Vasc Anesth* 2011; 25: 1141–53.

4. Assaad S, Popescu W, Perrino A. Fluid management in thoracic surgery. *Curr Opin Anaesthesiol* 2013; 26: 31–9.

5. Grocott MPW, Mythen MG, Gan TJ. Perioperative fluid management and clinical outcomes. *Anesth Analg* 2005; 100: 1093–106.

6. Jacob M, Bruegger D, Rehm M, *et al.* Contrasting effects of colloid and crystalloid resuscitation fluids on cardiac vascular permeability. *Anesthesiology* 2006; 104: 1223–31.

7. Bruegger D, Jacob M, Rehm M, *et al.* Atrial natriuretic peptide induces shedding of endothelial glycocalyx in coronary vascular bed of guinea pig hearts. *Am J Physiol Heart Circ Physiol* 2005; 289: H1993–9.

8. Rehm M, Bruegger D, Christ F, *et al.* Shedding of the endothelial glycocalyx in patients undergoing major vascular surgery with global and regional ischemia. *Circulation* 2007; 116: 1896–906.

9. Bruegger D, Schwartz L, Chappell D, *et al.* Release of atrial natriuretic peptide precedes shedding of the endothelial glycocalyx equally in patients undergoing on- and off-pump coronary artery bypass surgery. *Basic Res Cardiol* 2011; 106: 1111–21.

10. Chappell D, Hofmann-Kiefer K, Jacob M, *et al.* TNF-alpha induced shedding of the endothelial glycocalyx is prevented by hydrocortisone and antithrombin. *Basic Res Cardiol* 2009; 104: 78–89.

11. Berg S, Engman A, Hesselvik JF Laurent TC. Crystalloid infusion increases plasma hyaluronan. *Crit Care Med* 1994; 22: 1563–7.

12. Ueda S, Nishio K, Akai Y, *et al.* Prognostic value of increased plasma levels of brain natriuretic peptide in patients with septic shock. *Shock* 2006; 26: 134–9.

13. Bark BP, Persson J, Grande PO. Importance of the infusion rate for the plasma expanding effect of 5% albumin, 6% HES 130/0.4, 4% gelatin, and 0.9% NaCl in the septic rat. *Crit Care Med* 2013; 41: 857–66.

14. Rehberg S, Yamamoto Y, Sousse L, *et al.* Selective V(1a) agonism attenuates vascular dysfunction and fluid accumulation in ovine severe sepsis. *Am J Physiol Heart Circ Physiol* 2012; 303: H1245–54.

15. Woodcock TE, Woodcock TM. Revised Starling equation and the glycocalyx model of transvascular fluid exchange: an improved paradigm for prescribing intravenous fluid therapy. *Br J Anaesth* 2012; 108: 384–94.

16. Levick JR, Michel CC. Microvascular fluid exchange and the revised Starling principle. *Cardiovasc Res* 2010; 87: 198–210.

17. Nicholson JP, Wolmarans MR, Park GR. The role of albumin in critical illness. *Br J Anaesth* 2000; 85: 599–610.

18. Finfer S, Bellomo R, Boyce N, *et al.* A comparison of albumin and saline for fluid resuscitation in the intensive care unit. *N Engl J Med* 2004; 350: 2247–56.

19. Maitland K, Kiguli S, Opoka RO, *et al.* Mortality after fluid bolus in African children with severe infection. *N Engl J Med* 2011; 364: 2483–95.

20. Caironi P, Tognoni G, Masson S, *et al.* Albumin replacement in patients with severe sepsis or septic shock. *N Engl J Med* 2014; 370: 1412–21.

21. van Rijen EA, Ward JJ, Little RA. Effects of colloidal resuscitation fluids on reticuloendothelial function and resistance to infection after hemorrhage. *Clin Diagn Lab Immunol* 1998; 5: 543–9.

22. Schramko A, Suojaranta-Ylinen R, Kuitunen A, *et al.* Hydroxyethylstarch and gelatin solutions impair blood coagulation after cardiac surgery: a prospective randomized trial. *Br J Anaesth* 2010; 104: 691–7.

23. Nielsen VG. Hydroxyethyl starch enhances fibrinolysis in human plasma by diminishing alpha2-antiplasmin-plasmin interactions. *Blood Coagul Fibrinolysis* 2007; 18: 647–56.

24. Ertmer C, Rehberg S, van Aken H, Westphal M. Relevance of non-albumin colloids in intensive care medicine. *Best Pract Res Clin Anaesthesiol* 2009; 23: 193–212.

25. Ljungstrom KG. Safety of dextran in relation to other colloids-ten years experience with hapten inhibition. *Infusionsther Transfusionsmed* 1993; 20: 206–10.

26. Guidet B, Soni N, Della Rocca G, *et al.* A balanced view of balanced solutions. *Crit Care* 2010; 14: 325.

27. de Felippe J, Timoner J, Velasco IT, Lopes OU, Rocha-e-Silva M. Treatment of refractory hypovolaemic shock by 7.5% sodium chloride injections. *Lancet* 1980; 2: 1002–4.

28. Strandvik GF. Hypertonic saline in critical care: a review of the literature and guidelines for use in hypotensive states and raised intracranial pressure. *Anaesthesia* 2009; 64: 990–1003.

29. Tisherman SA, Schmicker RH, Brase KJ, *et al.* Detailed description of all deaths in both the shock and traumatic brain injury hypertonic saline trials of the Resuscitation Outcomes Consortium. *Ann Surg* 2015; 261: 586–90.

30. Smorenberg A, Ince C, Groeneveld AJ. Dose and type of crystalloid fluid therapy in adult hospitalized patients. *Perioper Med (Lond)* 2013; 2: 17.

31. Myburgh JA, Finfer S, Bellomo R, *et al.* Hydroxyethyl starch or saline for fluid resuscitation in intensive care. *N Engl J Med* 2012; 367: 1901–11.

32. Perner A, Haase N, Guttormsen AB, *et al.* Hydroxyethyl starch 130/0.42 versus Ringer's acetate in severe sepsis. *N Engl J Med* 2012; 367: 124–34.

33. James MF, Michell WL, Joubert IA, *et al.* Resuscitation with hydroxyethyl starch improves renal function and lactate clearance in penetrating trauma in a randomized controlled study: the FIRST trial (Fluids in Resuscitation of Severe Trauma). *Br J Anaesth* 2011; 107: 693–702.

34. Siegemend M. BaSES trial: Basel Starch Evaluation in Sepsis. *ClinicalTrialsgov Identifier.* NCT00273728 2013.

35. Annane D, Siami S, Jaber S, *et al.* Effects of fluid resuscitation with colloids vs. crystalloids on mortality in critically ill patients presenting with hypovolemic shock: the CRISTAL randomized trial. *JAMA* 2013; 310: 1809–17.

36. O'Malley CM, Frumento RJ, Hardy MA, *et al.* A randomized, double-blind comparison of lactated Ringer's solution and 0.9% NaCl during renal transplantation. *Anesth Analg* 2005; 100: 1518–24.

37. Waters JH, Gottlieb A, Schoenwald P, *et al.* Normal saline versus lactated Ringer's solution for intraoperative fluid management in patients undergoing abdominal aortic aneurysm repair: an outcome study. *Anesth Analg* 2001; 93: 817–22.

38. Meybohm P, van Aken H, De Gasperi A, *et al.* Re-evaluating currently available data and suggestions for planning randomised controlled studies regarding the use of hydroxyethyl starch in critically ill patients – a multidisciplinary statement. *Crit Care* 2013; 17: R166.

39. Ghijselings I, Rex S. Hydroxyethyl starches in the perioperative period. A review on the efficacy and safety of starch solutions. *Acta Anaesthesiol Belg* 2014; 65: 9–22.

40. Teixeira C, Garzotto F, Piccinni P, *et al.* Fluid balance and urine volume are independent predictors of mortality in acute kidney injury. *Crit Care* 2013; 17: R14.

41. Qureshi SH, Rizvi SI, Patel NN, Murphy GJ. Meta-analysis of colloids versus crystalloids in critically ill, trauma and surgical patients. *Br J Surg* 2016; 103: 14–26. doi: 10.1002/bjs. 9943.

Chapter

23

Pediatrics

Robert Sümpelmann and Nils Dennhardt

Summary

The main aim of perioperative fluid therapy is to stabilize or normalize the child's homeostasis. Young infants have higher fluid volumes, metabolic rates, and fluid needs than adults. Therefore, short perioperative fasting periods are important to avoid iatrogenic dehydration, ketoacidosis, and misbehavior. Balanced electrolyte solutions with 1–2.5% glucose are favored for intraoperative maintenance infusion. Glucose-free balanced electrolyte solutions should then be added as needed to replace intraoperative fluid deficits or minor blood loss. Hydroxyethyl starch or gelatin solutions are useful in hemodynamically instable patients or those with major blood loss, especially when crystalloids alone are not effective or the patient is at risk of interstitial fluid overload. The monitoring should focus on the maintenance or restoration of a stable tissue perfusion. Also, in non-surgical or postoperative children, balanced electrolyte solutions should be used instead of hypotonic solutions, both with 5% glucose, as recent clinical studies and reviews showed a lower incidence of hyponatremia.

An adequate fluid therapy is essential for the perioperative stabilization of the homeostasis of children, whereas dosing errors or an inappropriate use of unphysiologically composed solutions may lead to life-threatening complications. As a consequence, it is important firstly to understand and respect the physiology of children, secondly to use suitably composed infusion solutions, and thirdly to monitor the patient carefully for close guidance of the fluid therapy. In the following, well-established strategies, based on physiology, scientific studies, and clinical experience in large pediatric centers, are presented, with safety and efficacy as first priorities.

Physiology

The total body water (TBW) consists of intracellular (ICF) and extracellular fluid (ECF), represents up to 90% of the body weight in neonates, and reaches adult levels of about 60% after one year of age. The ECF represents the main part of TBW and decreases in parallel from 40% in term neonates to adult levels of 20–25% after one year of age.[1] The composition of ECF or plasma is similar in neonates, children, and adults, but dehydration occurs more rapidly in the younger age groups because of the higher fluid need.

At birth, the kidneys are still undeveloped and the reabsorptive areas of the tubular cells are small. As a consequence, neonates cannot concentrate urine effectively or excrete large salt loads. After a month, the kidneys reach about 60% of their maturation, but the reabsorptive areas of the tubular cells are still small, and the capacity for glucose reabsorption or potassium excretion is lower than in adults. In the first 2 years, the maturity and function of the kidneys increase greatly and reach adult levels.[2]

The newborn heart has a lower density of contractile elements and therefore has less reserve than the adult heart and does not respond to stress as well. A higher percentage of non-contractile elements results in decreased ventricular compliance and less responsiveness to changes in vascular tone and preload. The cardiac output is tightly coupled with oxygen consumption, which is several times higher in neonates and infants than in adults. The stroke volume of the small hearts is limited, and therefore the high cardiac

Clinical Fluid Therapy in the Perioperative Setting, Second Edition, ed. Robert G. Hahn. Published by Cambridge University Press. © Cambridge University Press 2016.

output depends strongly on a high heart rate. Normally, the heart pumps all of the venous return (VR) it receives, and under most conditions the VR is the main determinant of cardiac output in all age groups. VR depends strongly on the intravascular volume. Underestimation of hypovolemia and bleeding are the most common causes of perioperative cardiac arrest in children.[3] Therefore, maintaining normovolemia is of paramount importance in young age groups to maintain circulatory function and to stabilize the high tissue perfusion needed.[4]

Perioperative fasting

The main aim of preoperative fasting is to minimize the volume of gastric contents to lessen the risk of vomiting and aspiration during induction of anesthesia. Many hospitalized children are suffering from prolonged fasting periods leading to dehydration, ketoacidosis, and uncooperative behavior.[5] Perioperatively, infants have a more stable acid–base balance and lower ketone bodies when the fasting periods recommended in current guidelines (clear fluids 2 hours, breast milk 4 hours, formula milk or solids 6 hours) are not exceeded for more than 2 hours.[6] Oral fluid uptake is generally preferable to intravenous fluid therapy whenever possible. A recent clinical study showed no increased incidence in pulmonary aspiration in more than 10,000 children allowed clear fluids until called to the operating suite.[7] With child-friendly shortened preoperative fasting periods, perioperative fluid therapy is then often not really necessary for very short surgical procedures (duration <1 hour). Postoperatively, a liberal fluid and food intake as wanted by the child should be favored, which leads to a better mental state without increasing the frequency of nausea and vomiting.[8]

Maintenance infusion

Maintenance fluid therapy in children should meet the normal needs of water, electrolytes, and glucose. For half a century this has been based on Holliday and Segar's recommendations, suggesting firstly the 4–2–1 rule for infusion rate and secondly the use of hypotonic fluids with 5% glucose added.[9] In recent years, many studies and case reports have shown that the routine use of such fluids may lead to serious hyponatremia and hyperglycemia, and may occasionally result in permanent neurological damage or death.[10–12] The two main factors for the development of perioperative

hyponatremia are firstly the stress-induced secretion of antidiuretic hormone leading to an impaired ability to excrete free water, and secondly the administration of hypotonic solutions as a source of free water.[13,14] Hyponatremia leads to an influx of water into the brain, primarily through glial cell swelling, initially largely preserving neuronal cell volume. This process will ultimately lead to cerebral edema, brain stem herniation, and death. Prepubescent children are a high-risk group for a poor outcome associated with hyponatremic encephalopathy because of the presence of a high ratio of brain size to cranial vault and reduced Na-K-ATPase activity compared with the adult brain.[14]

Infants are also at increased risk of perioperative lipolysis and hypoglycemia owing to a higher metabolic rate than in adults. If hypoglycemia does occur, this will induce a stress response as well as altering cerebral blood flow and metabolism.[15] Permanent neurodevelopmental impairment can result if hypoglycemia goes unrecognized and untreated. However, intraoperative administration of 5% glucose solutions for prevention of hypoglycemia will often result in hyperglycemia due to stress-induced insulin resistance.[16] Hyperglycemia may also be detrimental to the brain because of an accumulation of lactate, a decrease in intracellular pH, and subsequently compromised cellular function in the context of global or focal cerebral ischemia.[17] Lastly, the administration of glucose-free solutions increases the risk of lipolysis with the release of ketone bodies and free fatty acids.[18,19]

Against the above-mentioned background, the intraoperative maintenance infusion of isotonic balanced fluids with lower glucose concentrations (i.e. 1 to 2.5%) represents a well-accepted compromise in many European countries to avoid hyponatremia, hypoglycemia, lipolysis, and hyperglycemia in children (Table 23.1 [20–22]). A higher infusion rate than calculated by the 4–2–1 rule can be used intraoperatively to compensate pre- and postoperative fasting deficits in routine surgeries (i.e. 10–20 ml/kg per hour [23]). Infusion pumps are recommendable to prevent accidental fluid overload especially in neonates and small infants. In prolonged surgeries the maintenance infusion should be adapted, i.e. after one hour in accordance to the patient's needs.

In non-surgical or postoperative children, the current trend is also to use isotonic balanced electrolyte solutions instead of hypotonic solutions, both with

Table 23.1 Composition of extracellular fluid (ECF) and various intravenous fluids for children (in mmol/l)

	Cations				Anions					Theoretical osmolarity[a]
	Na+	K+	Ca2+	Mg2+	Cl−	HCO3−	Acetate	Lactate	Glucose	
ECF	142	4.5	2.5	1.25	103	24	−	1.5	2.78–5	291
BEL[b] + 1% glucose	140	4	2	2	118	−	30	−	55.5	296
Normal saline	154	−	−	−	154	−	−	−	−	308
RL[c]	130	5	1	1	112	−	−	27	−	276
2/3 HEG[d]	100	18	2	3	90	−	38	−	277.5	251
1/2 HEG[d]	70	2	1.25	0.5	55	−	22.5	−	277.5	151
1/3 HEG[d]	45	25	−	2.5	45	−	20	−	277.5	148

[a] Σ (cations+anions).
[b] Balanced electrolyte solution.
[c] Ringer's lactate.
[d] hypotonic electrolyte solutions with 5% glucose.

5% glucose, for maintenance infusion, as recent clinical studies and reviews have shown a lower incidence of hyponatremia and no change in hypernatremia.[24,25]

Fluid replacement therapy

Fluid replacement using crystalloid solutions aims to compensate an ECF deficit as a result of cutaneous, enteral, or renal fluid loss. Intraoperative bleeding also leads to a shift of interstitial fluid into the intravascular space (autotransfusion), and the resulting extracellular fluid deficit should be corrected by the infusion of crystalloid solutions as a first step. Theoretically, the intravascular volume effect of crystalloids depends on the ratio between the intravascular and the extracellular fluid volume (ECFV). The ECFV of neonates and infants is larger than in adults,[1] and the intravascular volume effect of crystalloids is therefore in theory lower in the younger age groups.

The composition of ECF is independent of age, and therefore similar crystalloid solutions can be used for fluid replacement in both pediatric and adult age groups. Ideally, the composition of crystalloid solutions should mimic the composition of ECF as closely as possible, and each deviation could have unwanted effects on the homeostasis of the patients. Assuming a normal plasma osmolarity between 275 and 290 mosmol/l, normal saline (NS, 308 mosmol/l) is *in vitro* slightly hypertonic and Ringer's lactate (RL, 276 mosmol/l) is isotonic. After infusion the *in vivo* osmolarity is lower because the infused electrolytes, especially sodium and chloride (osmotic coefficient 0.926), are partly absorbed on cell membranes and proteins. As a result, the *in vivo* osmolarity of NS is isotonic and that of RL is slightly hypotonic.[26]

NS contains no bicarbonate precursor and has an unphysiologically high chloride concentration. It therefore may cause unwanted bicarbonate dilution and hyperchloremic acidosis with renal vasoconstriction and impaired renal function. RL contains lactate as bicarbonate precursor but is slightly hyponatremic (130 mmol/l) and therefore may increase the intracranial pressure and may worsen cerebral edema when infused in high volumes. This can all be avoided by the use of balanced electrolyte solutions (BELs) containing a physiological osmolarity and electrolyte composition, and with metabolic anions (i.e. acetate, lactate, or malate) as bicarbonate precursors for acid–base stabilization (Table 23.1).[26–28]

Most cases with minor or moderate surgical procedures can be managed with maintenance infusion plus extra volumes of 10–20 ml/kg BEL as needed to replace ECF or blood loss. In major cases with significant blood loss and restrictive transfusion, the infusion of very high volumes of crystalloids may lead to unwanted intravascular hypovolemia and interstitial fluid overload which may worsen recovery and outcome.[29]

Volume replacement therapy

Volume replacement using colloid solutions aims to replace blood loss, and to maintain or restore hemodynamics and tissue perfusion, especially when the use of crystalloids alone is not effective and the patient is in

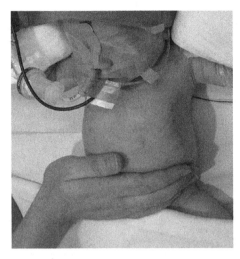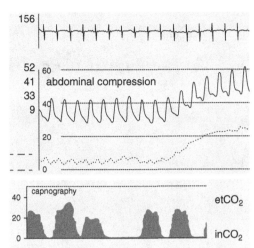

Figure 23.1 Abdominal pressure maneuver as test for fluid responsiveness in small children.

danger of interstitial fluid overload. In the past, human albumin (HA) was frequently used in children, but recently a number of gelatin and hydroxyethyl starch solutions (HES) have been shown in several clinical studies in children to be as effective and safe as HA, and less costly (review in [30]).

Gelatins have been in clinical use for more than 100 years, and studies from neonatology have shown high safety even when used in preterm infants.[31] The first generation of HES (molecular weight [MW] >450 kDa) was associated with significant adverse effects with regard to coagulation, organ function, and accumulation, but the second (MW 200 kDa) and especially the third generation of HES (MW 130 kDa) have an improved risk–benefit ratio and, therefore, the last should be the preferred HES solution for perioperative volume replacement in children (review in [32]).

Possible adverse drug reactions of artificial colloids include anaphylactoid reactions, coagulation disorders, renal function impairment, and tissue accumulation. In adults, anaphylactoid reactions occurred more frequently after gelatin than after HES, but generally the risk of severe anaphylactoid reactions seems to be lower in the younger age groups. Animal experiments and clinical studies in pediatric patients showed stable coagulation parameters after moderate doses (10–20 ml/kg) of gelatin or HES but significant impairment of clot formation after profound hemodilution of more than 50% of the estimated blood volume.[33,34]

Recent safety studies including high numbers of children with HES 130 infused perioperatively showed a very low incidence of adverse effects even in neonates, small infants, and high-risk patients undergoing cardiac surgery.[35,36] The acid–base balance was more stable when using HES in an acetate-containing BEL instead of NS. HES-related adverse effects were dose-dependent, and moderate doses of 10–20 ml/kg were very safe. High doses close to the maximum daily dose of 50 ml/kg should be used with more caution because they may lead to critical hemodilution, dilutional coagulopathy, or iatrogenic hypervolemia. HES-induced renal insufficiency could not be detected perioperatively in animals or children with normal renal function.[35–37] Iatrogenic hypervolemia may damage the endothelial surface layer (glycocalyx) of the capillaries; thus, carefully maintaining intravascular volume without hypervolemic peaks was hypothesized to be the most promising concept.[38]

Monitoring

Conscious children, especially neonates and small infants, manage to maintain blood pressure for long periods of time through vasoconstriction in the presence of larger fluid deficits even if a shock situation has already occurred. In deeply anesthetized children, however, some or all of the regulation mechanisms are suppressed so that hypotension is more likely to occur in the presence of reduced blood volume. Shallow anesthesia, on the other hand, may mask hypovolemia. As a consequence, a low normal blood pressure and a normal oxygen saturation are no guarantees of sufficient tissue perfusion. Also, the leg-raise test for evaluation of fluid responsiveness is not effective in small children because of their limited body height. Therefore, apart from standard parameters of heart rate and arterial blood pressure, other parameters need to be used to estimate a child's volume status and tissue perfusion.[39] A short manual pressure on the liver can be used to shift blood volume from intra-abdominal to intrathoracic and to analyze the consequences of the change in venous return on blood flow or expiratory carbon dioxide tension (Figure 23.1). Other possible parameters to evaluate fluid responsibility are respiratory-synchronous changes in the invasive blood pressure curve or perfusion/pleth variability index calculated by recent pulse oximeter algorithms. Stable base excess values and lactate concentrations reflect stable tissue perfusion perioperatively. Major surgical procedures should therefore be accompanied by regular blood gas analyses on induction of anesthesia and at hourly intervals thereafter for early detection of negative trends. When a central venous catheter is inserted, measurement of central venous oxygen saturation is very useful to evaluate the ratio between oxygen consumption and oxygen delivery. Other useful parameters for estimating volume status and tissue perfusion include recapillarization time or direct measurement of cardiac output or blood flow (such as echocardiography or transpulmonary thermodilution).

Clinical recommendations

The objectives of perioperative fluid therapy are to maintain a normal blood volume, normal tissue perfusion, normoglycemia, and normal water–acid–base–electrolyte balance. In line with current recommendations, children should be allowed to drink clear fluids until 2 hours before induction of anesthesia unless other considerations mandate otherwise. For preterm infants, neonates, and toddlers, it is advisable to compensate at least the deficit from preoperative fasting and the intraoperative maintenance requirements using BELs with 1–2% glucose. If such solutions are not available commercially, they can be prepared extemporaneously in the hospital pharmacy or by users themselves (i.e. by adding 6–12 ml of glucose 40% to 250 ml of i.v. fluid).[23,40] To compensate preoperative deficits (i.e. from fasting), the overall infusion rate in the first hour may be 10–20 ml/kg per hour. As blood glucose concentrations increase, glucose-containing i.v. fluids should be reduced or stopped, infusing correspondingly more glucose-free

Table 23.2 Suggested perioperative intravenous fluid therapy for neonates, infants, and toddlers

Before surgery:	Minimize fasting periods (milk up to 4 h preop, clear fluids up to 2 h preop)
Minor procedures	Intraop maintenance infusion of 10–20 ml/kg per hour of a balanced electrolyte solution with 1–2% glucose (add 6–12 ml of glucose 40% to 250 ml of balanced electrolyte solution); older toddlers and school-age children may also be given glucose-free balanced electrolyte solutions
Larger procedures	Adapt maintenance infusion to patient's need after one hour, use additional balanced electrolyte solution for fluid replacement; consider artificial colloids in case of persistent hypovolemia – the objective is to achieve normal blood volume, normal tissue perfusion, normoglycemia, and normal water–acid–base–electrolyte balance
Major procedures	Same as larger procedures; administer blood products in cases of critical hemodilution
After surgery	Permit oral fluid as soon after surgery as wanted by the children

BEL. Older toddlers and school-age children may also be given glucose-free BEL within the recommended fasting periods. In case of hemodynamic instability or bleeding, repetitive doses of BEL (single bolus dose 10–20 ml/kg) first and HES or gelatin (single bolus dose 5–10 ml/kg) thereafter may additionally be administered as required. Postoperatively, children should be allowed to take oral fluids again as wanted unless other considerations mandate otherwise (Table 23.2).

References

1. Friis-Hansen B. Body water compartments in children: changes during growth and related changes in body composition. *Pediatrics* 1961; 28: 169–81.

2. Bissonnette B. *Pediatric Anesthesia*. Shelton: People's Medical Publishing House-USA, 2011.

3. Bhananker SM, Ramamoorthy C, Geiduschek JM, *et al.* Anesthesia-related cardiac arrest in children: update from the Pediatric Perioperative Cardiac Arrest Registry. *Anesth Analg* 2007; 105: 344–50.

4. Nichols D, Ungerleider R, Spevak P. *Critical Heart Disease in Infants and Children*. Philadelphia: Mosby Elsevier, 2006.

5. Engelhardt T, Wilson G, Horne L, *et al.* Are you hungry? Are you thirsty? Fasting times in elective outpatient pediatric patients. *Paediatr Anaesth* 2011; 21: 964–8.

6. Dennhardt N, Beck C, Huber D, *et al.* Preoperative fasting times and ketone bodies in children under 36 months of age. *Eur J Anaesthesiol* 2015; 32: 857–61.

7. Andersson H, Zaren B, Frykholm P. Low incidence of pulmonary aspiration in children allowed intake of clear fluids until called to the operating suite. *Paediatr Anaesth* 2015; 25: 770–7.

8. Radke OC, Biedler A, Kolodzie K, *et al.* The effect of postoperative fasting on vomiting in children and their assessment of pain. *Paediatr Anaesth* 2009; 19: 494–9.

9. Holliday MA, Segar WE. The maintenance need for water in parenteral fluid therapy. *Pediatrics* 1957; 19: 823–32.

10. Duke T, Molyneux EM. Intravenous fluids for seriously ill children: time to reconsider. *Lancet* 2003; 362: 1320–3.

11. Moritz ML, Ayus JC. Hospital-acquired hyponatremia: why are there still deaths? *Pediatrics* 2004; 113: 1395–6.

12. Fraser CL, Arieff AI. Epidemiology, pathophysiology, and management of hyponatremic encephalopathy. *Am J Med* 1997; 102: 67–77.

13. Arieff AI. Postoperative hyponatraemic encephalopathy following elective surgery in children. *Paediatr Anaesth* 1998; 8: 1–4.

14. Ayus JC, Achinger SG, Arieff A. Brain cell volume regulation in hyponatremia: role of sex, age, vasopressin, and hypoxia. *Am J Physiol Renal Physiol* 2008; 295: F619–24.

15. Sieber FE, Traystman RJ. Special issues: glucose and the brain. *Crit Care Med* 1992; 20: 104–14.

16. Welborn LG, McGill WA, Hannallah RS, *et al.* Perioperative blood glucose concentrations in pediatric outpatients. *Anesthesiology* 1986; 65: 543–7.

17. Bailey AG, McNaull PP, Jooste E, *et al.* Perioperative crystalloid and colloid fluid management in children: where are we and how did we get here? *Anesth Analg* 2010; 110: 375–90.

18. Nishina K, Mikawa K, Maekawa N, Asano M, Obara H. Effects of exogenous intravenous glucose on plasma glucose and lipid homeostasis in anesthetized infants. *Anesthesiology* 1995; 83: 258–63.

19. Mikawa K, Maekawa N, Goto R, *et al.* Effects of exogenous intravenous glucose on plasma glucose and lipid homeostasis in anesthetized children. *Anesthesiology* 1991; 74: 1017–22.

20. Dubois MC, Gouyet L, Murat I, Saint-Maurice C. Lactated Ringer with 1% dextrose: an appropriate solution for peri-operative fluid therapy in children. *Paediatr Anaesth* 1992; 2: 99–104.

21. Berleur MP, Dahan A, Murat I, Hazebroucq G. Perioperative infusions in paediatric patients: rationale for using Ringer-lactate solution with low dextrose concentration. *J Clin Pharm Ther* 2003; 28: 31–40.

22. Sümpelmann R, Becke K, Crean P, *et al.* European consensus statement for intraoperative fluid therapy in children. *Eur J Anaesthesiol* 2011; 28: 637–9.

23. Sümpelmann R, Mader T, Eich C, *et al.* A novel isotonic-balanced electrolyte solution with 1% glucose for intraoperative fluid therapy in children: results of a prospective multicentre observational post-authorization safety study (PASS). *Paediatr Anaesth* 2010; 20: 977–81.

24. McNab S, Duke T, South M, *et al.* 140 mmol/L of sodium versus 77 mmol/L of sodium in maintenance intravenous fluid therapy for children in hospital (PIMS): a randomised controlled double-blind trial. *Lancet* 2015; 385: 1190–7.

25. Foster BA, Tom D, Hill V. Hypotonic versus isotonic fluids in hospitalized children: a systematic review and meta-analysis. *J Pediatr* 2014; 165: 163–9.

26. Zander R. *Fluid Management*. Melsungen: Bibliomed, 2009.

27. Witt L, Osthaus WA, Bunte C, *et al.* A novel isotonic-balanced electrolyte solution with 1% glucose for perioperative fluid management in children – an animal experimental preauthorization study. *Paediatr Anaesth* 2010; 20: 734–40.

28. Disma N, Mameli L, Pistorio A, *et al.* A novel balanced isotonic sodium solution vs. normal saline during major surgery in children up to 36 months: a multicenter RCT. *Paediatr Anaesth* 2015; 24: 980–6.

29. Arikan AA, Zappitelli M, Goldstein SL, *et al.* Fluid overload is associated with impaired oxygenation and morbidity in critically ill children. *Pediatr Crit Care Med* 2011; 13: 253–8.

30. Saudan S. Is the use of colloids for fluid replacement harmless in children? *Curr Opin Anaesthesiol* 2010; 23: 363–7.

31. Northern Neonatal Nursing Initiative Trial Group. Randomised trial of prophylactic early fresh-frozen plasma or gelatin or glucose in preterm babies: outcome at 2 years. *Lancet* 1996; 348: 229–32.

32. Westphal M, James MF, Kozek-Langenecker S, *et al.* Hydroxyethyl starches: different products–different effects. *Anesthesiology* 2009; 11: 187–202.

33. Osthaus WA, Witt L, Johanning K, *et al.* Equal effects of gelatin and hydroxyethyl starch (6% HES 130/0.42) on modified thrombelastography in children. *Acta Anaesthesiol Scand* 2009; 53: 305–10.

34. Witt L, Osthaus WA, Jahn W, *et al.* Isovolaemic hemodilution with gelatin and hydroxyethylstarch 130/0.42: effects on hemostasis in piglets. *Paediatr Anaesth* 2012; 22: 379–85.

35. Sümpelmann R, Kretz FJ, Luntzer R, *et al.* Hydroxyethyl starch 130/0.42/6:1 for perioperative plasma volume replacement in 1130 children: results of an European prospective multicenter observational postauthorization safety study (PASS). *Paediatr Anaesth* 2012; 22: 371–8.

36. van der Linden P, Dumoulin M, Van Lerberghe C, *et al.* Efficacy and safety of 6% hydroxyethyl starch 130/0.4 (Voluven) for perioperative volume replacement in children undergoing cardiac surgery: a propensity-matched analysis. *Crit Care* 2015; 19: 87.

37. Witt L, Glage S, Schulz K, *et al.* Impact of 6% hydroxyethyl starch 130/0.42 and 4% gelatin on renal function in a pediatric animal model. *Paediatr Anaesth* 2014; 24: 974–9.

38. Chappell D, Jacob M, Hofmann-Kiefer K, Conzen P, Rehm M. A rational approach to perioperative fluid management. *Anesthesiology* 2008; 109: 723–40.

39. Osthaus WA, Huber D, Beck C, *et al.* Correlation of oxygen delivery with central venous oxygen saturation, mean arterial pressure and heart rate in piglets. *Paediatr Anaesth* 2006; 16: 944–7.

40. Sümpelmann R, Mader T, Dennhardt N, *et al.* A novel isotonic balanced electrolyte solution with 1% glucose for intraoperative fluid therapy in neonates: results of a prospective multicentre observational postauthorisation safety study (PASS). *Paediatr Anaesth* 2011; 21: 1114–18.

Chapter

24

Obstetric, pulmonary, and geriatric surgery

Kathrine Holte

Summary

This chapter focuses on fluid management in obstetric, pulmonary, and geriatric surgery. In obstetrics, the fluid administration debate largely centers on the relevance of fluid infusions to counteract hypotension in conjunction with regional anesthesia administered for pain relief during labor or as anesthesia for Cesarean section, where both colloids and sympathomimetics reduce maternal hypotension. Particular to pulmonary surgery, a positive fluid balance is found to correlate with postoperative lung injury and should be strictly controlled. Elderly patients, while being at increased risk for postoperative complications, may also be more susceptible to perioperative fluid disturbances including preoperative dehydration.

In summary, evidence suggests that fluid management should be individualized and integrated into perioperative care programs. Both insufficient and excessive fluid administration may increase complications, and while determining fluid status is still a challenge, individualized fluid therapy to obtain certain hemodynamic goals may be recommended.

The limited knowledge of both pathophysiology and clinical outcomes of perioperative fluid management has precluded formation of evidence-based, rational guidelines. While plenty of studies have focused on fluid therapy in critically ill patients, clinical research into fluid administration in elective (not to mention emergency) surgical procedures has, until recently, been largely absent.[1] However, the past decade has seen a growing interest in perioperative fluid management, shifting focus from the (still unresolved) question of *which type* of fluid to administer to *how much* fluid should be administered (Box 24.1). Attention has increasingly focused on the avoidance of both insufficient fluid administration and fluid excess (more commonly seen), by individualizing the perioperative fluid administration.[2]

The perioperative patient is predisposed to fluid retention and thus potential postoperative fluid overload, as sodium and water are retained as a consequence of the physiological stress response to surgery as well as fluid accumulation in peripheral tissues.[3] Historically, this saline conservation has been essential to survival, and only recent practices of intravenous saline administration have made the capacity to excrete saline important. Thus, even healthy, non-operated volunteers may not readily excrete 1–3 liters of intravenous crystalloid.[1]

Currently, no available technique may reliably determine perioperative fluid status, a fact no doubt contributing greatly to the controversy of how much fluid should be administered perioperatively.[4] While weighing the patient may reflect overall fluid status, weight gain – the essential parameter – may easily exist in the presence of hypovolemia.

It is well known that pressure-guided cardiovascular monitoring (such as blood pressure and central venous pressures) are not adequate determinants of intravascular volume and have generally been disappointing when applied to guide fluid administration in clinical trials.[5] On the contrary, guiding intraoperative fluid administration by individual flow-directed cardiovascular monitoring (so-called goal-directed fluid administration) has been shown to improve outcome in some but not all studies.[4,6] The

---

Clinical Fluid Therapy in the Perioperative Setting, Second Edition, ed. Robert G. Hahn. Published by Cambridge University Press. © Cambridge University Press 2016.

Box 24.1 Perioperative fluid management – current controversial issues

Geriatric surgery

Similar issues to non-geriatric surgery:
"Liberal" vs. "restrictive" vs. goal-directed fluid
Administration:
Which type of fluid to administer

Pulmonary surgery

Role of fluid administration in
post-pneumonectomy pulmonary edema

Obstetrics

Preload to alleviate hypotension in regional
analgesia for labor

The terms "liberal" vs. "restrictive," or "high" vs. "low" fluid (internationally accepted in the medical literature), simply describe two different levels of fluid administration and do not imply conclusions about the suitability of either regimen. However, these terms have contributed to confusion in the literature and, whenever possible, the actual amounts of fluid administered are mentioned. The term "fluid administration" refers to intravenous crystalloid administration unless stated otherwise.

only goal-directed fluid administration strategy sufficiently evaluated in clinical trials consists of colloid infusions guided by cardiac filling pressures obtained via a trans-esophageal Doppler device, but other techniques are available.[5] Both hypovolemia and fluid overload may obviously lead to impaired outcomes; however, these issues have not been systematically investigated.

Regarding the type of fluid to administer, a systematic review of all (80) randomly controlled trials (RCTs) in elective, non-cardiac surgery concluded that available data offered no conclusions on the choice of fluid to administer, mainly owing to most studies being underpowered (very few studies with >100 patients) as well as the failure to report relevant outcomes.[7] Furthermore, perioperative care was generally not standardized, and the follow-up period tended not to include the postoperative period.

A multimodal revision of principles of perioperative care (so-called fast-track surgery) has been found to shorten hospital stay and improve convalescence in various surgical procedures.[8] Core components of this concept are opioid-sparing analgesia, early enteral feeding and mobilization, as well as preoperative patient education and standardized postoperative care protocols. There is an overall decrease in intravenous

fluid administration in fast-track protocols; as early oral intake without restrictions is encouraged, intravenous fluid therapy is given on special indications only.

Geriatric surgery

Despite an increasing number of surgical procedures being performed in the elderly population, few studies have been specifically concerned with elderly patients. Furthermore, elderly patients are often excluded from investigational trials, leaving very little specific evidence on the care of the elderly surgical patient, which is unfortunate as age >65 years is a major risk factor for in-hospital mortality.[9]

The propensity for fluid retention described above applies for elderly patients as well, as infusion of ~3 liters of crystalloids results in a significant although small (~5–7%) decrease in pulmonary function in addition to a significant weight gain over 24 hours in non-operated elderly (median 63 years) volunteers.[10]

Preoperative fluid management

Preoperatively, bowel preparation has been found to lead to a decrease in functional cardiovascular capacity in the elderly (median 63 years), despite a daily oral fluid intake above 2.5 liters.[11] As this functional impairment presumably is caused by dehydration, it may very well be even more pronounced in older patients with a documented decreased capacity for oral intake. In patients undergoing colonic and rectal surgery, 28% were estimated to be dehydrated preoperatively, which led to increased postoperative complications.[12] Thus, in elderly patients, especially those undergoing preoperative bowel preparation, correction of a preoperative fluid deficit, if present, seems warranted.[4]

Intraoperative fluid management

As mentioned previously, very few studies have specifically investigated elderly patients. Nevertheless, in many of the available studies, mostly conducted in the area of abdominal and/or colorectal surgery, most of the participants, despite the lack of a formal age limit, may be considered elderly (>65 years).

Several randomized studies in abdominal surgery suggest that both so-called "restrictive" fluid administration and regimens leading to fluid overload worsen outcome,[13–15] and a meta-analysis found individualized fluid administration based on hemodynamic goals superior to "liberal" fluid regimens without hemodynamic goals, but with uncertain effects compared with restrictive fluid regimens.[6] In patients undergoing radical prostatectomy, goal-directed fluid administration did not reduce the postoperative orthostatic intolerance, which often limits mobilization and thus early recovery.[16] In summary, it would seem that both fluid overload and a too restrictive perioperative fluid regimen may worsen outcome.[4]

In elective orthopedic surgery, a randomized study in knee replacement surgery (fast-track), found "liberal" (4,250 ml) vs. "restrictive" (1,740 ml) intraoperative crystalloid-based fluid administration to result in significant hypercoagulability (confirming previous reports in healthy volunteers) although with no differences in morbidity or recovery.[17] Following proximal femoral fracture, a disease typical of the elderly population, a Cochrane review found no evidence that fluid optimization strategies improved outcome.[18]

A systematic review of various types of fluids administered in a general (not age-restricted) surgical population failed to find differences between the various types of fluid administered.[7] A Cochrane review also found no outcome differences between administration of buffered vs. non-buffered fluids,[19] although the available studies are of insufficient volume and/or quality to allow firm conclusions to be drawn.

Postoperative fluid management

No studies have specifically targeted the elderly population postoperatively, and generally the literature on postoperative fluid management is very sparse. In the context of fast-track surgery, immediate reuptake of normal food intake combined with the absence of ileus greatly diminishes the need for postoperative intravenous fluid administration, and less than 10% of patients undergoing fast-track colonic surgery receive postoperative intravenous fluid supplements.[8]

Obstetric surgery

The debate on fluid management in obstetrics largely centers on the relevance of fluid infusions to counteract hypotension in conjunction with regional anesthesia administered for pain relief during labor or as anesthesia for Cesarean section. The theory is that regional anesthesia (spinal, epidural, or combined spinal–epidural) may induce hypotension, which again may cause fetal heart rate abnormalities owing to a decrease in intrauterine blood flow. However, both the underlying mechanism and the clinical significance of these heart rate abnormalities are unclear.

A Cochrane review from 2004 [20] included six trials with 473 patients in which 500–1,000 ml crystalloid vs. none was administered for preload before regional analgesia in labor. The authors concluded that the overall effects of preloading were questionable: In one (of two) studies applying high-dose local anesthetics, preload reduced maternal hypotension and fetal heart rate abnormalities, while no effects of preload were seen in the other trial applying high-dose local anesthetic or in the remaining four trials of low-dose local anesthetics or combined spinal–epidural anesthesia.[20] For Cesarean section performed under spinal anesthesia, a Cochrane review from 2006 concluded preload with colloids to be more efficient than crystalloids, which again were more effective than placebo in preventing maternal hypotension.[21] The superior effects of colloids were confirmed in a large RCT with 167 parturients.[22] Even though both colloids and sympathomimetics reduced maternal hypotension, no intervention has been found to alleviate it entirely. The lack of fluid efficacy may be attributed to the relatively short volume expansion and a possibly concomitant increase in atrial natriuretic peptide secretion.[3]

Pulmonary surgery

The obligatory decrease in pulmonary function after surgery may theoretically be amplified by fluid overload, predisposing to pneumonia and respiratory failure.[3] Several studies have consistently shown the incidence of lung injury/pulmonary edema after pulmonary surgery to correlate with the amounts of fluid administered perioperatively, and it may not be recommended to exceed a positive fluid balance of 1.5 liters.[23] The pathophysiology is complex, however, including multiple factors such as impaired lymphatic drainage and ischemia/reperfusion injury.[24] Thus, theoretically, patients subjected to lung surgery may be at particular risk of complications related to fluid overload, but no randomized clinical trials have been performed in pulmonary surgery investigating the influence of perioperative fluid administration.

References

1. Holte K. Pathophysiology and clinical implications of peroperative fluid management in elective surgery. *Dan Med Bull* 2010; 57: B4156.

2. Doherty M, Buggy, DJ. Intraoperative fluids: how much is too much? *Br J Anaesth* 2012; 109: 69–79.

3. Holte K, Sharrock NE, Kehlet H. Pathophysiology and clinical implications of perioperative fluid excess. *Br J Anaesth* 2002; 89: 622–32.

4. Navarro LH, Bloomstone JA, Auler JO Jr, *et al.* Perioperative fluid therapy: a statement from the perioperative fluid optimization group. *Perioper Med (Lond)* 2015; 4: 3.

5. Bundgaard-Nielsen M, Holte K, Secher NH, *et al.* Monitoring of peri-operative fluid administration by individualized goal-directed therapy. *Acta Anaesthesiol Scand* 2007; 51: 331–40.

6. Corcoran T, Rhodes JE, Clarke S, *et al.* Perioperative fluid management strategies in major surgery: a stratified meta-analysis. *Anesth Analg* 2012; 104: 640–51.

7. Holte K, Kehlet H. Fluid therapy and surgical outcomes in elective surgery: a need for reassessment in fast-track surgery. *J Am Coll Surg* 2006; 202: 971–89.

8. Kehlet H, Wilmore DW. Evidence-based surgical care and the evolution of fast-track surgery. *Ann Surg* 2008; 248: 189–98.

9. Masoomi H, Kang CY, Chen A, *et al.* Predictive factors of in-hospital mortality in colon and rectal surgery. *J Am Coll Surg* 2012; 215: 255–61.

10. Holte K, Jensen P, Kehlet H. Physiologic effects of intravenous fluid administration in healthy volunteers. *Anesth Analg* 2003; 96: 1504–9.

11. Holte K, Nielsen KG, Madsen JL, *et al.* Physiologic effects of bowel preparation. *Dis Colon Rectum* 2004; 47: 1397–402.

12. Moghadamyeghaneh Z, Phelan MJ, Carmichael JC, *et al.* Preoperative dehydration increases risk of postoperative acute renal failure in colon and rectal surgery. *J Gastrointest Surg* 2014; 18: 2178–85.

13. Holte K, Foss NB, Andersen J, *et al.* Liberal or restrictive fluid administration in fast-track colonic surgery: a randomized, double-blind study. *Br J Anaesth* 2007; 99: 500–8.

14. Wenkui Y, Ning L, Jianfeng G, *et al.* Restricted peri-operative fluid administration adjusted by serum lactate level improved outcome after major elective surgery for gastrointestinal malignancy. *Surgery* 2010; 147: 542–52.

15. Brandstrup B, Tonnesen H, Beier-Holgersen R, *et al.* Effects of intravenous fluid restriction on postoperative complications: comparison of two perioperative fluid regimens: a randomized assessor-blinded multicenter trial. *Ann Surg* 2003; 238: 641–8.

16. Bundgaard-Nielsen M, Jans Ø, Müller RG, *et al.* Does goal-directed fluid therapy affect postoperative orthostatic intolerance? A randomized trial. *Anesthesiology* 2013; 119: 813–23.

17. Holte K, Kristensen BB, Valentiner L, *et al.* Liberal versus restrictive fluid management in knee arthroplasty: a randomized, double-blind study. *Anesth Analg* 2007; 105: 465–74.

18. Brammar A, Nicholson A, Trivella M, *et al.* Perioperative fluid volume optimization following proximal femoral fracture. *Cochrane Database Syst Rev* 2013; CD003004.

19. Burdett E, Dushianthan A, Benett-Guerrero E, *et al.* Perioperative buffered versus non-buffered fluid administration for surgery in adults. *Cochrane Database Syst Rev* 2012; CD004089.

20. Hofmeyr G, Cyna A, Middleton P. Prophylactic intravenous preloading for regional analgesia in labour. *Cochrane Database Syst Rev* 2004; CD000175.

21. Cyna AM, Andrew M, Emmett RS, *et al.* Techniques for preventing hypotension during spinal anaesthesia for caesarean section. *Cochrane Database Syst Rev* 2006; CD002251.

22. Mercier FJ, Diemunsch P, Ducloy-Bouthors AS, *et al.* 6% Hydroxyethyl starch (130/0.4) vs. Ringer's lactate preloading before spinal anaesthesia for Caesarean delivery: The randomized, double-blind, multicentre CAESAR trial. *Br J Anaesth* 2014; 113: 459–67.

23. Evans RG, Naidu B. Does a conservative fluid management strategy in the perioperative management of lung resection patients reduce the risk of acute lung injury? *Interact Cardiovasc Thorac Surg* 2012; 15: 498–504.

24. Chau EH, Slinger P. Perioperative fluid management for pulmonary resection surgery and esophagectomy. *Semin Cardiothorac Vasc Anesth* 2014; 18: 36–44.

Chapter 25

Transplantations

Laurence Weinberg

Summary

Patients with end-stage liver disease have a hyper-dynamic resting circulation with high cardiac output states and low systemic vascular resistance and tachycardia. During liver transplantation, this state is amplified. The potential for massive bleeding is common and can result in sudden and catastrophic hypovolemia. Massive blood transfusion results in large volumes of citrated blood being administered. With limited or no hepatic function to metabolize citrate, citrate intoxication can occur, and calcium chloride should be administered when appropriate. Mild to moderate acidosis can be safely tolerated. Albumin is the most common colloid used, while the use of lactate-based crystalloid solutions can result in hyperlactatemia as lactate anions are ineffectively metabolized. Acetate-buffered solutions should be preferred. The most common cause of death in fulminant liver failure is intractable intracranial hypertension from cerebral edema, present in approximately 50–80% of patients with fulminant liver failure. Therefore, permissive hypernatremia and use of hypertonic saline solutions are frequently treatment options in this setting.

Crystalloids are the mainstay and first choice of perioperative fluid intervention in renal transplantation. Conventionally, 0.9% saline is widely advocated because of concerns about hyperkalemia from the balanced/buffered solutions, which all contain potassium. However, this fear has not been confirmed in clinical trials.

Hydroxyethyl starch should be avoided owing to increased risk of a delayed graft function.*

With improvements in surgical skills, anesthetic techniques, graft preservation, and perioperative management, liver and renal transplantation have become established treatments for patients with end-stage acute and chronic hepatic failure, as well as in advanced and irreversible chronic kidney disease. In this context, transplantation is a therapeutic intervention that improves survival and quality of life, and controls and/or reverses many of the comorbidities associated with organ failure.

The scientific literature provides little evidence-based guidance on amount (quantitative fluid intervention) or type (qualitative fluid intervention) of fluid to optimize outcomes during liver and renal transplantation. Fluid intervention and vasoactive pharmacological support of transplantation depend on attending clinician preference, institutional resources, and practice culture. This chapter provides a contemporary overview of the fundamental principles underpinning fluid intervention for adult liver and renal transplantation.

Fluid intervention for liver transplantation

Factors influencing postoperative graft function and patient outcomes in liver transplantation are complex and multifactorial. Donor factors include but are not limited to advanced age, increase in transaminases, requirement for catecholamines, intensive care time, cold and warm ischemia times, and histology and macroscopic graft appearance. Recipient

* Summary compiled by the Editor.

factors included Child–Pugh classification, Model for End-Stage Liver Disease (MELD) scores, pre-operative gastrointestinal bleeding, mechanical ventilation, hemodialysis, and requirement for cate-cholamines.[1,2] Recently combined donor–recipient risk index models have allowed prediction of outcomes that provide a more complete picture of overall risk and allow benchmarking of graft survivals between centers and regions.[3]

The goal of optimum fluid intervention for liver transplantation is to maintain adequate tissue perfusion to the new graft and other organs, and ensure adequate tissue oxygenation. Optimal fluid intervention is dependent on a thorough understanding of the phases of the surgery, which are conveniently divided into three stages. A fundamental understanding of each stage is paramount to guide optimum quantitative and qualitative fluid intervention. Patients should be managed on an individualized basis, and whilst no single approach will be effective in all cases, the principles of fluid intervention for each surgical stage are summarized in Table 25.1.

Factors influencing volume and type of fluid for liver transplantation

As liver transplantation imposes a major pathophysiological insult on the patient, the volume and type of fluid intervention depends on the presence and severity of the following perioperative sequelae.

Hemodynamic changes

Management of the patient's hemodynamic status depends on both the severity of the derangement and its etiology. Patients with end-stage liver disease have a hyperdynamic resting circulation with high cardiac output states, low systemic vascular resistance, and tachycardia. Intraoperatively this state is amplified. The potential for massive bleeding is common and can result in sudden and catastrophic hypovolemia. This can be compounded by obstruction or clamping of the inferior vena cava, or surgical manipulation of the liver that decreases venous return and cardiac output. In addition, profound vasoplegia is common, particularly at reperfusion. Patients with end-stage liver disease suffer from glycocalyx alterations, and ischemia reperfusion injury during transplantation further exacerbates endothelial damage.[4] The endothelial glycocalyx participates in the

maintenance of vascular integrity, and its perturbations cause capillary leakage, loss of vascular responsiveness, and enhanced adhesion of leukocytes and platelets. Reperfusion syndrome can result in profound hemodynamic embarrassment and cardiac arrest [5,6] as outlined in Table 25.1.

Biochemical derangements

Severe biochemical derangements are common and include citrate toxicity, metabolic acidosis, hypocalcemia, osmolality changes, and rapid potassium influx. Massive blood transfusion results in large volumes of citrated blood being administered and the development of a metabolic acidosis. There is limited or no hepatic function to metabolize citrate, therefore citrate intoxication can occur and resultant hypocalcemia is frequent. Ionized calcium levels must be frequently monitored and calcium chloride should be administered when appropriate. Mild to moderate acidosis can be safely tolerated during transplantation; however, in the author's institution, for a base deficit of greater than −15 or a pH less than 7.1, titration of 8.4% sodium bicarbonate is administered to reduce the risk of reperfusion arrhythmias and impaired myocardial contractility. Sodium bicarbonate must be used cautiously, as aggressive correction of pre-existing hyponatremia can impose a risk of serious neurological complications from pontine and extrapontine myelinosis. Intravenous sterile water is frequently administered to control hypernatremia.

Coagulopathy

Fluid intervention for the management of coagulopathy is beyond the scope of this review; however, there are multiple causes of coagulopathy during liver transplantation.[7–9] These include pre-existing coagulopathy due to chronic liver insufficiency and reduced synthesis of clotting factors, pre-existing enhanced fibrinolytic activity thrombocytopenia, variable disseminated intravascular coagulopathy, and coagulopathy from hemodilution and massive blood transfusion. Pediatric patients, and patients with primary biliary cirrhosis, primary sclerosing cholangitis, or underlying hepatoma, may have a hypercoagulable state; in contrast, patients with advanced cirrhosis often present with pre-existing enhanced fibrinolytic activity. During Stages 2 and 3 of the surgery, there is lack of hepatic clearance of tissue plasminogen activator and progressive thrombocytopenia reaching a nadir post reperfusion. In addition, if University of Wisconsin

Table 25.1 Stages of liver transplantation and associated hemodynamic challenges

Surgical phase	Surgical technique	Challenges	Hemodynamic and fluid goals
Stage 1: Pre-anhepatic or dissection phase	Commences with surgical incision and extends until the portal vessels are clamped Mobilization and dissection of native liver	Hemodynamic instability can be pronounced owing to: • Decompression of ascites • Bleeding from extensive collateral circulation due to portal hypertension • Bleeding from adhesions due to previous surgery • Effects of liver retraction of the inferior venae cava with compromised venous return to the right atrium	Maintenance of baseline vascular filling pressures with a combination of vasoactive pharmacotherapy (e.g. noradrenaline) and fluids Some centers advocate restrictive fluid therapy, with low central venous pressure to minimize Stage 1 blood loss Most cirrhotic patients have increased blood volumes and cardiac output, therefore will tolerate 15–20% blood loss with little volume intervention or vasoactive support needed Volume reduction of this magnitude can be tolerated if mean arterial pressure is greater than 65 mmHg and cardiac index is above 2.0 liter/min/m^2 **Advantages of Stage 1 restrictive fluid intervention:** • Less bleeding may lower venous pressure and intravascular volume of abdominal collateral vessels • In cases of caval injury, less brisk bleeding can facilitate faster control and repair **Disadvantages of Stage 1 restrictive fluid intervention:** • Increased risk of air embolism • May result in impaired organ perfusion rather than decreased venous pressures • Increase risk of postoperative acute renal failure

Stage 2: Anhepatic phase	• Begins with transection of the portal vessels and ends with reperfusion	• Portal vein clamping can induce portal hypertension and splanchnic congestion making dissection more difficult
		• Splanchnic congestion can cause renal congestion and subsequent renal dysfunction
		• Surgeons frequently apply side clamps to inferior vena cava to facilitate surgery
		• Depending on extent, type, and duration of surgical clamping of the inferior vena cava, venous return will be compromised
		• Temporary portal caval shunts associated with preservation of the inferior vena cava have been used safely without the need for veno-venous bypass and associated with better hemodynamic stability
		• If hemodynamically unstable, veno-venous bypass can be considered
			• IVC clamp reduces venous return by 50%
			• Consider judicious volume loading prior to inferior vena cava clamp
			• Once inferior vena cava clamp is applied, avoid aggressive volume loading unless replacing ongoing blood losses
			• Aggressive volume loading can precipitate volume overload and right heart failure on reperfusion
			• Aggressive volume loading can result in high central venous pressure during Stage 3 increasing venous congestion in the new graft
			• As the portal vein anastomosis is nearing completion ensure:
			  · Calcium > 1.1 mmol/l
			  · Potassium < 5.0 mmol/l

Table 25.1 (*cont.*)

Surgical phase	Surgical technique	Challenges	Hemodynamic and fluid goals

Stage 3: Reperfusion and neohepatic phase	• Begins with removal of caval clamps and passive washout from hepatic veins
	• Surgical testing of the caval hepatic anastomoses is then performed with back pressure before portal venous flow is restored
	• After reperfusion of the liver with portal venous blood, the hepatic arterial anastomosis is completed
	• Biliary anastomosis is finally completed (either a duct to duct anastomosis connection or a Roux-en-Y choledo-chojejunostomy
	• After the vascular and biliary anastomosis, perfect surgical hemostasis must be achieved prior to closure
		• Reperfusion results in release of CO_2, tumor necrosis factor, and other active mediators and cytokines
		• Reperfusion syndrome: diagnosed by sustained reduction in mean arterial pressure by 30% for greater than 1 min
		• Reperfusion syndrome occurs in 8–30% of transplants and is caused by acidemia, metabolic derangements, emboli of air and microthrombus, and release of vasoactive substances from the ischemic liver
		• Throughout the neohepatic phase, signs of improving graft function include:
		  - Improvements in coagulation
		  - Falling potassium
		  - Improving acid–base physiology
		  - Falling lactate
		  - Improved urine output
		  - Improvement in hemodynamics
		  - Production of bile from new graft
			• Significant hemodynamic changes occur in ∼30–50% of patients including arrhythmias and hypotension
			• Reperfusion mediators are negative inotropes and can result in acute right cardiac dysfunction, elevated pulmonary artery pressures, and increased right ventricular afterload
			• Right ventricular distension limits left ventricular filling and can cause profound hemodynamic embarrassment
			• Reperfusion can result in life-threatening hyperkalemia
			• Drugs used to treat reperfusion syndrome and hyperkalemia include adrenaline, noradrenaline calcium, atropine, insulin/dextrose, and bicarbonate
			• Vasopressin and methylene blue can be used for refractory vasoplegia
			• If right cardiac dysfunction is present, large volume fluid intervention/ resuscitation may increase central venous pressure, and precipitate right cardiac failure and cardiac arrest. Use of trans-esophageal echocardiography is useful to guide fluid intervention and assess the hemodynamic state in this scenario

solution is used for graft preservation, platelet aggregation due to the adenosine can occur post reperfusion. Heparin activity can also occur post reperfusion owing to release of exogenous heparin from the graft and the release of endogenous heparinoids from damaged endothelium. Hypothermia slows enzymatic reactions and also prolongs factor reaction time and reduces platelet aggregation.

Renal dysfunction

The incidence of acute renal failure post liver transplantation varies between 48% and 94%, with 8% to 17% of patients requiring renal replacement therapy.[10,11] Whilst the etiology is multifactorial, common causes include pre-existing ischemic acute tubular necrosis, cyclosporine toxicity, and sepsis. Patients with acute renal failure from hepato-renal syndrome will recovery in most cases, although recovery may be delayed up to 6 months. The risk of chronic kidney disease is approximately 18% at 5 years and increases to approximately 25% by 10 years after transplantation. Although preoperative, intraoperative, and post-transplant factors may contribute to the development of post-transplantation chronic renal failure, pre-transplant chronic renal failure appears to be one of the most important risk factors.[12]

Physicochemical considerations for choice of fluids

The liver plays a vital function in acid–base regulation, and severe metabolic derangements during transplantation are common and frequently profound. Choice of fluid for liver transplantation should take into account the important role that the liver plays in the maintenance of acid–base homeostasis. The physicochemical composition of the commonly available crystalloid solutions used in liver transplantation are summarized in Table 25.2.

Metabolic acidosis

Accumulating data and expert opinion suggest that large volumes of saline 0.9% result in hyperchloremic metabolic acidosis.[13–15] Severe acidemia can

Table 25.2 Characteristics of common crystalloid solutions compared with human plasma

	Human plasma	0.9% saline (unbuffered solution)	Compound sodium lactate (lactate buffered solution)	Ringer's lactate (lactate buffered solution)	Ionosteril® (acetate buffered solution)	Sterofundin ISO® (acetate and malate buffered solution)	Plasma-Lyte-148® (acetate and gluconate buffered solution)
Sodium (mmol/l)	136–145	154	129	130	137	145	140
Potassium (mmol/l)	3.5–5.0		5	4	4	4	5
Magnesium (mmol/l)	0.8–1.0				1.25	1	1.5
Calcium (mmol/l)	2.2–2.6		2.5	3	1.65	2.5	
Chloride (mmol/l)	98–106	154	109	109	110	127	98
Acetate (mmol/l)					36.8	24	27
Gluconate (mmol/l)							23
Lactate (mmol/l)			29	28			
Malate (mmol/l)						5	
eSID (mEq/l)	42	0	27	28	36.8	25.5	50
Theoretical osmolarity (mosmol/l)	291	308	278	273	291	309	295
Actual or measured[a] osmolality (mosmol/kg H_2O)	287	286	256	256	270	Not stated	271
pH	7.35–7.45	4.5–7	5–7	5–7	6.9–7.9	5.1–5.9	4–8

[a] Freezing point depression.
eSID, effective strong ion difference.
Plasma-Lyte-148 manufactured by Baxter Healthcare, Toongabie, NSW, Australia.
Ringer's lactate manufactured by Baxter Healthcare, Deerfield, IL, USA.
Hartmann's solution manufactured by Baxter Healthcare, Toongabie, NSW, Australia.
Ionosteril manufactured by Fresenius Medical Care, Schweinfurt, Germany.
Sterofundin ISO manufactured by B. Braun Melsungen AG, Melsungen, Germany.

result in impaired cardiac contractility, arrhythmias, pulmonary hypertension, renal and splanchnic vasoconstriction, and impaired coagulation,[16] all of which are common during liver transplantation. Correction of acidemia during liver transplantation is contentious, as the physiological benefits of acidemia include improved oxygen delivery via the Bohr effects and protection against hypoxic stress.[16] Experimental evidence has shown that the optimal strong ion difference for an intravenous fluid not to influence blood pH should be approximately 24 mEq/l.[17,18] Saline (0.9%), with its equal concentrations of sodium and chloride, has a strong ion difference of zero. Use of 0.9% saline during transplantation will significantly reduce the strong ion difference of plasma and exacerbate the severity of any metabolic acidosis. Use of buffered solutions with a high effective strong ion difference composition can minimize the severity of metabolic acid–base disturbances in this setting, whilst restoring intravascular volume deficit.

Inorganic anions

The liver plays a vital role in its capacity to metabolize various organic anions, which results in consumption of hydrogen ions and regeneration of the extracellular bicarbonate buffer. Anions may be exogenous (e.g. citrate in blood transfusion, or gluconate, acetate, and lactate from buffered crystalloid solutions), or endogenous such as lactate from active glycolysis or anaerobic metabolism. During liver transplantation, hepatic metabolism is severely or completely compromised, and therefore organic anions present in delivered buffered fluid solutions may not be adequately metabolized to generate bicarbonate.

Theoretically, the use of acetate-buffered solutions confers several advantages over the lactate-buffered solutions in the setting of liver transplantation.[19] Use of lactate-based crystalloid solutions can result in hyperlactatemia, as lactate anions are ineffectively metabolized. Lactate levels may therefore be an unreliable index of the severity of graft function. Hyperlactatemia has also been shown to be an important prognostic marker after liver resection,[20] shock states, and critical illness,[21,22] correlating strongly with increased risks of complications and death. Unlike lactate, acetate is metabolized widely throughout the body and not reliant entirely on hepatic metabolism.

A canine study showed that acetate metabolism is well-preserved in profound shock while lactate metabolism was significantly impaired.[23] Acetate is metabolized more rapidly than lactate, with an increase in bicarbonate levels evident after 15 min after the start of an acetate infusion.[24,25] Acetate is also more alkalinizing than lactate, which may be advantageous for patients undergoing liver transplantation.

More recently, in a larger clinical trial of 78 critically ill trauma patients resuscitated with sodium acetate as an alternative to 0.9% saline or lactated Ringer's, patients receiving acetate had hemodynamic profiles without evidence of hemodynamic instability. Normalization of hyperchloremia and metabolic acidosis occurred faster in the patients who received acetate.[26] Acetate turnover shows no age-related differences,[27] and acetate may protect against malnutrition by replacing fat as an oxidative fuel without affecting glucose oxidation or causing hyperglycemia.[28,29] Finally, acetate metabolism

does not change the glucose or insulin concentrations,[30] whereas exogenously administered lactate can be converted to glucose via gluconeogenesis, resulting in significant hyperglycemia.[31] In diabetic patients, intraoperative glucose levels have been shown to double following administration of exogenous lactate solutions.[30] Compared with bicarbonate, lactate, or acetate, the alkalizing effect of gluconate is almost zero,[32,33] so its clinical effects *in vivo* as a metabolizable anion appear to be limited.

Historically, adverse effects of acetate have been observed with high doses and high rates of acetate infusions, particularly in the setting of hemodialysis. The generalizability of these findings to liver transplantation is unknown. Small quantity of acetate present in various dialysis fluids (usually 35 mmol/l) has resulted in plasma acetate concentration of 10 to 40 times physiological levels.[34–36] Kirkendol et al. reported that sodium acetate produced a direct dose-related decrease in myocardial contractility and blood pressure in a dog model, but that a slow infusion of sodium acetate did not result in adverse hemodynamic effects.[33,37] Hypoxia and hypotension have been reported in patients with end-stage renal disease dialyzed against solutions containing acetate.[38–40]

In a crossover study involving 12 patients undergoing hemofiltration randomized to either acetate or bicarbonate (acetate free) dialysate, Selby et al. demonstrated that exposure to acetate-free dialysate was associated with less deterioration in systemic hemodynamics and less suppression of myocardial contractility.[41] Similarly, Jacob et al. examined the effect of acetate on cardiac energy metabolism using the isovolumic isolated perfused heart model.[42] Exposure of myocardial tissue to acetate concentrations as low as 5 mmol/l selectively impaired fatty acid metabolism in cardiac tissue, and decreased ATP production and tissue ATP concentrations, which in turn resulted in impaired contractile function. Whilst the authors cautioned that this finding could be due to other parenterally administered acetate-containing solutions, there have been no human studies to support the findings in the isolated heart model. In contrast, Nitenberg et al. evaluated the effects of acetate on left ventricular contractility and function before and after a 20-min sodium acetate infusion during dialysis where heart rate was controlled by atrial pacing.[43] Angiographically determined left ventricular volumes and pressures were used to calculate the ventricular function indices. A plasma acetate concentration of

3.13 mmol/l increased ejection fraction and cardiac index.

Hyperchloremia

Use of fluid solutions with physiological concentrations of chloride during liver transplantation may be beneficial, but hyperchloremia has been linked to adverse clinical outcomes in several animal and human studies. McCluskey *et al.* reviewed the datasets of 22,851 surgical patients undergoing non-cardiac surgery with normal preoperative serum chloride concentration and renal function.[44] Acute postoperative hyperchloremia was associated with postoperative renal dysfunction and 30-day mortality. Yunos *et al.* reported that the implementation of a chloride-restrictive strategy decreased the incidence of acute kidney injury and use of renal replacement therapy.[45] Finally, a recent systematic review and meta-analysis assessed the relationship between the chloride content of intravenous resuscitation fluids and patient outcomes in the perioperative and intensive care settings. A weak but significant association between higher chloride content fluids and unfavorable outcomes was found, although mortality was unaffected.[46] Mechanisms of hyperchloremic-induced renal injury include inability of the proximal tubule capacity to reabsorb chloride, resulting in greater chloride delivery to the thick ascending limb of the distal tubule from inactivation of tubuloglomerular feedback by the macula densa and a reduction in glomerular filtration,[47–49] hyperchloremic-induced thromboxane release with associated vasoconstriction,[50] and an alteration in the expression of inflammatory cytokines.[51]

Plasma osmolality

An understanding of the osmolality of intravenous solutions is important during liver transplantation. Hartmann's solution or Ringer's lactate are hypotonic solutions with a calculated *in vivo* osmolality (tonicity) of approximately 254 mosmol/kg H_2O (Table 25.2). Hypotonic fluids must be used cautiously, if at all, in patients undergoing liver transplantation with fulminant liver failure. The most common cause of death in fulminant liver failure is intractable intracranial hypertension from cerebral edema, present in approximately 50–80% of these patients with fulminant liver failure.

Permissive hypernatremia and use of hypertonic saline solutions are choices of treatment in this specific setting. Saline (0.9%) is considered a relatively hypertonic solution because the sum of its osmotically active components gives a theoretical *in vitro* osmolality of 308 mosmol/kg H_2O (154 mmol/l sodium plus 154 mmol/l chloride). However, 0.9% saline is an isotonic solution as its constituents, sodium and chloride, are only partially active, with an osmotic coefficient of 0.926.[52] The calculated *in vivo* osmolality (tonicity) of saline is 285 mosmol/kg H_2O, which is the same as plasma osmolality (tonicity). Saline may therefore be a more appropriate fluid in the setting of transplantation for fulminant liver failure. Finally, administration of hypotonic fluids can represent a significant free water load that may not be easily excreted in the presence of the high antidiuretic hormone concentrations commonly associated with physiological stress.[53] Failure to excrete water in a timely fashion may result in postoperative transplantation positive fluid balance, edema, and weight gain.

Colloids in liver transplantation

Schumann *et al.* recently conducted a survey evaluating the use of fluids during liver transplantation.[54] Representative samples of 61 US academic institutions with a comprehensive liver transplant anesthesia program were studied. Among the different types of colloids available for intraoperative fluid replacement and volume expansion, albumin was the most common (85%), followed by the synthetic colloids hydroxyethyl starch (HES) in saline (Hespan) or HES in balanced electrolyte solution (Hextend) in 48% and 52% of programs, respectively. High-volume programs (>100 transplants annually) were less inclined to use albumin intraoperatively. Routine perioperative blood product utilization demonstrated the frequent use of packed red blood cells, fresh frozen plasma, cryoprecipitate, and platelets.

There are no large-scale prospective studies guiding the efficacy and safety of any colloids in the setting of liver transplantation. In a small single-center study, 40 patients undergoing living donor liver transplantation were prospectively randomized to receive albumin or HES. The use of HES as an alternative to human albumin resulted in equivalent renal outcomes.[55] More recently, in a larger single-center observational study, Zhou *et al.* evaluated the influence of HES on renal function in 394 patients undergoing orthotopic liver transplantation. Perioperative use of HES had no significant effect on renal function in the first postoperative week.[56] In contrast, Hand *et al.* performed a retrospective cross-sectional analysis of 147 adult patients who underwent orthotopic liver transplantation and reported that patients receiving HES had an increased odds of acute kidney injury compared with patients receiving 5% albumin.[57]

There is a paucity of data on the safety of HES in patients undergoing liver transplantation, despite HES being commonly used. Whilst HES is generally the most common type of colloid administered to resuscitate critically ill patients,[58] emerging data has recently questioned its safety, and there is strong expert opinion of no beneficial effect of HES in any subgroup of critically ill patients [59] (which would include patients undergoing liver transplantation). In 2012, two landmark studies – The Crystalloid versus Hydroxyethyl Starch Trial (CHEST) [60] and the Scandinavian Starch for Severe Sepsis/Septic Shock Trial (6S) [61] addressed the issue of whether resuscitation with HES affects kidney function differently from resuscitation with a crystalloid solution. The CHEST study recruited over 7,000 patients admitted to intensive care and demonstrated an association between more severe acute kidney injury or need for renal replacement therapy and use of HES. The 6S study also found an association between HES and mortality. Conclusions of these studies are supported by a meta-analysis examining HES solutions for resuscitation of patients with sepsis [62] and in critically ill patients requiring volume resuscitation.[63] A recent re-analysis of a Cochrane collaboration analysis of trials examining colloids versus crystalloids for fluid resuscitation in critically ill patients concluded that HES solutions are associated with increased risk of acute kidney injury, and recommended against use in the critically ill.[64]

In 2013, Bagshaw *et al.* evaluated the efficacy and safety of HES or 0.9% saline for fluid resuscitation in critically ill patients with a focus on survival and kidney function.[58] There was no significant difference in 90-day mortality between HES or 0.9% saline. Renal replacement therapy was needed in 7.0% of the HES group vs. 5.8% of the saline group ($p = 0.04$), although RIFLE Class I was less frequent in the HES group, and amounted to 34.6% compared with 38.0% in the saline group ($p = 0.005$). Hydroxyethyl starch was associated with a decrease in new cardiovascular organ failure compared with saline (36.5% vs. 39.9%, $p = 0.03$), but an increase in new hepatic organ failure compared with saline (1.9% vs. 1.2%, $p = 0.03$), which

has direct relevance for patients undergoing liver transplantation.

Inappropriate daily positive fluid balance may, however, be an important source of heterogeneity in many of the trials reporting the association of HES with excess mortality in septic patients.[65] In an updated Cochrane review, which was first published in 2010,[66] Mutter *et al.* reviewed the current evidence and suggested that all HES products increase the risk of acute kidney injury and renal replacement therapy (in all patient populations), and that a safe volume of any HES solution has yet to be determined. The review concluded that in most clinical situations it is likely that these risks outweigh any benefits, and alternate volume replacement therapies should be used in place of HES products.[67] There is no clear evidence that HES solutions are harmful outside critical illness, but in the context of liver transplantation there is also no evidence that HES solutions provide any clinically important benefits. As safer alternatives exist, HES is no longer used in patients undergoing liver transplantation in the author's institution.

There is a greater paucity of data regarding the use of gelatin-based solutions in liver transplantation. The associations of gelatins and adverse effects on hemostasis and coagulation have been the main detractions for its use in liver transplantation given that coagulopathy during transplantation is common, pronounced, and often refractory.[68–70] Both gelatin and HES solutions have been associated with adverse effects on blood coagulation.[69,71] There are fewer effects on blood coagulation using crystalloids compared with colloids, and it is possible that adverse coagulation effects of both gelatin and HES solutions may be similar. There appear to be no differences in adverse coagulation effects between balanced HES 130/0.42 and non-balanced HES 130/0.4.[71] Gelatin causes more impairment in renal function in elective living-donor liver transplantation than HES solutions do.[72] Despite years of clinical use, there is insufficient quality of clinical trials to confirm both the safety and efficacy of gelatin in the setting of liver transplantation.[73] Finally, in the Australian Consultative Council for Morbidity and Mortality report for the Triennium 2003–2005, 27 cases of anesthesia-related anaphylactic reactions to HES solutions and gelatin were reported, 5 of which were fatal.[74] This again has specific relevance to patients undergoing liver transplantation, given the severe hemodynamic challenges faced with each case.

Albumin is the most common colloid used in liver transplantation. Advantages specific to liver transplantation include maintenance of colloid osmotic pressure, preservation of kidney function, pleiotropic physiological benefits on endothelial integrity, improving the endothelial integrity by substantially protecting the glycocalyx of endothelial cells,[75,76] facilitation of negative fluid balance in hypoproteinemia states that are common in transplant patients, and maintenance of glomerular filtration via hemodynamic and oncotic mechanisms.[77–79] Biological plausibility, freedom from nephrotoxicity (safety), and reduction of renal morbidity in liver cirrhosis (effectiveness) support the use of albumin in liver transplantation.[80] In contrast to other colloids, fluid resuscitation with human albumin is not considered nephrotoxic.

Albumin has been extensively reappraised as a resuscitation fluid by Finfer.[81] Available as iso-oncotic and iso-osmolar 4–5% solutions and hyper-oncotic 20–25% solutions, albumin is both suspended in sodium chloride and contains octanoate as the anion stabilizer. It remains an attractive colloid for liver transplantation with 4–5% albumin, providing plasma volume expansion by an amount approximately equal to the volume infused, whilst concentrated albumin expands the plasma volume by approximately 4–5 times the volume infused.[81] However, albumin might be harmful in patients with traumatic brain injury.[82] Therefore, large volumes of albumin should be used cautiously in fulminant liver transplant recipients with raised intracranial pressure.

The pooled analysis of mortality data from large studies of volume therapy with human albumin in sepsis, namely SAFE and ALBIOS, confirms that administration of albumin could significantly reduce mortality in patients with severe sepsis or septic shock.[60,83] In the ALBIOS study, patients in the albumin group not only achieved more frequently hemodynamic stabilization but also had prognostically favorable negative fluid balance.[83] A meta-analysis by Patel et al. confirmed that albumin appears to be safe in the settings of critical illness.[84]

Crystalloids in liver transplantation

In the survey by Schumann et al. evaluating the use of fluids during liver transplantation,[54] in the same representative sample of 61 US academic institutions with a comprehensive liver transplant program,

0.9% saline was the most frequent crystalloid used (81%), followed by a pH-adjusted buffered/balanced crystalloid solution, Plasma-Lyte-148 (74%). Least favored were glucose-containing normal saline solutions (43%). Such practice variation is related to the paucity of prospective evidence regarding the comparative safety and efficacy of available crystalloid solutions for both fluid resuscitation and maintenance therapy in the perioperative setting.

Existing data from observational studies in the perioperative and critical care settings suggest that the use of high-chloride, unbuffered crystalloid fluid may be associated with major complications and increased mortality.[45,85,86] However, owing to the retrospective nature of these studies and potential for unmeasured confounding, it is not possible to establish whether using balanced/buffered crystalloid fluid instead of 0.9% saline is beneficial or harmful during liver transplantation on the basis of observational studies alone.

Until 2015, all interventional studies comparing 0.9% saline to buffered crystalloid had a small sample ($n < 100$) and focused primarily on short-term physiological or biochemical outcomes. A systemic review and meta-analysis published in 2014 identified 28 prospective, randomized control trials with at least 20 adult participants that had compared the effects of different crystalloid fluids.[87] Use of 0.9% saline was associated with decreased serum pH, elevated serum chloride levels, and decreased bicarbonate levels. In studies that examined renal outcomes, no significant differences were found between fluids. In three surgical studies that evaluated volume of red blood cells transfused, patients who had received Ringer's lactate required a significantly lower volume of red blood cells than those that received 0.9% saline. No differences were found between Ringer's lactate and 0.9% saline in requirements for transfusion or operative blood loss, except in an exploratory subgroup analysis of "high-risk" patients that showed increased blood loss with the use of 0.9% saline in patients that were at increased risk of bleeding.

Fluid intervention for renal transplantation

Crystalloids in renal transplantation

The ideal intravenous fluid for renal transplantation has also not been defined. Traditionally, crystalloids are the mainstay and first choice of perioperative fluid intervention in renal transplantation. Conventionally, 0.9% saline is widely advocated because of concerns about hyperkalemia from the balanced/buffered solutions, which all contain potassium. To date, there have been four clinical trials comparing buffered crystalloid solutions to 0.9% saline in living donor kidney transplant recipients. In 2005, O'Malley et al. conducted a prospective, randomized, double-blind clinical trial comparing 0.9% saline against Ringer's lactate for intraoperative fluid therapy for patients undergoing renal transplantation.[88] The study was terminated for safety reasons after interim analysis of data from 51 patients. Whilst 0.9% saline did not have adverse effects on graft function, Ringer's lactate was associated with less hyperkalemia and acidosis compared with saline, and was considered a safe alternative for fluid intervention in kidney transplantation.

Hadimioglu et al. performed a randomized controlled trial comparing Plasma-Lyte-148, Hartmann's solution, and 0.9% saline as intraoperative fluid replacement in 90 patients undergoing renal transplantation.[89] Those receiving 0.9% saline had higher chloride concentration, lower pH, and lower base excess than the other two groups. Patients receiving Hartmann's had elevated lactate levels. Potassium level, urine output, serum urea and creatinine, and creatinine clearance were not significantly different between the groups. The authors concluded that all three fluids appear safe in short-duration uncomplicated renal transplant surgery, but the metabolic profile was best maintained with Plasma-Lyte-148.

Khajavi et al. then conducted a smaller double-blinded randomized prospective clinical trial comparing 0.9% saline to Ringer's as intraoperative intravenous fluid replacement therapy in living related kidney transplantation.[90] Compared with those receiving 0.9% saline, patients receiving Ringer's lactate had lower serum potassium levels and were less acidemic, but had a higher incidence of graft thrombosis. Finally Kim et al. compared the effects of 0.9% saline and Plasma-Lyte-148 on acid–base balance during living donor kidney transplantation using the Stewart and base excess methods. Patients receiving 0.9% saline had significantly lower values of pH, base excess, and effective strong ion differences during the post-reperfusion period compared with Plasma-Lyte.[91]

In the setting of cadaveric renal transplantation, where delayed graft function is more common, a larger randomized clinical trial in 150 patients was recently conducted by Potura et al., comparing the effect of 0.9% saline to that of a chloride-reduced, acetate-buffered crystalloid on the incidence of hyperkalemia.[92] The incidence of metabolic acidosis and kidney function were secondary aims. There were no significant differences in hyperkalemia between groups. Use of buffered crystalloid resulted in less hyperchloremia and metabolic acidosis. Significantly more patients in the saline group required administration of catecholamines for circulatory support. These randomized controlled trials are underpowered to address clinical endpoints such as immediate or delayed graft function, longer-term graft function, and patient survival.

Colloids and renal transplantation

Many of the adverse effects of colloid solutions outlined in the section "Colloids in liver transplantation" above are relevant to patients undergoing kidney transplantation. Specific to renal transplantation, there have been historical concerns regarding the use of HES solutions and impaired renal function.[93] An early prospective randomized trial in 1993 comparing HES and gelatin for plasma volume expansion in brain-dead organ donors found that HES was associated with impaired immediate renal function in kidney transplant recipients.[94] Renal biopsies demonstrated osmotic, nephrosis-like lesions in the HES-treated group.[95] Similar findings have been reported by other investigators.[96]

In the absence of direct chemical toxicity, the most likely attributed mechanism for HES-induced renal dysfunction is swelling and vacuolization of tubular cells and tubular obstruction due to the production of hyperviscous urine. Renal dysfunction from high plasma colloid osmotic pressure is thought to increase with repeated doses of concentrated HES of high molecular weight and high degree of substitution.[97] Findings from these older studies have been recently confirmed by Patel et al. who evaluated the impact of HES in organ donors after neurological determination of death on recipient renal graft outcomes. Nine hundred and eighty-six kidneys were transplanted from 529 donors. Forty-two percent received HES and 35% developed delayed graft function. Hydroxyethyl starch use during donor management was independently associated with a 41% increase in the risk of delayed graft function.[98]

Conclusions

Fluid prescription and intervention for liver and renal transplantation is complex. Whilst there are physiologically rational and biologically plausible data to suggest that certain fluids may confer metabolic, organ, and outcome benefits, there are no unequivocal data to support the use of any single fluid. Clinicians should have a fundamental understanding of the physicochemical properties of the available crystalloid and colloid solutions in order to individualize therapy to the patient's underlying pathophysiological condition. It is imperative to continue to conduct large-scale clinical trials to determine both the optimal type and dose of fluid for patients undergoing either liver or renal transplantation.

References

1. Mueller AR, Platz KP, Krause P, *et al.* Perioperative factors influencing patient outcome after liver transplantation. *Transpl Int* 2013; 13 Suppl 1: S158–61.

2. Gruenberger T, Steininger R, Sautner T, *et al.* Influence of donor criteria on postoperative graft function after orthotopic liver transplantation. *Transpl Int* 1994; 7 Suppl 1: S672–4.

3. Blok JJ, Putter H, Rogiers X, *et al.* Eurotransplant Liver Intestine Advisory Committee (ELIAC). Combined effect of donor and recipient risk on outcome after liver transplantation: Research of the Eurotransplant database. *Liver Transpl* 2015; 21: 1486–93. doi:10.1002/lt.24308.

4. Schiefer J, Lebherz-Eichinger D, Erdoes G, *et al.* Alterations of endothelial glycocalyx during orthotopic liver transplantation in patients with end-stage liver disease. *Transplantation* 2015; 99: 2118–23.

5. Bukowicka B, Akar RA, Olszewska A, *et al.* The occurrence of postreperfusion syndrome in orthotopic liver transplantation and its significance in terms of complications and short-term survival. *Ann Transplant* 2011; 16: 26–30.

6. Paugam-Burtz C, Kavafyan J, Merckx P, *et al.* Postreperfusion syndrome during liver transplantation for cirrhosis: outcome and predictors. *Liver Transpl* 2009; 15: 522–9.

7. Sabate A, Dalmau A, Koo M, *et al.* Coagulopathy management in liver transplantation. *Transplant Proc* 2012; 44: 1523–5.

8. Porte RJ. Coagulation and fibrinolysis in orthotopic liver transplantation: current views and insights. *Semin Thromb Hemost* 1993; 19: 191–6.

9. Massicotte L, Lenis S, Thibeault L, *et al.* Effect of low central venous pressure and phlebotomy on blood product transfusion requirements during liver transplantations. *Liver Transpl* 2006; 12: 117–23.

10. Sirivatanauksorn Y, Parakonthun T, Premasathian N, *et al.* Renal dysfunction after orthotopic liver transplantation. *Transplant Proc* 2014; 46: 818–21.

11. Yalavarthy R, Edelstein CL, Teitelbaum I. Acute renal failure and chronic kidney disease following liver transplantation. *Hemodial Int* 2007; 11 Suppl 3: S7–12.

12. Tinti F, Umbro I, Giannelli V, *et al.* Acute renal failure in liver transplant recipients: role of pretransplantation renal function and 1-year follow-up. *Transplant Proc* 2011; 43: 1136–8.

13. Scheingraber S, Rehm M, Sehmisch C, Finsterer U. Rapid saline infusion produces hyperchloremic acidosis in patients undergoing gynecologic surgery. *Anesthesiology* 1999; 90: 1265–70.

14. Waters JH, Miller LR, Clack S, Kim JV. Cause of metabolic acidosis in prolonged surgery. *Crit Care Med* 1999; 27: 2142–6.

15. Prough DS, Bidani A. Hyperchloremic metabolic acidosis is a predictable consequence of intraoperative infusion of 0.9% saline. *Anesthesiology* 1999; 90: 1247–9.

16. Morgan TJ. The ideal crystalloid – what is 'balanced'? *Curr Opin Crit Care* 2013; 4: 299–307.

17. Morgan TJ, Venkatesh B. Designing 'balanced' crystalloids. *Crit Care Resusc* 2003; 5: 284–91.

18. Omron EM. Omron RM. A physicochemical model of crystalloid infusion on acid–base status. *J Intensive Care Med* 2010; 25: 271–80.

19. Zander R. *Fluid Management*. 2nd edn. http://www.bbraun.com/documents/Knowledge/Fluid_Management_0110.pdf (accessed 14 April 2015).

20. Watanabe I, Mayumi T, Arishima T, *et al.* Hyperlactaemia can predict the prognosis after liver resection. *Shock* 2007; 28: 35–8.

21. Jansen TC, van Bommel J, Bakker J. Blood lactate monitoring in critically ill patients: a systematic health technology assessment. *Crit Care Med* 2009; 37: 2827–39.

22. Kveim M, Nesbakken R, Bakker J, *et al.* Serial blood lactate levels can predict the development of multiple organ failure following septic shock. *Am J Surg* 1996; 171: 221–6.

23. Nakatani T. Utilization of exogenous acetate during canine haemorrhagic shock. *Scand J Clin Lab Invest* 1979; 39: 653–8.

24. Mudge GH, Manning JA, Gilman A. Sodium acetate as a source of fixed base. *Proc Soc Exp Biol Med* 1949; 71: 136–8.

25. Hamada T, Yamamoto M, Nakamura K, *et al.* The pharmacokinetics of D-lactate, L-lactate and acetate in humans. *Masui* 1997; 46: 229–36.

26. McCague A, Dermendjieva M, Hutchinson R, Wong DT, Dao N. Sodium acetate infusion in critically ill trauma patients for hyperchloremic acidosis. *Scand J Trauma Resusc Emerg Med* 2011; 19: 24.

27. Skutches CL, Holroyde CP, Myers RN, *et al.* Plasma acetate turnover and oxidation. *J Clin Invest* 1979; 64: 708–13.

28. Akanji AO, Bruce MA, Frayn KN. Effect of acetate infusion on energy expenditure and substrate oxidation rates in non-diabetic and diabetic subjects. *Eur J Clin Nutr* 1989; 43: 107–15.

29. Akanji AO, Hockaday TDR. Acetate tolerance and the kinetics of acetate utilization in diabetic and nondiabetic subjects. *Am J Clin Nutr* 1990; 51: 112–18.

30. Thomas DJ, Alberti KG. Hyperglycaemic effects of Hartmann's solution during surgery in patients with maturity onset diabetes. *Br J Anaesth* 1978; 50: 185–8.

31. Arai K, Mukaida K, Fujioka Y, *et al.* A comparative study of acetated Ringer's solution and lactated Ringer's solution as intraoperative fluids. *Hiroshima J Anesth* 1989; 25: 357–63.

32. Naylor JM, Forsyth GW. The alkalinizing effects of metabolizable bases in the healthy calf. *Can J Vet Res* 1986; 50: 509–16.

33. Kirkendol PL, Starrs J, Gonzalez FM. The effect of acetate, lactate, succinate and gluconate on plasma pH and electrolytes in dogs. *Trans Am Soc Artif Intern Organs* 1980; 26: 323–7.

34. Coll E, Perez-Garcia R, Rodriguez-Benitez P, *et al.* Clinical and analytical changes in hemodialysis without acetate. *Nefrologia* 2007; 27: 742–8.

35. Bottger I, Deuticke U, Evertz-Prusse E, Ross BD, Wieland O. On the behavior of the free acetate in the miniature pig. Acetate metabolism in the miniature pig. *Z Gesamte Exp Med* 1968; 145: 346–52.

36. Fournier G, Potier J, Thebaud HE, *et al.* Substitution of acetic acid for hydrochloric acid in the bicarbonate buffered dialysate. *Artif Organs* 1998; 22: 608–13.

37. Kirkendol NW, Gonzalez FM, Devia CJ. Cardiac and vascular effects of infused sodium acetate in dogs. *Trans Am Soc Artif Intern Organs* 1978; 24: 714–18.

38. Thaha M, Yogiantoro M, Soewanto P. Correlation between intradialytic hypotension in patients undergoing routine hemodialysis and use of acetate compared in bicarbonate dialysate. *Acta Med Indones* 2005; 37: 145–8.

39. Veech RL, Gitomer WL. The medical and metabolic consequences of administration of sodium acetate. *Adv Enzyme Regul* 1988; 27: 313–43.

40. Quebbeman EJ, Maierhofer WJ, Piering WF. Mechanisms producing hypoxemia during hemodialysis. *Crit Care Med* 1984; 12: 359–63.

41. Selby NM, Fluck RJ, Taal MW, McIntyre CW. Effects of acetate-free double-chamber hemodiafiltration and standard dialysis on systemic hemodynamics and troponin T levels. *ASAIO J* 2006; 52: 62–9.

42. Jacob AD, Elkins N, Reiss OK, Chan L, Shapiro JI. Effects of acetate on energy metabolism and function in the isolated perfused rat heart. *Kidney Int* 1997; 52: 755–60.

43. Nitenberg A, Huyghebaert MF, Blanchet F, Amiel C. Analysis of increased myocardial contractility during sodium acetate infusion in humans. *Kidney Int* 1984; 26: 744–51.

44. McCluskey SA, Karkouti K, Wijeysundera D, *et al.* Hyperchloremia after noncardiac surgery is independently associated with increased morbidity and mortality: a propensity-matched cohort study. *Anesth Analg* 2013; 117: 412–21.

45. Yunos NM, Bellomo R, Hegarty C, *et al.* Association between a chloride-liberal vs. chloride-restrictive intravenous fluid administration strategy and kidney injury in critically ill adults. *JAMA* 2012; 308: 1566–72.

46. Krajewski ML, Raghunathan K, Paluszkiewicz SM, Schermer CR, Shaw AD. Meta-analysis of high- versus low-chloride content in perioperative and critical care fluid resuscitation. *Br J Surg* 2015; 102: 24–36.

47. Wilcox CS. Regulation of renal blood flow by plasma chloride. *J Clin Invest* 1983; 71: 726–35.

48. Salomonsson M, Gonzalez E, Kornfeld M, Persson AE. The cytosolic chloride concentration in macula densa and cortical thick ascending limb cells. *Acta Physiol Scand* 1993; 147: 305–13.

49. Hashimoto S, Kawata T, Schnermann J, Koike T. Chloride channel blockade attenuates the effect of angiotensin II on tubuloglomerular feedback in WKY but not spontaneously hypertensive rats. *Kidney Blood Press Res* 2004; 27: 35–42.

50. Bullivant EM, Wilcox CS, Welch WJ. Intrarenal vasoconstriction during hyperchloremia: role of thromboxane. *Am J Physiol* 1989; 256: F152–7.

51. Zhou F, Peng ZY, Bishop JV, *et al.* Effects of fluid resuscitation with 0.9% saline versus a balanced electrolyte solution on acute kidney injury in a rat model of sepsis. *Crit Care Med* 2014; 42: e270–8.

52. Guidet B, Soni N, Della Rocca G, *et al.* A balanced view of balanced solutions. *Crit Care* 2010; 14: 325.

53. McCloughlin PD, Bell DA. Hartmann's Solution – osmolality and lactate. *Anaesth Intensive Care* 2010; 38: 1135–6.

54. Schumann R, Mandell S, Michaels MD, Klinck J, Walia A. Intraoperative fluid and pharmacologic management and the anesthesiologist's supervisory role for nontraditional technologies during liver transplantation: a survey of US academic centers. *Transplant Proc* 2013; 45: 2258–62.

55. Mukhtar A, Aboulfetouh F, Obayah G, *et al.* The safety of modern hydroxyethyl starch in living donor liver transplantation: a comparison with human albumin. *Anesth Analg* 2009; 109: 924–30.

56. Zhou ZB, Shao XX, Yang XY, *et al.* Influence of hydroxyethyl starch on renal function after orthotopic liver transplantation. *Transplant Proc* 2015; 47: 1616–19.

57. Hand WR, Whiteley JR, Epperson TI, *et al.* Hydroxyethyl starch and acute kidney injury in orthotopic liver transplantation: a single-center retrospective review. *Anesth Analg* 2015; 120: 619–26.

58. Bagshaw SM, Chawla LS. Hydroxyethyl starch for fluid resuscitation in critically ill patients. *Can J Anaesth* 2013; 60: 709–13.

59. Haase N, Perner A. Hydroxyethyl starch for resuscitation. *Curr Opin Crit Care* 2013; 19: 321–5.

60. Myburgh JA, Finfer S, Bellomo R, *et al.* Hydroxyethyl starch or saline for fluid resuscitation in intensive care. *N Engl J Med* 2012; 367: 1901–11.

61. Perner A, Haase N, Guttormsen AB, *et al.* Hydroxyethyl starch 130/0.42 versus Ringer's acetate in severe sepsis. *N Engl J Med* 2012; 367: 124–34.

62. Haase N, Perner A, Hennings LI, *et al.* Hydroxyethyl starch 130/0.38–0.45 versus crystalloid or albumin in patients with sepsis: systematic review with meta-analysis and trial sequential analysis. *BMJ* 2013; 346: 839.

63. Zarychanski R, Abou-Setta AM, Turgeon AF, *et al.* Association of hydroxyethyl starch administration with mortality and acute kidney injury in critically ill patients requiring volume resuscitation: a systematic review and meta-analysis. *JAMA* 2013; 309: 678–88.

64. Perel P, Roberts I, Ker K. Colloids versus crystalloids for fluid resuscitation in critically ill patients. *Cochrane Database Syst Rev* 2013; 28: CD000567.

65. Ma PL, Peng XX, Du B, *et al.* Sources of heterogeneity in trials reporting hydroxyethyl starch 130/0.4 or 0.42 associated excess mortality in septic patients: a systematic review and meta-regression. *Chin Med J* 2015; 128: 2374–82.

66. Dart AB, Mutter TC, Ruth CA, Taback SP. Hydroxyethyl starch (HES) versus other fluid therapies: effects on kidney function. *Cochrane Database Syst Rev* 2010; 20: CD007594.

67. Mutter TC, Ruth CA, Dart AB. Hydroxyethyl starch (HES) versus other fluid therapies: effects on kidney function. *Cochrane Database Syst Rev* 2013; 7: CD007594.

68. Niemi TT, Suojaranta-Ylinen RT, Kukkonen SI, Kuitunen AH. Gelatin and hydroxyethyl starch, but not albumin, impair hemostasis after cardiac surgery. *Anesth Analg* 2006; 102: 998–1006.

69. Konrad C, Markl T, Schuepfer G, Gerber H, Tschopp M. The effects of *in vitro* hemodilution with gelatin, hydroxyethyl starch, and lactated Ringer's solution on markers of coagulation: an analysis using SONOCLOT. *Anesth Analg* 1999; 88: 483–8.

70. Hartog CS, Reuter D, Loesche W, Hofmann M, Reinhart K. Influence of hydroxyethyl starch (HES) 130/0.4 on hemostasis as measured by viscoelastic device analysis: a systematic review. *Intensive Care Med* 2011; 37: 1725–37.

71. Casutt M, Kristoffy A, Schuepfer G, Spahn DR, Konrad C. Effects on coagulation of balanced (130/0.42) and non-balanced (130/0.4) hydroxyethyl starch or gelatin compared with balanced Ringer's solution: an *in vitro* study using two different viscoelastic coagulation tests ROTEM™ and SONOCLOT™. *Br J Anaesth* 2010; 105: 273–81.

72. Demir A, Aydınlı B, Toprak HI, *et al.* Impact of 6% starch 130/0.4 and 4% gelatin infusion on kidney function in living-donor liver transplantation. *Transplant Proc* 2015; 47: 1883–9.

73. Thomas-Rueddel DO, Vlasakov V, Reinhart K, *et al.* Safety of gelatin for volume resuscitation – a systematic review and meta-analysis. *Intensive Care Med* 2012; 38: 1134–42.

74. Victorian Consultative Council on Anaesthetic Mortality and Morbidity. 10th Report of the Victorian Consultative Council on Anaesthetic Mortality and Morbidity, May 2011, Melbourne, Victoria: Department of Health. http://www.health.vic.gov.au/vccamm/vccamm-reports.htm (accessed 21 June 2015).

75. Jacob M, Paul O, Mehringer L, *et al.* Albumin augmentation improves condition of guinea pig hearts after 4 hr of cold ischemia. *Transplantation* 2009; 87: 956–65.

76. Kozar RA, Peng Z, Zhang R, *et al.* Plasma restoration of endothelial glycocalyx in a rodent model of hemorrhagic shock. *Anesth Analg* 2011; 112: 1289–95.

77. Dawidson IJ, Sandor ZF, Coorpender J, *et al.* Intraoperative albumin administration affects the outcome of cadaver renal transplantation. *Transplantation* 1992; 53: 774–82.

78. Pockaj BA, Yang JC, Lotze MT, *et al.* A prospective randomized trial evaluating colloid versus crystalloid

resuscitation in the treatment of the vascular leak syndrome associated with interleukin-2 therapy. *J Immunother Tumor Immunol* 1994; 15: 22–8.

79. Stevens AP, Hlady V, Dull RO. Fluorescence correlation spectroscopy can probe albumin dynamics inside lung endothelial glycocalyx. *Am J Physiol Lung Cell Mol Physiol* 2007; 293: L328–35.

80. Wiedermann CJ, Joannidis M. Nephroprotective potential of human albumin infusion: a narrative review. *Gastroenterol Res Pract* 2015; 2015: 912839.

81. Finfer S. Reappraising the role of albumin for resuscitation. *Curr Opin Crit Care* 2013; 19: 315–20.

82. The SAFE Study Investigators. Saline or albumin for fluid resuscitation in patients with traumatic brain injury. *N Engl J Med* 2007; 357: 874–84.

83. Caironi P, Tognoni G, Masson S, *et al.* Albumin replacement in patients with severe sepsis or septic shock. *N Engl J Med* 2014; 370: 1412–21.

84. Patel A, Laffan MA, Waheed U, Brett SJ. Randomised trials of human albumin for adults with sepsis: systematic review and meta-analysis with trial sequential analysis of all-cause mortality. *BMJ* 2014; 349: g4561.

85. Raghunathan K, Shaw A, Nathanson B, *et al.* Association between the choice of IV crystalloid and in-hospital mortality among critically ill adults with sepsis. *Crit Care Med* 2014; 42: 1585–91.

86. Shaw AD, Perner SM, Goldstein SL, *et al.* Major complications, mortality, and resource utilization after open abdominal surgery: 0.9% saline compared to Plasma-Lyte. *Ann Surg* 2012; 255: 821–9.

87. Orbegozo Cortés D, Rayo Bonor A, Vincent JL. Isotonic crystalloid solutions: a structured review of the literature. *Br J Anaesth* 2014; 112: 968–81.

88. O'Malley CM, Frumento RJ, Hardy MA, *et al.* A randomized, double-blind comparison of lactated Ringer's solution and 0.9% NaCl during renal transplantation. *Anesth Analg* 2005; 100: 1518–24.

89. Hadimioglu N, Saadawy I, Saglam T, Ertug Z, Dinckan A. The effect of different crystalloid solutions on acid–base balance and early kidney function after kidney transplantation. *Anesth Analg* 2008; 107: 264–9.

90. Khajavi MR, Etezadi F, Moharari RS, *et al.* Effects of normal saline vs. lactated Ringer's during renal transplantation. *Ren Fail* 2008; 30: 535–9.

91. Kim SY, Huh KH, Lee JR, *et al.* Comparison of the effects of normal saline versus Plasmalyte on acid–base balance during living donor kidney transplantation using the Stewart and base excess methods. *Transplant Proc* 2013; 45: 2191–6.

92. Potura E, Lindner G, Biesenbach P, *et al.* An acetate-buffered balanced crystalloid versus 0.9% saline in patients with end-stage renal disease undergoing cadaveric renal transplantation: a prospective randomized controlled trial. *Anesth Analg* 2015; 120: 123–9.

93. Schnuelle P, Johannes van der Woude F. Perioperative fluid management in renal transplantation: a narrative review of the literature. *Transpl Int* 2006; 19: 947–59.

94. Legendre C, Thervet E, Page B, *et al.* Hydroxyethylstarch and osmotic-nephrosis-like lesions in kidney transplantation. *Lancet* 1993; 342: 248–9.

95. Cittanova ML, Leblanc I, Legendre C, *et al.* Effect of hydroxyethylstarch in brain-dead kidney donors on renal function in kidney-transplant recipients. *Lancet* 1996; 348: 1620.

96. Bernard C, Alain M, Simone C, Xavier M, Jean-Francois M. Hydroxyethylstarch and osmotic nephrosis-like lesions in kidney transplants. *Lancet* 1996; 348: 1595.

97. Baron JF. Adverse effects of colloids on renal function. In: Vincent JL, ed. *Yearbook of Intensive Care and Emergency Medicine*. Berlin: Springer, 2000: 486–93.

98. Patel MS, Niemann CU, Sally MB, *et al.* The impact of hydroxyethyl starch use in deceased organ donors on the development of delayed graft function in kidney transplant recipients: a propensity-adjusted analysis. *Am J Transplant* 2015; 15: 2152–8.

Neurosurgery

Hemanshu Prabhakar

Summary

Fluid administration is one of the basic components in the management of neurosurgical patients. Despite advances and extensive research in the field of neurosciences, there is still a debate on the ideal fluid. Issues related to adequate volume replacement and effects on the intracranial pressure persist. Studies have demonstrated the harmful effects of colloids over crystalloids. Normal saline has remained a fluid of choice, but there is now emerging evidence that it too is not free from its harmful effects. Hypertonic saline has also been accepted by many practitioners, but its use and administration requires close monitoring and vigilance. There is now growing evidence on the use of balanced solutions for neurosurgical patients. However, this evidence comes from a small number of studies. This chapter tries to briefly cover various clinical situations in neurosciences with respect to fluid administration.

Introduction

Neurosurgical patients form a special population that poses challenges to anesthetists and intensivists when it comes to fluid administration. Issues pertaining to elevated intracranial pressure (ICP) and intraoperative blood losses have to be dealt with more compositely. Earlier, it was believed that fluid intake restriction up to 1 liter daily in patients undergoing craniotomy maintains good homeostasis. Larger volumes may result in expansion of the extracellular space and may result in brain edema,[1] although it was cautioned that fluid restriction might be dangerous in patients receiving hyperoncotic fluids,

diuretics, and dexamethasone. However, the practice has changed over the years, and it is now believed that a generally restrictive fluid strategy could be dangerous as these neurosurgical patients so often receive mannitol and diuretics to prevent rise in ICP and reduce brain edema. The effect of anesthetics may be additive in causing systemic hypotension, which risks compromising the cerebral perfusion pressure (CPP), reducing the cerebral oxygenation and producing intracranial complications. These neurosurgical patients are also not excluded from the controversy over colloids versus crystalloids.[2]

This chapter deals with various neurosurgical situations in which fluid administration is vital to the overall management of the patient. Although the main focus of the chapter is on perioperative fluid management in different clinical scenarios, it also discusses the therapeutic roles of fluid aimed at reduction of ICP and improving CPP.

General principles

Crystalloids or colloids along with blood and blood products are routinely used during neurosurgical procedures. It has, in general, become common practice in neuroanesthesia to avoid fluids that are hypo-osmolar or contain glucose, because of the view that the free water produced by hypo-osmolar and glucose-containing solutions results in brain edema. Thus the fluids of choice include 0.9% normal saline and lactated Ringer's solution, both being nearly equiosmolar to normal plasma. For the purpose of achieving brain relaxation in the intraoperative period, hypertonic fluids such as mannitol and hypertonic saline are frequently used. It is by virtue of these hypertonic fluids that water is drawn from intracellular and interstitial compartments into the intravascular compartment. This results in relaxation of the brain and increased compliance. However, it is essential that the blood–brain barrier be intact for hypertonic fluids to produce their effect on the brain.[3]

In general, sufficient fluids should be administered to neurosurgical patients to maintain good cardiac output and hemodynamic stability. It is accepted that respiratory variations in arterial pressure during mechanical ventilation reflect volume status and fluid responsiveness of the patients.[4] These "dynamic" hemodynamic parameters, such as the stroke volume, arterial pulse pressure, and the variations during positive pressure mechanical ventilation, are considered accurate by many authors in predicting volume status.[5]

In the following, we describe some of the situations in neurosurgery in which fluid administration requires special considerations.

Supratentorial tumor surgery

Administration of fluids in patients undergoing craniotomy for supratentorial surgery is not only for the purpose of replacement but also to provide brain relaxation. Whereas mannitol and hypertonic saline are popular fluids used for providing brain relaxation, normal saline remains the choice of fluid for maintaining the volume status of the patients. There remains a controversy over which fluid to use for intraoperative brain relaxation: mannitol or hypertonic saline. In a recent meta-analysis, the authors found that hypertonic saline significantly reduced the risk of tense brain, but the quality of evidence was low and the findings were from a limited number of studies.[6] Normal saline remains the fluid of choice to maintain intraoperative volume status. However, amidst the controversy of crystalloid versus colloid for neurosurgical patients, a recent study by Xia and colleagues compared goal-directed crystalloid and goal-directed colloid therapy in patients undergoing craniotomy.[7] Based on a study conducted on 40 patients, the authors concluded that goal-directed hydroxyethyl starch therapy was not superior to goal-directed lactate Ringer's solution therapy for brain relaxation and cerebral metabolism. The authors found that less fluid volume was needed to maintain the target stroke volume variation in the colloid group when compared with the crystalloid group.

Subarachnoid hemorrhage

Fluid management in patients with subarachnoid hemorrhage (SAH) aims to maintain a good fluid balance and correction of hyponatremia, which accompanies the cerebral salt wasting syndrome often associated with SAH. This also formed the basis of "triple-H" therapy. The standard triple-H therapy consisted of hypervolemia, hemodilution, and hypertension. However, in a recent exploratory analysis on 413 patients enrolled in the CONSCIOUS-1 trial, the authors found that administration of colloid and maintenance of a positive fluid balance during the period of vasospasm after SAH was associated with poor outcome.[8] In a systematic review by Dankbaar and colleagues, the authors concluded that controlled studies did not offer evidence that supported the use of triple-H therapy or any of its components in improving cerebral blood flow. They also found from uncontrolled studies that "hypertension" was possibly the most effective component of triple-H therapy in increasing cerebral blood flow.[9]

When considering patients with severe brain injury, a pilot study demonstrated that balanced solutions reduced the incidence of hyperchloremic acidosis when compared with administration of chloride-rich solutions.[10] Similar findings have also been reported by Lehmann and colleagues, who found that in the management of patients with SAH, saline-based fluids resulted in a greater proportion of patients with hyperchloremic acidosis, hyperosmolality, and positive fluid balance when compared with balanced solutions.[11] Although evidence is accumulating in favor of balanced solutions rather than normal saline, it is still too early for any conclusive statement to be made in support of any type of fluid to be recommended for patients with SAH.

Pituitary surgery

Surgical procedures related to the pituitary pose challenges in terms of fluid and electrolyte imbalance, which may frequently be related. Diabetes insipidus (DI) may be observed both during the intraoperative and postoperative period. Fluid balance needs close monitoring to avoid fluid overload, electrolyte imbalance, and complications. Syndrome of inappropriate antidiuretic hormone secretion (SIADH) is another postoperative complication associated with pituitary surgery.[12] The management of these syndromes is beyond the scope of this chapter; however, it cannot be

Table 26.1 Salient differential features between diabetes insipidus (DI) and syndrome of inappropriate antidiuretic hormone secretion (SIADH)

Clinical parameters	DI	SIADH
Urine output	>30 ml/kg per hour	Decreased
Fluid balance (intravascular)	Reduced	Neutral or slightly positive
Serum osmolality	Increased	Decreased
Serum Na⁺ concentration	Increased	Decreased
Urine osmolality	Decreased	Increased (>100 mosmol/kg)
Urinary Na⁺ concentration	<15 mEq/l	>20 mEq/l
Fluid replacement	Half normal saline or 5% dextrose	Fluid restriction

overemphasized that fluid and electrolyte disturbances occur during the treatment of patients with pituitary tumors. Half normal saline and 5% dextrose are fluids of choice in cases of DI, whereas, in the case of SIADH, fluid restriction is the most appropriate treatment. A comparison of these two conditions is given in Table 26.1. It is important to check serum osmolality frequently, to guide the administration of amount and type of fluid.

Traumatic brain injury

Most of the work in the field of fluid management related to neurosurgery is probably carried out in the group of patients suffering from traumatic brain injury. The need for early restoration of intravascular fluid status and maintenance of hemodynamics predicts the outcome of these patients by preventing secondary injuries to the brain. Euvolemia is the mainstay in managing head-injured patients. Hypovolemia must be avoided and so must fluid overload, as it can worsen cerebral edema. In the popular study by the Saline versus Albumin Fluid Evaluation (SAFE) investigators, the authors found that higher rates of mortality were associated with use of albumin as resuscitating fluid when compared with saline.[13] Small-volume fluid resuscitation with hypertonic saline had been actively popularized earlier, and success was reported even in pediatric patients.[14] Soon these fluids, hypertonic saline and colloids, fell into controversy, and the debate continues. Discussing the types of fluids used for resuscitation in traumatic brain injury, Van Aken and colleagues have rightly said that it is the osmolality of an infusion solution rather than the colloid osmotic pressure that represents the key determinant in the pathogenesis of cerebral edema formation.[15] In a systematic review

on the use of crystalloids versus colloids for prehospital fluid management in traumatic brain injury, Tan and colleagues found that neither was superior to the other.[16] In general, hypotonic fluids and glucose-containing fluids have to be avoided during management of patients with traumatic brain injury. Maintaining the iso-osmolality (using fluid having osmolality around 300 mosmol/kg) is suggested when administering large amounts of fluid for resuscitation.

Spinal surgery

Surgeries on the spine may be extensive, involving many sections of the vertebral column, especially when instrumentation is planned. Massive blood loss and blood transfusions may be expected. It is important to maintain adequate fluid status without producing fluid overload, which may lead to venous congestion and at the same time compromising the blood flow and oxygenation of the spinal cord.[17] A study revealed that there was a correlation between the total amount of fluid administered and length of hospital stay and pulmonary complications.[18] With each increase of 1,000 ml of crystalloids, the odds for having a pulmonary complication increased by 30%.

Conclusion

A strategic approach in fluid management is essential for all neurosurgical procedures and perioperative management of neurological patients. Optimum fluid administration is essential for maintenance of perfusion pressures through the brain and the spinal cord. It appears logical to use isotonic crystalloids and avoid colloids as far as possible. Data supporting the use of balanced solutions are limited, although the results with their use are encouraging. Hyperglycemia or hypoglycemia must be avoided under all circumstances.

References

1. Shenkin HA, Bezier HS, Bouzarth WF. Restricted fluid intake. Rational management of the neurosurgical patient. *J Neurosurg* 1976; 45: 432–6.

2. Perel P, Roberts I, Ker K. Colloids versus crystalloids for fluid resuscitation in critically ill patients. *Cochrane Database Syst Rev* 2013; 2: CD000567.

3. Tommasino C. Fluids in the neurosurgical patient. *Anesthesiology Clin N Am* 2002; 20: 329–46.

4. Perel A, Pizov R, Cotev S. Respiratory variations in the arterial pressure during mechanical ventilation reflect volume status and fluid responsiveness. *Intensive Care Med* 2014; 40: 798–807.

5. Zimmermann M, Feibicke T, Keyl C, et al. Accuracy of stroke volume variation compared with pleth variability index to predict fluid responsiveness in mechanically ventilated patients undergoing major surgery. *Eur J Anaesthesiol* 2010; 27: 555–61.

6. Prabhakar H, Singh GP, Anand V, Kalaivani M. Mannitol versus hypertonic saline for brain relaxation in patients undergoing craniotomy. *Cochrane Database Syst Rev* 2014; 7: CD010026.

7. Xia J, He Z, Cao X, et al. The brain relaxation and cerebral metabolism in stroke-volume variation-directed fluid therapy during supratentorial tumor resection: crystalloid solution versus colloid solution. *J Neurosurg Anesthesiol* 2014; 26: 320–7.

8. Ibrahim GM, Macdonald RL. The effects of fluid balance and colloid administration on outcomes in patients with aneurysmal subarachnoid hemorrhage: a propensity score-matched analysis. *Neurocrit Care* 2013; 19: 140–9.

9. Dankbaar JW, Slooter AJ, Rinkel GJ, Schaaf IC. Effect of different components of triple-H therapy on cerebral perfusion in patients with aneurysmal subarachnoid haemorrhage: a systematic review. *Crit Care* 2010; 14: R23.

10. Roquilly A, Loutrel O, Cinotti R, et al. Balanced versus chloride-rich solutions for fluid resuscitation in brain-injured patients: a randomised double-blind pilot study. *Crit Care* 2013; 17: R77.

11. Lehmann L, Bendel S, Uehlinger DE, et al. Randomized, double-blind trial of the effect of fluid composition on electrolyte, acid–base, and fluid homeostasis in patients early after subarachnoid hemorrhage. *Neurocrit Care* 2013; 18: 5–12.

12. Verbalis JG. Management of disorders of water metabolism in patients with pituitary tumors. *Pituitary* 2002; 5: 119–32.

13. SAFE Study Investigators. Saline or albumin for fluid resuscitation in patients with traumatic brain injury. *N Engl J Med* 2007; 357: 874–84.

14. Simma B, Burger R, Falk M, Sacher P, Fanconi S. A prospective, randomized, and controlled study of fluid management in children with severe head injury: lactated Ringer's solution versus hypertonic saline. *Crit Care Med* 1998; 26: 1265–70.

15. Van Aken HK, Kampmeier TG, Ertmer C, Westphal M. Fluid resuscitation in patients with traumatic brain injury: what is a SAFE approach? *Curr Opin Anaesthesiol* 2012; 25: 563–5.

16. Tan PG, Cincotta M, Clavisi O, et al. Prehospital fluid management in traumatic brain injury. *Emerg Med Australas* 2011; 23: 665–76.

17. Zheng F, Cammisa FP, Sandhu HS, Girardi FP, Khan SN. Factors predicting hospital stay, operative time, blood loss and transfusion in patients undergoing revision posterior lumbar spine decompression, fusion, and segmental instrumentation. *Spine* 2002; 15: 818–24.

18. Siemionow K, Cywinski J, Kusza K, Lieberman I. Intraoperative fluid therapy and pulmonary complications. *Orthopedics* 2012; 35: e184–91.

Intensive care

Alena Lira and Michael R. Pinsky

Summary

Fluid infusions are an essential part of the management of the critically ill, and include maintenance fluids to replace insensible loss and resuscitation efforts to restore blood volume. This chapter is on fluid resuscitation. Fluid administration is a vital component of resuscitation therapy, with the aim being to restore cardiovascular sufficiency. Initial resuscitation aims to restore a minimal mean arterial pressure and cardiac output compatible with immediate survival. This is often associated with emergency surgery and associated life-saving procedures. Then, optimization aims to rapidly restore organ perfusion and oxygenation before irreversible ischemic damage occurs. Stabilization balances fluid infusion rate with risks of volume overload, and finally de-escalation promotes polyuria as excess interstitial fluid is refilled into the circulation. There is no apparent survival benefit of colloids over crystalloids. Hydroxyethyl starch solutions have deleterious effects in certain patient populations, for example in sepsis. Balanced salt solutions are superior to normal saline. Further fluid resuscitation should be guided by the patient's need for increased blood flow and by their volume-responsiveness.

Introduction

Fluid infusions are an essential part of the management of the critically ill patient. There is a large pool of clinical evidence to guide resuscitation and fluid administration.[1,2] Yet the actual choice for fluids across physicians, hospitals, and counties varies widely.[3] Some of these differences may be driven by economic considerations,[4] whereas others probably reflect habit and lack of familiarity with recent findings and their associated recommendations. Fluid therapy in the intensive care unit can be separated into those fluids infused in patients unable to take fluid orally as maintenance fluids, and those fluids used in resuscitation. The former can become quite complex as insensible fluid losses can vary widely in patients with burns, open wounds, peritonitis, diarrhea, and polyuria. The latter refers to use of fluid therapy as part of resuscitation from circulatory shock. This chapter focuses on fluids in resuscitation.

The resuscitative management of the critically ill patient presenting with circulatory shock can be separated into four phases: rescue, optimization, stabilization, and de-escalation.[5] Rescue or salvage focuses on achieving a minimal arterial pressure and cardiac output compatible with immediate survival. This is often associated with performing appropriate life-saving interventions to treat the underlying cause of circulatory shock. Importantly, fluid resuscitation alone may not restore arterial pressure if either systolic pump function or arterial vasodilation co-exist. In these cases, inotrope and vasopressor therapies, respectively, need to be used. Still, rapid fluid infusion, independent of fluid type, is often indicated because of the presumed decrease in effective circulating blood volume. Importantly, approximately half the patients presenting in circulatory shock are not volume-responsive.[6] Presumably, the causes of shock in those cases include severe cardiac pump dysfunction of various etiologies. Following this short rescue interval, circulatory optimization begins, focusing on restoring global tissue perfusion and oxygenation. This phase often requires invasive hemodynamic monitoring. During this phase, serial measures of arterial and either mixed venous or central venous O_2 and CO_2 levels, blood lactate, and acid–base status are often used to track resuscitation effectiveness at achieving tissue blood flow and oxygenation adequate to meet the demands of tissue aerobic metabolism. These early phases are often marked by significant violation of integrity of the vascular endothelium with significant capillary leakage, and movement of fluid from the intravascular space to the interstitium resulting in edema, manifesting as a patient who is overloaded in total body fluid yet intravascularly depleted. These phenomena occur commonly in states associated with profound inflammatory response accompanied by cytokine release, such as severe sepsis, trauma, burns, and pancreatitis. Once the circulation has been optimized to reverse tissue hypoperfusion (and there is debate as to what defines such optimization), the stabilization phase commences with the aim of minimizing organ dysfunction due to iatrogenic factors, such as overhydration, with the goal of sustaining organ-system function. The de-escalation phase aims at promoting diuresis as the initial fluid resuscitation needed in the first two phases to maintain an effective circulating blood volume is now mobilized from the tissues and interstitium and returning to the bloodstream. This results in an autoregulatory polyuric response, but occasionally during this phase diuretics or dialysis can be needed to remove this newly resorbed fluid. Within each phase, fluid infusions are usually a central aspect of therapy. However, also important is the choice of which fluid to give as part of resuscitation.

Pathophysiology of cardiovascular insufficiency

Acute cardiovascular insufficiency or shock can be caused by processes that are often grouped into four pathological processes: cardiogenic, hypovolemic, obstructive, and distributive shock.[7] Clinical history and hemodynamic monitoring often allow for both the diagnosis of the shock etiology and monitoring of response to therapy. Importantly, if systemic hypotension co-exists with circulatory shock, vital tissue hypoperfusion will also be present, presenting a medical emergency. This hypotension needs to be rapidly reversed independent of fluid management. In practice, depending on the etiology of shock, a combination of intravenous fluids and vasopressors (e.g. noradrenaline) are used to restore mean arterial pressure. Although a complete description of the diagnosis and management of circulatory shock is beyond the scope of this chapter, some specific concepts are central to fluid management.

Acute cardiogenic shock is usually not associated with volume overload. Volume overload when present in heart failure is a chronic adaptive condition, caused by reactive renal sodium and water retention. Thus, any acute cardiogenic pulmonary edema is due to pump failure (e.g. acute coronary or acute valvular insufficiency) and its resultant elevated pulmonary venous back pressure. The initial resuscitative treatment is systemic arterial afterload reduction and increased inotropy if organ flow is reduced, and fluid resuscitation to sustain adequate filling pressures in the setting of left ventricular diastolic dysfunction, while simultaneously addressing the primary cause of pump failure (e.g. coronary angioplasty for coronary thrombosis, or valvular repair in the setting of acute mitral regurgitation due to papillary muscle rupture). Importantly, heart failure with preserved left ventricular ejection fraction, otherwise known as diastolic dysfunction, occurs commonly. The decreased left ventricular diastolic compliance makes fluid management difficult, with slight decreases in filling pressure causing hypovolemia and slight increases in filling inducing cardiogenic pulmonary edema. Examples of diastolic dysfunction include cor pulmonale secondary to pulmonary hypertension or vascular obstruction and left ventricular hypertrophy due to arterial hypertension or aortic stenosis.

Hypovolemic shock is usually due to hemorrhage, although excess fluid loss from the gut or kidneys, or insensible loss during prolonged surgical interventions with open abdomen or chest, can also cause profound hypovolemia. Importantly, cellular and interstitial fluids move into the vascular space, resulting in a whole-body volume deficiency proportional to the rate of volume loss and its duration. The longer that patients are hypovolemic, the greater their overall fluid deficiency. The normal adaptive response to acute intravascular volume loss is to increase sympathetic tone, decrease fractional excretion of sodium and water from the kidneys and divert blood flow away from less vital organs such as the skin and non-exercising muscle, and eventually causing profound hypoperfusion to the liver, gut, and kidney.[8] Rapid fluid administration (20–30 ml/kg) of crystalloid solution often restores arterial pressure because these patients usually have a high vasomotor tone and normal volume-responsive hearts. If arterial pressure is not restored rapidly to ≥ 65 mmHg, in an otherwise non-hypertensive patient, then vasopressor therapy needs to be started to reach this minimal arterial pressure target.[9]

Obstructive shock (e.g. massive pulmonary embolism and cardiac tamponade) require, vasopressors to sustain mean arterial pressure and treatments directed at the primary problem (e.g. thrombolysis, pericardiocentesis). Fluid resuscitation is usually only transiently effective in restoring cardiovascular sufficiency and if acute cor pulmonale is present, it can cause further deterioration by dilating further the stressed over-distended right ventricle. In these cases, fluid management needs to be closely titrated by cardiovascular monitoring, including echocardiography and hemodynamic monitoring so as to avoid irreversible right ventricular failure.

Distributive shock is caused by dysregulation of normal autonomic control of the circulation. The classic example is septic shock, although other etiologies such as anaphylaxis and high grade spinal anesthesia, as well as frank right ventricular failure, can present with a similar picture. With non-specific vasodilation, the unstressed blood volume greatly increases, making the patient appear to be hypovolemic because the driving pressure for venous return is markedly decreased. Here initial aggressive fluid resuscitation (20–30 ml/kg) to restore venous return and central venous pressure, combined with vasopressor therapy, if needed to maintain a mean arterial pressure >65 mmHg, is often required.[9] Once initial rescue has occurred, further aggressive resuscitation to optimize organ blood flow is required, driven by end-organ function and evidence of tissue hypoperfusion. Importantly, septic shock usually has elements of hypovolemia along with loss of vasomotor tone.

As listed above, loss of vascular endothelial tight junction integrity often occurs in septic shock, leading to markedly increased plasma transudation into the interstitium, leading to secondary hypovolemic shock. Thus, the fluid requirements in severe sepsis and septic shock are often much greater than would be the case if pure vasodilation alone without associated inflammatory component were present. Indirect estimates of tissue hypoperfusion include venous O_2 saturation (SvO_2) and the veno-arterial PCO_2 gradient.[10]

Since loss of vascular endothelial integrity commonly accompanies septic shock, referring to the Starling forces principle, many clinicians prefer using colloid solutions for resuscitation in an effort to retain the infused fluid in the intravascular space. However, recent work calls into question completeness of the initial Starling forces principle.[11] In sepsis and markedly altered circulatory states, the transvascular barrier, which comprises the endothelial glycocalyx layer and endothelial basement membrane, with tight junctions between cells and extracellular matrix, is damaged.[12] When the vascular barrier is intact, transcapillary movement of fluid is unidirectional, as there is no absorption of fluid from the interstitium back to the intravascular space, and drainage of the interstitium is accomplished primarily by lymphatic clearance. Transcapillary movement is then dependent on capillary pressure. Increasing capillary pressures increases edema formation. Under the same conditions, infusion of crystalloid solutions also increases capillary pressure, but by dilution decreases oncotic pressure, thus resulting in more transcapillary movement than colloids. At subnormal capillary pressures, however, transcapillary movement nears zero; thus both crystalloids and colloids result in increase in capillary pressure, but neither sufficient to result in change in transcapillary movement. Indeed, when physicians were blinded to the infusion of solution when managing patients in septic shock, they gave the same amounts of albumin and of crystalloid solution during resuscitation,[13] suggesting that the hemodynamic response to albumin and crystalloids infusion in a septic patient is not clinically significantly different.

Although much attention focuses on the rescue and optimization phases of resuscitation, management during stabilization and de-escalation is also important, because it is in those times that the deleterious effects of fluids become most manifest, presumably because the risks of the pathological process that caused the initial illness subsides. Still, those fluid-associated risks are probably present throughout all resuscitation phases.

Choice of resuscitation fluids

Primary decisions for fluid administration include the use of colloid or crystalloid, and which specific colloid or crystalloid to use within each family. The goal of resuscitation is initially to support intravascular volume and promote tissue perfusion, while minimizing causing interstitial edema.[14] All resuscitation fluids will expand the intravascular space.[15] The available colloids include albumin, hydroxyethyl starch (HES), gelatin, and dextran. Available crystalloids include 0.9% normal saline (NS), lactated Ringer's (LR), Hartmann's solution, and several similar balanced salt solutions (e.g. Plasma-Lyte, Normo-Sol). As clinical trials expand, analysis has switched from the colloid versus crystalloid debate to which colloid or crystalloid to use.[16] It should be noted that intraoperative choices of resuscitation fluids follow different physiology, and the discussion becomes altered when one considers resuscitation fluid choices in the ICU.

Crystalloids

Crystalloids are aqueous fluids that contain low-molecular-weight crystal-forming elements (electrolytes), which easily pass through vascular endothelial membrane barriers followed by water, leading to their equilibration between the intravascular and extracellular space.[17]

Crystalloid solutions can contain a variety of inorganic cations, such as K^+, Ca^{2+}, Mg^{2+}, and organic anions such as lactate, acetate, gluconate, or bicarbonate as well as Cl^-, allowing the Na^+, Cl^-, and K^+ values to vary independent of each other. The term "normal" saline is a misnomer which was coined because its concentration 0.9% w/v is "normal" or about 3,000 mOsmol/l (or 9 g/l), not because its composition is normal or "physiological" as an electrolyte solution. Normal saline (NS) is slightly hypertonic and has equal amounts of Na^+ and Cl^-, making it both hypernatremic and hyperchloremic relative to plasma. Thus, NS infusions promote hypernatremia and hyperchloremic metabolic acidosis, resulting in renal vasoconstriction.[18] NaCl is available in varying degrees of non-hyperosmolar dilution (0.9, 0.45, and 0.225 NaCl) alone or with 5% dextrose. NaCl solutions are compatible with co-infusion of blood products. LR and other balanced salt solutions containing Ca^{2+} are not. Crystalloid alternatives to NS represent fluids more closely resembling the electrolyte composition of plasma, including LR, Hartmann's solution, Normo-Sol, and Plasma-Lyte.

Studies have compared different crystalloid solutions in resuscitation, specifically chloride-liberal (i.e. NS) versus chloride-restricted (balanced salt) solutions.[19] These results come primarily from perioperative literature including mainly trauma patients and in-patients undergoing major abdominal surgery, and suggest that the use of balanced salt solutions in some patient populations decreases mortality and the incidence of acute kidney injury (AKI) when compared with NS. Subsequent studies of 2,012 patients demonstrated a decrease in incidence of AKI and in use of renal replacement therapy (RRT) in ICU patients with implementation of chloride-restricted strategy.[19] The use of NS has long been known to be associated with increased risk of hyperchloremic metabolic acidosis,[20] but it has only recently been shown that these metabolic changes can result in decreased renal blood flow and renal cortical hypoperfusion, as demonstrated in healthy volunteers.[18] These data suggest that the choice of crystalloid solution should be guided by individual patient characteristics so as to decrease use of NS in patients in whom its metabolic profile can cause harm.

Colloids

Colloids are aqueous solutions that contain both large organic macromolecules and electrolytes. These molecules are retained within the intravascular space to a greater degree than pure crystalloids under normal conditions owing to their higher oncotic pressure.

The first colloid solution used clinically was albumin. It is available in several concentrations (4%, 5%, 20%, and 25%). The greatest barrier to its use has been its cost. Synthetic colloids, in particular starches (hydroxyethyl starch, HES), gelatins, and dextran, present more economical alternatives. Gelatins are derived from bovine gelatin, and their colloid base is protein. HES are derived from potato or maize starch, and their colloid base is large carbohydrate. Solutions of various molecular weight are available (130, 200, and 450 kilodaltons, kDa). Dextran is also a polysaccharide-based colloid, made by bacteria during ethanol fermentation. The oncotic pressure of these solutions varies depending on the molecular weight and concentration, and both hypo-oncotic (gelatins, 4% and 5% albumin) and hyperoncotic solutions (20% or 25% albumin, dextran, and HES 6% and 10%) are available. Although albumin is degraded, the hydroxylation of starches in HES and dextran results in their accumulation in skin, kidney, and liver, resulting in organ-specific clinical manifestations and potential morbidities such as AKI or liver injury.[20–22] There is significant evidence that the use of HES in the ICU increases morbidity. Its use as a resuscitation fluid increases both serum creatinine and use of RRT in clinical trials [23,24] and in meta-analyses.[25–32] These effects likely result from the tissue accumulation with prolonged or repeated use, and based on these data, HES use in Europe has recently been limited to use only for routine intraoperative volume expansion.

Colloid versus crystalloid

Although, during conditions of normal capillary pressure, colloids result in transient greater increase in intravascular volume, it has not been shown that greater intravascular volume expansion translates to improvement in mortality outcomes.

Several studies focused on albumin as the comparator colloid. The large multicenter SAFE trial [13] showed no difference in mortality with the use of albumin versus NS, with the exception of the subgroup of traumatic brain injury patients whose outcomes were worse with albumin.[13] Recent meta-analysis suggests that in sepsis, albumin is superior to other colloids and NS but not to other balanced crystalloid solutions.[30] Still, the ALBIOS trial,[33] which compared 20% albumin with crystalloid in 1,800 severe sepsis and septic shock patients, does not corroborate this finding. Albumin-treated patients had higher serum albumin level and higher mean arterial pressure, but no differences in mortality at 28 or 90 days. A *post-hoc* subgroup analysis of only septic shock patients (>1,100 of the 1,800) showed a 90-day survival benefit in the albumin-treated patients, whereas the albumin-treated group in patients without septic shock had an increased mortality.

Multiple studies (Table 27.1) [19,23–25,33,34] and recent meta-analyses (Table 27.2) [26–32] evaluated the outcomes associated with the use of synthetic colloids, showing no benefit of individual synthetic colloids over other colloids or over crystalloids. Resuscitation with HES comes to question on the basis of mortality risk as well as risk of renal insult. HES resuscitation increased 90-day mortality when compared with LR in 800 patients with severe sepsis in the 6S trial.[23] The CHEST trial [24] showed no difference in mortality between HES and NS in a 7,000-patient general ICU population, and Bagshaw and Chawla [25] showed no mortality difference in a 7,000-patient multicenter randomly controlled trial comparing HES with NS. Similarly, a study evaluating goal-directed fluid therapy in colorectal surgery showed no mortality benefit of HES over balanced crystalloid solution.[34] Three recent meta-analyses [27,28,30] support the conclusion that use of HES in resuscitation does not reduce mortality when compared with other resuscitation fluids. In contrast, the recent CRISTAL trial, which studied 2,857 patients with hypovolemic shock, sepsis, and trauma,[35] and compared administration of colloids (of which HES was the most used) with crystalloids (of which NS was the most used), showed better 90-day survival in the colloid group. Although this study has been criticized amply, its conclusions leave unresolved the question of mortality risk of HES alone, rather than all colloids. Furthermore, given that the data regarding HES vary with variables such as molecular weight in ways that are not consistent with any particular hypothesis, this suggests that confounding factors may exist that are not being accounted for. One such confounding factor may in fact be the electrolyte composition of solution used for preparation of the starches.

However, despite the fact that the mortality data on HES use in resuscitation remain equivocal, its deleterious effects on renal function, development of AKI, and increase in the need for the used RRT have been established repeatedly and unequivocally.[24–28,31,32] In conjunction, the above data have given us clearer resuscitation consensus guidelines,[14] taking into consideration pathophysiological principles associated with resuscitation context as well as individual patient characteristics.

Goal-directed therapy

Perioperative fluid management has long been dictated by a generalized formulaic approach, rather than physiological and homeostatic needs. However, both perioperative fluid under-resuscitation and over-resuscitation can have deleterious effects and lead to increased morbidity and mortality.[36]

Goal-directed fluid resuscitation therapy targets physiological goals of hemodynamic stabilization, and benefit of such approach has been shown in multiple studies and recent meta-analyses.[37,38] The main goal of such therapy is maintenance of end-organ perfusion, achieved by adequate circulating volume as well as adequate function of the cardiovascular system. All of these components can be altered by sedatives, analgesics, and body temperature. Thus, fluid resuscitation should be used to achieve these specific goals when monitoring suggests the patient to be in need of fluids and fluid responsive.[39] The counterargument is raised by studies evaluating fluid resuscitation in the septic patient. As recommended by the Surviving Sepsis Campaign,[40] aggressive initial fluid resuscitation

Table 27.1 Colloids versus crystalloids: results of large prospective multicenter randomized ICU clinical trials

Author, year, (trial), reference	n	Population	Type of fluid				Outcomes	Conclusion
			Intervention	n	Control	n		
Finfer 2004 (SAFE) [13]	6,997	ICU patients requiring fluid resuscitation	4% albumin	3,497	Saline	3,500	28-day all-cause mortality	No difference in 28-day mortality, amount of fluid infused, LOS, or MV duration
Perner 2012 (6S) [23]	798	ICU patients with severe sepsis	6% HES (130/0.42)	398	Ringer's acetate	400	90-day mortality, RRT	Increased 90-day mortality with HES, increased use of RRT with HES
Myburgh 2012 (CHEST) [24]	6,651	ICU patients	6% HES (130/0.4)	3,315	Saline	3,336	90-day mortality, AKI, RRT	No mortality difference; increased AKI and RRT use with HES
Annane 2013 (CRISTAL) [35]	2,857	ICU patients with hypovolemic shock	Colloid (gelatin, dextran, HES, 4% or 20% albumin)	1,414	Crystalloid (isotonic or hypertonic saline, Ringer's lactate)	1,443	28- and 90-day mortality; days alive without the need for RRT, MV, or vasopressors	No difference in 28-day mortality; 90-day mortality lower in colloid group
Caironi 2014 (ALBIOS) [33]	1,810	ICU patients with severe sepsis or septic shock	20% albumin and crystalloid	903	Crystalloid	907	28- and 90-day mortality; organ dysfunction, LOS	No difference in mortality or other outcomes

AKI, acute kidney injury; HES, hydroxyethyl starch; ICU, intensive care unit; LOS, length of stay (ICU or hospital); MV, mechanical ventilation; n, number of patients; RRT, renal replacement therapy.

should be used (i.e. 2–3 liters of fluid within the first few hours) and further fluids thereafter. The effectiveness of this approach was recently addressed by three large multicenter randomized clinical trials: ProCESS, ARISE, and ProMISe.[38,41,42] Importantly, all these large multicenter clinical trials showed no difference in outcome of sepsis patients treated in an emergency department with highly detailed protocols for early goal-directed therapy versus two types of usual care: one requiring a central line placement and initial large fluid infusions for resuscitation, and the other without specific guidance. Importantly, all arms of all studies received roughly the same amount of fluid therapy both in the initial few hours and over the first day. Thus, it is not clear how much fluid should be given during the acute resuscitation from septic shock, but it is not mandatory to insert a central venous catheter for that infusion, nor to monitor either central venous O_2 saturation or serial serum lactate levels, to be effective.

It is not just the volume, but mostly the ability to stabilize the critically ill patient with that volume that defines outcome.[43,44] Volume responsiveness is only one of the components of the perioperative or septic physiological state, the others being need and

responsiveness to vasoactive agents and inotropic support. Therefore, fluid resuscitation therapy should not be used in isolation, since the goals of therapy are to make the patient cardiovascular status sufficient. This approach stresses the importance of understanding pathophysiological principles and how they contribute to each individual's acute pathophysiological state.[45] The sole objective of resuscitation should be to provide perfusion adequate to sustain tissue metabolic demands and promote aerobic metabolism. Fluid therapy therefore should be used only in volume-responsive patients, and only when end-organ perfusion goals are not met. It is not sufficient to target volume administration to attainment of a high arterial pressure. In a clinical trial of vasopressor-dependent septic shock patients, improved arterial blood pressure was not associated with better outcomes.[9] Hence, determining fluid need is dependent on dynamic parameters of hemodynamic monitoring, and should be individualized to each patient.[46] In support of this conclusion, studies comparing goal-directed fluid administration strategies with fluid liberal strategies show improved outcomes with goal-directed therapies.[47,48]

Table 27.2 Colloid versus crystalloid during acute ICU resuscitation: meta-analyses and systematic reviews

Author, year, reference	Number of trials	Number of patients	Population	Intervention	Control	Outcomes	Conclusion
Thomas-Rueddel 2012 [29]	40	3,275	Adult and pediatric, primarily elective surgery, as well as ICU and ED	Gelatin	Albumin or crystalloid	Mortality, blood products administration, AKI, RRT	Unable to determine safety owing to small studies and large heterogeneity
Perel 2013 [1]	70	22,392	Cochrane review	Colloid	Crystalloid	Mortality	Colloids do not decrease mortality, HES may increase mortality
Zarychanski 2013 [27]	38	10,880	Critically ill, including sepsis, trauma, burn, hypovolemic shock	HES	Crystalloid, gelatin, albumin	Mortality, AKI, LOS, MV,	After exclusion of Boldt studies HES increased mortality, AKI, and RRT
Gattas 2013 [31]	35	10,391	Critically ill or surgical patients	6% HES 130/0.4–0.42	Other fluid	Mortality, RRT, AKI, transfusion, bleeding	Increased risk of RRT with HES
Haase 2013 [32]	9	3,456	ICU patients with sepsis	6% HES 130/0.38–0.45	Crystalloid or albumin	All cause mortality, RRT, AKI, bleeding, and transfusion, adverse effects as defined in the individual studies	HES increased RRT, increased blood transfusion, increased incidence of adverse effects
Gillies 2013 [16]	19	1,567	Surgical patients	6% HES	Other colloid or crystalloid	Postoperative in hospital mortality, AKI, RRT	No difference in measured outcomes, no demonstrable benefit of HES
Mutter 2013 [26]	42	11,399	Cochrane review	HE	Other fluid	Renal function	Increased need for RRT with all HES products in all patient populations
Serpa Neto 2014 [28]	10	4,624	Septic patients	HES	Crystalloid	28- and 90-day mortality, AKI, RRT, transfusion, LOS, fluid intake	HES shows increase in AKI, RRT, need for RBC transfusion, and 90-day mortality

AKI, acute kidney injury; ED, emergency department; HES, hydroxyethyl starch; ICU, intensive care unit; LOS, length of stay (ICU or hospital); MV, mechanical ventilation; RBC, red blood cell; RRT, renal replacement therapy.

References

1. Perel P, Roberts I, Ker K. Colloids versus crystalloids for fluid resuscitation in critically ill patients. *Cochrane Database Syst Rev* 2013; 2: CD000567.

2. Reinhart K, Perner A, Sprung CL, *et al.* Consensus statement of the ESICM task force on colloid volume therapy in critically ill patients. *Intensive Care Med* 2012; 38: 368–83.

3. Finfer S, Bette L, Colman T, *et al.* Resuscitation fluid use in critically ill adults: an international cross sectional study in 391 intensive care units. *Crit Care* 2010; 14: R185.

4. Singer M. Management of fluid balance: a European perspective. *Curr Opin Anaesthesiol* 2012; 25: 96–101.

5. Vincent JL, De Backer D. Circulatory shock. *N Engl J Med* 2013; 369: 1726–34.

6. Michard F, Teboul JL. Predicting fluid responsiveness in ICU patients: a critical analysis of the evidence. *Chest* 2002; 121: 2000–8.

7. Weil MH, Shubin H. Proposed reclassification of shock states with special reference to distributive defects. *Adv Exp Med Biol* 1971; 23: 13–23.

8. Schlichtig R, Kramer D, Pinsky MR. Flow redistribution during progressive hemorrhage is a determinant of critical O_2 delivery. *J Appl Physiol* 1991; 70: 169–78.

9. Asfar P, Meziani F, Hamel JF, *et al.* High versus low blood pressure target in patients with septic shock. *N Engl J Med* 2014; 370: 1583–93.

10. Vallet B, Pinsky MR, Cecconi M. Resuscitation of patients with septic shock: please "Mind the Gap"! *Intensive Care Med* 2013; 39: 1653–5.

11. Woodcock TE, Woodcock TM. Revised Starling equation and the glycocalyx model of transvascular fluid exchange: an improved paradigm for prescribing intravenous fluid therapy. *Br J Anaesth* 2012; 108: 384–94.

12. Clough G. Relationship between microvascular permeability and ultrastructure. *Prog Biophys Mol Biol* 1991; 55: 47–69.

13. Finfer S, Bellomo R, Boyce N, *et al.* A comparison of albumin and saline for fluid resuscitation in the intensive care unit. *N Engl J Med* 2004; 350: 2247–56.

14. Cecconi M, De Backer D, Antonelli M, *et al.* Consensus on circulatory shock and hemodynamic monitoring, Task Force of the European Society of Intensive Care Medicine. *Intensive Care Med* 2014; 49: 1795–815.

15. Severs D, Hoorn EJ, Rookmaaker MB. A critical appraisal of intravenous fluids: from the physiological basis to clinical evidence. *Nephrol Dial Transplant* 2014; 10: 1–10.

16. Gillies MA, Habicher M, Jhanji S, *et al.* Incidence of postoperative death and acute kidney injury associated with i.v. 6% hydroxyethyl starch use: systematic review and meta-analysis. *Br J Anaesth* 2013; 112: 25–34.

17. Myburgh JA, Mythen MG. Resuscitation fluids. *N Engl J Med* 2013; 369: 1243–51.

18. Chowdhury AH, Cox EF, Francis ST, *et al.* A randomized, controlled, double-blind crossover study on the effects of 2-L infusion of 0.9% saline and Plasma-Lyte(R) 148 on renal blood flow velocity and renal cortical tissue perfusion in healthy volunteers. *Ann Surg* 2012; 256: 18–24.

19. Yunos NM, Bellomo R, Hegarty C, *et al.* Association between a chloride liberal versus chloride restrictive intravenous fluid administration strategy and kidney injury in critically ill adults. *JAMA* 2012; 308: 1566–72.

20. Wiedermann CJ, Joannidis M. Accumulation of hydroxyethyl starch in human and animal tissues: a systematic review. *Intensive Care Med* 2014; 40: 160–70.

21. Christidis C, Mal F, Ramos J, *et al.* Worsening of hepatic dysfunction as a consequence of repeated hydroxyethyl starch infusion. *J Hepatol* 2001; 35: 726–32.

22. Bork K. Pruritus precipitated by hydroxyethyl starch: a review. *Br J Dermatol* 2005; 152: 3–12.

23. Perner A, Haase N, Guttormsen AB, *et al.* Hydroxyethyl starch 130/0.42 versus Ringer's acetate in severe sepsis. *N Engl J Med* 2012; 367: 124–34.

24. Myburgh JA, Finfer S, Bellomo R, *et al.* Hydroxyethyl starch or saline for fluid resuscitation in intensive care. *N Engl J Med* 2012; 367: 1901–11.

25. Bagshaw SM, Chawla LS. Hydroxyethyl starch for fluid resuscitation in critically ill patients. *Can J Anaesth* 2013; 60: 709–13.

26. Mutter TC, Ruth CA, Dart AB. Hydroxyethyl starch versus other fluid therapies: effect on kidney function. *Cochrane Database Syst Rev* 2013; 7: CD007594.

27. Zarychanski R, Abou-Setta AM, Turgeon AF, *et al.* Association of hydroxyethyl starch administration with mortality and acute kidney injury in critically ill patients requiring volume resuscitation: a systematic review and meta-analysis. *JAMA* 2013; 309: 678–88.

28. Serpa Neto A, Veelo D, Peireira VG, *et al.* Fluid resuscitation with hydroxyethyl starches in patients with sepsis associated with an increased incidence of acute kidney injury and use of renal replacement therapy: a systematic review and meta-analysis of the literature. *J Crit Care* 2014; 29: 185e1–7.

29. Thomas-Rueddel DO, Vlasakov V, Reinhart K, *et al.* Safety of gelatin for volume resuscitation: a systematic review and meta-analysis. *Intensive Care Med* 2012; 38: 1134–42.

30. Rochwerg B, Alhazzani W, Sindi A, *et al.* Fluid resuscitation in sepsis: a systematic review and network meta-analysis. *Ann Intern Med* 2014; 161: 347–55.

31. Gattas JD, Dan A, Myburgh J, *et al.* Fluid resuscitation with 6% hydroxyethyl starch (130/0.4 and 130/0.42) in acutely ill patients: systematic review of effects on mortality and treatment with renal replacement therapy. *Intensive Care Med* 2013; 39: 558–68.

32. Haase N, Perner A, Hennings LI, *et al.* Hydroxyethyl starch 130/0.38–0.45 versus crystalloid or albumin in patients with sepsis: systematic review with meta-analysis and trial sequential analysis. *BMJ* 2013; 346: f839.

33. Caironi P, Tognoni G, Masson S, *et al.* Albumin replacement in patients with severe sepsis or septic shock. *N Engl J Med* 2014; 370: 1412–21.

34. SAFE Study Investigators. Impact of albumin compared to saline on organ function and mortality of patients with severe sepsis. *Intensive Care Med* 2011; 37: 86–96.

35. Annane D, Siami S, Jaber S, *et al.* Effects of fluid resuscitation with colloids vs. crystalloids on mortality in critically ill patients presenting with hypovolemic shock: the CRISTAL trial. *JAMA* 2013; 310: 1809–17.

36. Boyd JH, Forbes J, Nakada T, *et al.* Fluid resuscitation in septic shock: a positive fluid balance and elevated central venous pressure are associated with increased mortality. *Crit Care Med* 2011; 39: 259–65.

37. Hamilton MA, Cecconi M, Rhodes A. A systematic review and meta-analysis on the use of preemptive hemodynamic intervention to improve postoperative outcomes in moderate and high-risk surgical patients. *Anesth Analg* 2011; 112: 1392–402.

38. The ARISE Investigators and the ANZICS Clinical Trials Group. Goal-directed resuscitation for patients with early septic shock. *N Engl J Med* 2014; 371: 1496–506.

39. Marik PE, Cavalazzi R, Vasu T. Stroke volume variations and fluid responsiveness. A systematic review of literature. *Crit Care Med* 2009; 37: 2642–7.

40. Dellinger RP, Levy MM, Rhodes A, *et al.* The Surviving Sepsis Campaign Guidelines Committee including The Pediatric Subgroup. Surviving Sepsis Campaign: international guidelines for management of severe sepsis and septic shock, 2012. *Intensive Care Med* 2013; 39: 165–228.

41. Yealy DM, Kellum JA, Huang DT, *et al.* A randomized trial of protocol-based care for early septic shock. *N Engl J Med* 2014; 370: 1683–93.

42. Mouncey PR, Osborn TM, Power GS, *et al.* Trial of early, goal-directed resuscitation for septic shock. *N Engl J Med* 2015; 372: 1301–11.

43. Marik PE, Lemson J. Fluid responsiveness: an evolution of our understanding. *Br J Anaesth* 2014; 112: 617–20.

44. Bartels K, Thiele RH, Gan TJ. Rational fluid management in today's ICU. *Crit Care* 2013; 17: S6.

45. Cecconi M, Corredor C, Arulkumaran N, *et al.* Clinical review: goal-directed therapy-what is the evidence in surgical patients? The effect on different risk groups. *Crit Care* 2013; 17: 209.

46. Marik PE, Monnet X, Teboul JL. Hemodynamic parameters to guide fluid therapy. *Ann Intensive Care* 2011; 1: 1.

47. Noblett SE, Snowden CP, Shenton BK, *et al.* Randomized clinical trial assessing the effect of Doppler-optimized fluid management on outcome after elective colorectal resection. *Br J Surg* 2006; 93: 1069–76.

48. Feldheiser A, Pavlova V, Bonomo T, *et al.* Balanced crystalloid compared with balanced colloid solution using a goal-directed haemodynamic algorithm. *Br J Anaesth* 2013; 110: 231–40.

Severe sepsis and septic shock

28

Palle Toft and Else Tønnesen

Summary

Sepsis is a systemic disorder with a protean clinical picture and a complex pathogenesis characterized by the release of both pro- and anti-inflammatory elements. The organ dysfunction and organ failure occurring in the early phase of severe sepsis are believed to result from an excessive inflammatory response. Degradation or destruction of the glycocalyx layer causes transudation of fluid from the vascular space into extravascular tissue. Such capillary leakage makes the patient hypovolemic and promotes a generalized edema in the lungs, heart, gut, brain, and other tissues, which impairs organ function and sometimes causes excessive weight gain. Early, aggressive goal-directed therapy (EGDT) based on the protocol by Rivers et al.[1] from 2001 stresses that adequate volume replacement is a cornerstone in management, as restoration of flow is a key component in avoiding tissue ischemia or reperfusion injury. It is the speed with which septic patients are fluid resuscitated that makes the difference. Deep general anesthesia should be avoided and noradrenaline might be needed to prevent circulatory shock before sufficient amounts of fluid have been administered.

Survival improves from EGDT only if optimization is instituted before organ failure is manifested. Most patients require continuous aggressive fluid resuscitation during the first 24 hours of management. In the later course of the disease, between 2 and 7 days, a more restricted fluid management strategy should be instituted. Not all patients who are "fluid responders" should automatically receive fluids.*

Patients subjected to infections, trauma, burns, or surgery are characterized by *systemic inflammatory response syndrome* (SIRS) or *sepsis* in cases with suspected or documented infection. These complex syndromes are defined as the presence of at least two of the following criteria:

- Temperature <36 °C or >38 °C
- Heart rate >90 beats/min
- Respiratory rate >20 breaths/min or $PaCO_2$ <4.3 kPa (32 mmHg)
- White blood cell count >12,000/mm^3 or <4,000/mm^3 or 10% immature (band) forms

Severe sepsis is defined as sepsis associated with hypoperfusion or dysfunction of at least one organ system, and *septic shock* is associated with acute circulatory failure defined as persistent hypotension despite "adequate" volume resuscitation.[2] Severe sepsis and septic shock carry mortality rates of 30% and 40–70%, respectively.

Sepsis is a systemic disorder with a protean clinical picture and a complex pathogenesis characterized by the release of both pro- and anti-inflammatory elements. The organ dysfunction and organ failure occurring in the early phase of severe sepsis is believed to result from an excessive inflammatory response.

The critically ill patient

The development of septic complications is usually prolonged, taking days to develop into organ dysfunction and, in the worst cases, multi-organ dysfunction

---

* Summary compiled by the Editor.

and septic shock. The acute phase is different from the prolonged phase with respect to the inflammatory and hemodynamic response.

In severe sepsis and septic shock, all organ systems are affected, although acute kidney injury is especially frequent. The etiology of organ dysfunction in response to critical illness is multifactorial and may include hypoperfusion, ischemia-reperfusion injuries, a dysfunctional immune system, and coagulopathies. The microcirculation is compromised by massive vasodilatation, making the clinical picture of the patient with septic shock (*warm* shock) quite different from the patient with cardiogenic or hemorrhagic shock (*cold* shock).

The vascular endothelial wall is covered with a biologically active barrier, 0.5 to 1 μm thick, called the endothelial glycocalyx. It is composed of proteins and polysaccharides, and its constituents are shed into the circulation in conditions when the glycocalyx is degraded.

Soluble components of the plasma, especially albumin, are trapped in the glycocalyx, and it has been estimated that up to 25% of the plasma volume is trapped as a non-circulating part of the intravascular space. An intact endothelial glycocalyx is necessary for the integrity of the microcirculation. Degradation or destruction of the glycocalyx is manifested as capillary leakage, which is central in the pathogenesis of sepsis. Capillary leakage is manifested as transudation of fluid from the vascular space into extravascular tissue. It contributes to a generalized edema in the lungs, heart, gut, brain, and other tissues, and it contributes to the impairment of organ function and sometimes to excessive weight gain. Capillary leakage may also make the patient hypovolemic.

Critically ill patients are often elderly with significant comorbidity, with the presence of disorders such as ischemic heart disease, diabetes, cancer, and alcohol-related organ dysfunction in addition to the acute illness.

Another complicating factor that influences fluid and electrolyte therapy is acute renal dysfunction/failure, meaning that fluid therapy must be restricted until renal replacement therapy has been initiated. Ongoing intravenous treatments in the intensive care unit (ICU) comprise nutrition, sedatives, analgesics, vasoactive drugs, and insulin infusion – all contributing to a considerable fluid load, which must be included in the calculation of intraoperative fluid management.

The principles of perioperative fluid therapy have traditionally been based on the assumption that preoperative deficit, maintenance, and blood loss require replacement by crystalloids or colloids. However, the principles of fluid therapy used for patients undergoing elective surgery are not applicable in critically ill patients.

Anesthesia for septic patients

Surgery performed on critically ill septic patients is often acute, and fluid therapy is fundamentally different from fluid treatment in relation to elective surgery.[3,4] Perioperative fluid therapy in patients with severe sepsis and septic shock must follow the principles applied for critically ill patients in general.

Deep general anesthesia should also be avoided in patients with severe sepsis or septic shock. Patients are often more or less sedated to tolerate ventilator therapy, and even without sedation, they may not be fully awake, owing to septic encephalopathy. Even a smaller amount of anesthetic agents may have a detrimental effect on their hemodynamic stability. Postoperative patient-controlled analgesia may be an approach in some septic patients. Reducing the amount of postoperative sedation improves fluid balance, increases diuresis, and improves renal function.[5]

Early versus late septic shock

The fluid therapy used in septic patients undergoing surgery depends on where in the course of the septic disease the patient is. Moreover, fluid management in the early course of sepsis or septic shock should be modified if organ failure has already developed.

As described by Cuthbertson nearly 60 years ago,[6] the inflammatory response in the very early ebb-phase is characterized by low cardiac output, reduced tissue perfusion, and profound peripheral vasoconstriction. According to Cuthbertson, this phase is followed by a flow phase characterized by increased cardiac output and normalization of tissue perfusion.

Early fluid resuscitation

During the initial phase of sepsis or inflammation, adequate volume replacement is a cornerstone in management as restoration of flow is a key component in avoiding tissue ischemia or reperfusion injury. In 2001, Rivers *et al.* [1] performed a randomized study and described the beneficial effect of early, aggressive, goal-directed therapy (EGDT) in the acute treatment of severe sepsis and septic shock.

The principles of EGDT

- Within the first 6 hours after admission to hospital, patients with severe sepsis or septic shock were hemodynamically optimized. All the patients were intubated, mechanically ventilated, and had a central venous line and arterial catheter.
- When the central venous pressure (CVP) was <8 mmHg, crystalloids and colloids were infused to achieve CVP between 8 and 12 mmHg. The Surviving Sepsis Campaign recommends an even higher target CVP of 12–15 mmHg.
- If the mean arterial pressure (MAP) was >65 mmHg, fluid resuscitation alone would be enough while patients with MAP <65 mmHg were also treated with noradrenaline to obtain MAP >65 mmHg.
- The central venous oxygen saturation (ScvO$_2$) was monitored. If ScvO$_2$ was <70%, a blood transfusion was initiated until a hematocrit >30% was achieved. In cases where the ScvO$_2$ was below 70%, inotropic agents were given.

A clinically important finding was that the beneficial effect of EGDT was not related to the total amount of fluid given. It was the *speed* with which the septic patients were fluid resuscitated that made the difference. The importance of rapid and early fluid resuscitation has also been confirmed in pediatric septic shock cases. Hence, early fluid optimization, before organ failure is manifested, is of major importance.

The goal-directed approach to stabilization of the hemodynamics resulted in a mortality of only 30.5% in the intervention group compared with 46% in the control group receiving "standard therapy." The EGDT also resulted in a lower serum lactate concentration, a smaller base deficit, higher pH, and a significantly lower APACHE II score.

Rivers' study has been the subject of much discussion, but there is no doubt that implementation of the principles of EGDT has improved and optimized the acute treatment of patients with severe sepsis and septic shock. Owing to better treatment of the control group influenced by EGDT, the striking beneficial effect demonstrated in Rivers' study cannot be reproduced today.[7]

Fluid resuscitation of a patient with severe sepsis and septic shock must start as early as possible. The tissue perfusion will suffer for every minute or hour that the resuscitation is delayed, and cellular dysfunction and cell death will develop. It is unclear when the transition from reversible to irreversible cell dysfunction occurs, but it might be different in various tissues.

Other studies of EGDT

In 2002, Kern and Shoemaker reviewed 21 randomized clinical trials that described hemodynamic optimization in acutely ill patients.[8] They included different types of high-risk patients: those undergoing elective surgery and trauma and septic patients. *Early* optimization was defined as that occurring 8–12 hours postoperatively or before organ failure, and *late* was defined as later than 12 hours after surgery, 24 hours after injury, or after organ failure had developed.

There was a significantly lower mortality in those cases where early optimization was completed before organ failure occurred.

Survival did not improve significantly in six of the studies where optimization was instituted after organ failure was manifested. A confidential inquiry was made concerning the quality of care before admission to intensive care in the group of patients where care was assessed as suboptimal. This inquiry showed that circulatory support and monitoring most often were suboptimal.

Results from animal studies show that, in early septic shock, autoregulation of the microcirculatory blood flow is largely intact.[9] Videomicroscopy of the sublingual microcirculation of humans has shown that increased microcirculatory flow during resuscitation is associated with reduced organ failure without substantial differences in global hemodynamics.[10] However, it remains to be clarified whether the microcirculatory changes demonstrated sublingually are accompanied by similar changes at organ level.

While aggressive fluid resuscitation is beneficial early in the course of sepsis, it is of minor importance when organ dysfunction has occurred. It has been demonstrated that early fluid resuscitation in septic patients reduces the secretion of pro- and anti-inflammatory cytokines and the amount of apoptotic biomarker.[11]

Later course of sepsis

The EGDT principles focus on the initial fluid resuscitation within the first 6 hours. Severe sepsis and septic shock are, however, characterized by venous

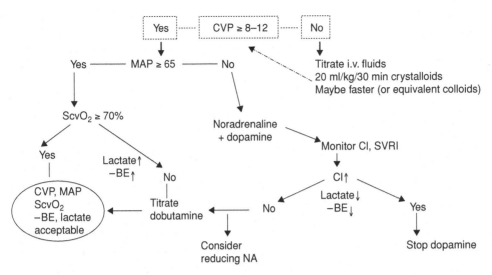

Figure 28.1 Fluid therapy in septic shock. BE, base excess; CI, cardiac index; CVP, central venous pressure; MAP, mean arterial pressure; NA, noradrenaline; ScvO$_2$, central venous oxygen saturation; SVRI, systemic vascular resistance index.

dilation and ongoing capillary leakage. Therefore, most patients require continuous aggressive fluid resuscitation during the first 24 hours of management (Figure 28.1). In most septic patients, early resuscitation transforms a hypovolemic and hypodynamic circulation into a hyperdynamic, low-resistance circulation where oxygen delivery/transport is normal or high, at least in the macrocirculation.

In the course of sepsis, unnecessary fluid might aggravate degradation of the endothelial glycocalyx and thus contribute to edema due to capillary leakage and not enhance perfusion. A continuous positive fluid balance lasting for days is a significant predictor of mortality.[12] However, it is possible that a positive fluid balance is only a marker of the severity of illness.

In the "fluids and catheter treatment trial," 1,000 patients with acute lung injury or acute respiratory distress syndrome were randomized to a conservative fluid administration strategy compared with a more liberal strategy.[13] The trial lasted for 7 days, and the liberal group was brought into a positive fluid balance of 1 liter/day. In the conservative group, the fluid balance was nearly 0. The conservative strategy improved oxygenation, increased the number of ventilator-free days, and reduced the length of stay in the ICU. Patients were relatively young (average about 50 years), and those with overt renal failure were excluded from the trial. However, fluid therapy in this trial was started on average 43 hours after admission to the ICU and 24 hours after the

establishment of acute lung injury. These patients were, in other words, already optimized with early fluid administration.

This study underlines that what is beneficial in the early course of sepsis might not be beneficial later. In the later course of the disease, between 2 and 7 days, a more restricted fluid management strategy should be instituted. Not all critically ill patients who are fluid responders should automatically receive fluids. The intensivist should always consider whether the fluid bolus would be beneficial for the patients. Thus, it is prudent to treat patients with severe sepsis or septic shock with EGDT during the first 6–24 hours only.

Crystalloids versus colloids

The "Surviving Sepsis Campaign" recommends administering crystalloids as the initial fluid.[14] Subgroup analysis of meta-analyses has demonstrated that crystalloid resuscitation was associated with a lower mortality in trauma patients. In contrast, albumin resuscitation in some subgroup analysis has been associated with a better outcome in patients with septic shock. This tendency was observed in two large prospective randomized trials.[15,16]

Fluid resuscitation with albumin results in a greater and faster increase in cardiac filling and cardiac output than crystalloid resuscitation in septic hypovolemia. Albumin remains in circulation for a longer time than the crystalloids, and crystalloids require that more fluid is used in a patient to attain the same goals, whereby more edema might develop.[17] Hydroxy-ethyl starch and dextran are no longer used in critically ill septic patients, owing to increased morbidity and mortality.[18]

The Surviving Sepsis Campaign recommends initial fluid resuscitation with crystalloid and consideration of the addition of albumin in patients who continue to require substantial amount of crystalloids to maintain adequate mean arterial pressure.[14]

Blood transfusions

Anemia is a common problem in critically ill patients. Harmful effects of anemia include increased risk of cardiac-related morbidity and mortality as well as a general decrease in oxygen-carrying capacity.[19].

The consequences of anemia may be deleterious in this population because critical illness is often associated with increased metabolic demands. A surgical procedure will accentuate metabolic demands, and intraoperative blood loss reduces oxygen delivery. Therefore, an optimal hemoglobin level must be maintained. However, the criteria for an optimal hemoglobin level in critical illness are not clearly defined. A Canadian study indicated that a liberal use of transfusions (100–120 g/l) might result in increased hospital mortality rates compared with a more restrictive transfusion regime (70–90 g/l).[20] A later observational multicenter study confirmed that there is an association between transfusions and diminished organ function as well as between transfusions and mortality.[21] A recent study showed no effect on mortality and morbidity between patients receiving liberal (9 g/l) versus restricted transfusion regimen (70 g/l).[22] There seems to be a very delicate balance between the harmful effects of anemia on organ function and the harmful effects of transfusion. In the future, treatment with blood transfusion should probably be individualized.

Fluid responsiveness in septic shock

It is important that the critically ill patient is hemodynamically stable and normovolemic before being transported from the ICU or emergency room to the operation theater. This is not always possible in, for example, patients with ongoing and uncontrolled bleeding.

Patients with severe sepsis or septic shock are often resuscitated with *fluid challenges*. In this process, a large amount of fluid is administered under close

monitoring to evaluate the hemodynamic response. The "Surviving Sepsis Campaign" recommends an initial fluid challenge of 20 ml/kg of crystalloids administered over 30 min. If the patient is in severe shock, a more rapid infusion might be necessary. Repeated fluid challenges are performed as long as the patient improves hemodynamically. Clinical signs of hemodynamic improvement might be increasing arterial pressure, decreasing heart rate, increasing urine output, or improvement in capillary refill time.

Adequate fluid resuscitation cannot, however, be based only on normalization of vital signs. Traditionally, physicians have used static hemodynamic values such as CVP or the pulmonary artery occlusion pressure (PAOP) to evaluate whether the patient would benefit from further fluid challenge. There is increasing evidence that estimates of intravascular volume based on CVP or PAOP do not reliably predict the patient's response to a fluid challenge [12,23].

In addition to the Swan–Ganz (SG) catheter, cardiac output can be measured by pulse contour analysis. This method also estimates the global end-diastolic volume and intrathoracic blood volume. These new static preload parameters correlate better with cardiac index than the traditionally measured CVP. However, static preload measurements are inaccurate and must be supplemented with more dynamic measures.

Functional hemodynamic parameters, such as systolic pressure variation (SPV), pulse pressure variation (PPV), and passive leg raising are more sensitive indices of fluid responsiveness. SPV and PPV can be used only in sedated, mechanically ventilated patients with rather large tidal volumes. With more invasive monitoring, cardiac output can be measured and used as an adjunct when evaluating the response to a fluid challenge. Cardiac output measurement may also help to identify the minority of patients who have a low cardiac output despite adequate fluid resuscitation.

After fluid resuscitation, septic shock is often hyperdynamic with high cardiac output, low systemic vascular resistance (SVR), and reduced MAP. This hyperdynamic state is, however, often confined to the large vessels, whereas the regional microcirculation is compromised.

As there is no perfect hemodynamic parameter, the patient's response to fluid administration must be evaluated together with other parameters, such as the $ScvO_2$. A multimodal monitoring approach has to be instituted. The goal of fluid resuscitation in the study by Rivers *et al.* [1] was a $ScvO_2$ greater than 70%. If a

SG catheter was used, a mixed venous oxygen saturation (SvO_2) greater than 65% could be the goal.

SvO_2 has been considered to be the gold standard to monitor whole-body perfusion. This might be true in hemorrhagic shock, but in septic shock the SvO_2 is often normal or even supernormal owing to reduced oxygen extraction at the microvascular level. In contrast, serum lactate is a useful measure of anaerobic metabolism, and base excess is often negative if the organs are not adequately perfused.[24] Monitoring serum lactate as well as the base excess improves the overall evaluation of the patient's response to fluid challenge.

Treatment with vasopressors and inotropic agents

The "Surviving Sepsis Campaign" recommends that noradrenaline is used as the initial vasopressor agent.[14] A new, large multicenter study was not able to show any significant difference in mortality in septic patients treated with noradrenaline compared with dopamine, although those treated with dopamine had more arrhythmic events.[25] There has also been some concern that the use of noradrenaline in patients who are inadequately fluid resuscitated would increase blood pressure because of vasoconstriction, and thereby reduce the blood flow to the organs.

It might be necessary to use noradrenaline to restore MAP during the early course of septic shock, before the patient is adequately fluid resuscitated. Some caution is recommended as animal studies have shown that noradrenaline-masked hypovolemia is associated not only with renal failure but also with cardiomyocyte necrosis.[26]

Echocardiography cannot provide continuous hemodynamic data but can be used initially to determine the type of shock or cardiac function when septic shock is evident. When the patient with septic shock does not respond to initial therapy, they should be monitored with a SG catheter or pulse contour analysis. Then cardiac output can be measured and SVR calculated. When this monitoring is instituted, the vasoconstrictor noradrenaline should be used to increase MAP guided by SVR, whereas dobutamine can be used to increase cardiac output, if necessary. When adequately fluid-resuscitated, the septic patient most often has hyperdynamic shock with high cardiac output and low SVR. Only in a minority of fluid-resuscitated septic patients is it necessary to administer dobutamine to increase cardiac output. In the study by Rivers et al. 15.4% of the patients who received EGDT were treated with dobutamine.[1] By administration of noradrenaline, the low SVR can be increased and a MAP ≥65 mmHg obtained. The goal is, however, not to normalize SVR.

Adrenaline is not used very often in septic patients as it can impair the splanchnic circulation in septic shock. Compared with noradrenaline there was no difference in mortality, but adrenaline was associated with more adverse effects.[27]

Key messages

Surgery performed on critically ill septic patients is often acute, and fluid therapy is fundamentally different from fluid treatment in relation to elective surgery.

Perioperative fluid therapy in patients with severe sepsis and septic shock must follow the principles applied for critically ill patients in general.

In septic patients, the institution of fluid therapy at an early stage is of vital importance to the outcome.

Early resuscitation might transform a hypovolemic and hypodynamic circulation into a hyperdynamic, low-resistance circulation where oxygen delivery/transport is normal or high.

The Surviving Sepsis Campaign recommends the combined use of noradrenaline as the first choice vasopressor to maintain MAP ≥65 mmHg, even when the patient is not yet adequately monitored.

When full monitoring is instituted, noradrenaline can be used to increase MAP guided by SVR, whereas dobutamine can be used to increase cardiac output, if necessary.

If the patient is anesthetized, the anesthetic agents will nearly always induce some vasodilatation, and it might be necessary to increase an ongoing noradrenaline infusion during the anesthesia, but the anesthetist should always be aware of the danger of noradrenaline-masked hypovolemia.

References

1. Rivers E, Nguyen B, Havstad S, et al. Early goal-directed therapy in the treatment of severe sepsis and septic shock. N Engl J Med 2001; 345: 1368–77.
2. Levy MM, Fink MP, Marshall JC, et al. 2001 SCCM/ESICM/ACCP/ATS/SIS International Sepsis Definitions Conference. Crit Care Med 2003; 31: 1250–6.

3. Brandstrup B, Tonnesen H, Beier-Holgersen R, *et al.* Effects of intravenous fluid restriction on postoperative complications: comparison of two perioperative fluid regimens: a randomized assessor-blinded multicenter trial. *Ann Surg* 2003; 238: 641–8.

4. Joshi GP. Intraoperative fluid restriction improves outcome after major elective gastrointestinal surgery. *Anesth Analg* 2005; 101: 601–5.

5. Strom T, Martinussen T, Toft P. A protocol of no sedation for critically ill patients receiving mechanical ventilation: a randomised trial. *Lancet* 2010; 375: 475–80.

6. Cuthbertson DP. Post-shock metabolic response. *Lancet* 1942; i: 433–47.

7. Mouncey PR, Osborn TM, Power S, *et al.* Trial of early goal-directed resuscitation for septic shock. *N Engl J Med* 2015; 372: 1301–11.

8. Kern JW, Shoemaker WC. Meta-analysis of hemodynamic optimization in high-risk patients. *Crit Care Med* 2002; 30: 1686–92.

9. Hiltebrand LB, Krejci V, tenHoevel ME, Banic A, Sigurdsson GH. Redistribution of microcirculatory blood flow within the intestinal wall during sepsis and general anesthesia. *Anesthesiology* 2003; 98: 658–69.

10. Trzeciak S, McCoy JV, Phillip DR, *et al.* Early increases in microcirculatory perfusion during protocol-directed resuscitation are associated with reduced multi-organ failure at 24 hours in patients with sepsis. *Intensive Care Med* 2008; 34: 2210–17.

11. Rivers EP, Kruse JA, Jacobsen G, *et al.* The influence of early hemodynamic optimization on biomarker patterns of severe sepsis and septic shock. *Crit Care Med* 2007; 35: 2016–24.

12. Durairaj L, Schmidt GA. Fluid therapy in resuscitated sepsis: less is more. *Chest* 2008; 133: 252–63.

13. Wiedemann HP, Wheeler AP, Bernard GR, *et al.* Comparison of two fluid-management strategies in acute lung injury. *N Engl J Med* 2006; 354: 2564–75.

14. Dellinger RP, Levy MM, Rhodes, *et al.* The Surviving Sepsis Campaign Guidelines Committee including The Pediatric Subgroup. Surviving Sepsis Campaign: international guidelines for management of severe sepsis and septic shock: 2012. *Crit Care Med* 2013; 41: 580–637.

15. Velanovich V. Crystalloid versus colloid fluid resuscitation: a meta-analysis of mortality. *Surgery* 1989; 105: 65–71.

16. Finfer S, Bellomo R, Boyce N, *et al.* A comparison of albumin and saline for fluid resuscitation in the intensive care unit. *N Engl J Med* 2004; 350: 2247–56.

17. Trof RJ, Sukul SP, Twisk JW, Girbes AR, Groeneveld AB. Greater cardiac response of colloid than saline fluid loading in septic and non-septic critically ill patients with clinical hypovolaemia. *Intensive Care Med* 2010; 36: 697–701.

18. Myburgh JA, Finfer S, Bellomo R, *et al.* CHEST Investigators; Australian and New Zealand Intensive Care Society Clinical Trials Group. Hydroxyethyl starch or saline for fluid resuscitation in intensive care. *N Engl J Med* 2012; 367: 1901–11.

19. Rao SV, Jollis JG, Harrington RA, *et al.* Relationship of blood transfusion and clinical outcomes in patients with acute coronary syndromes. *JAMA* 2004; 292: 1555–62.

20. Hebert PC, Wells G, Blajchman MA, *et al.* A multicenter, randomized, controlled clinical trial of transfusion requirements in critical care. Transfusion Requirements in Critical Care Investigators, Canadian Critical Care Trials Group. *N Engl J Med* 1999; 340: 409–17.

21. Vincent JL, Baron JF, Reinhart K, *et al.* Anemia and blood transfusion in critically ill patients. *JAMA* 2002; 288: 1499–507.

22. Holst LB, Haase N, Wetterslev J, *et al.* Lower versus higher hemoglobin threshold for transfusion in septic shock. *N Engl J Med* 2014; 371: 381–91.

23. Michard F, Teboul JL. Predicting fluid responsiveness in ICU patients: a critical analysis of the evidence. *Chest* 2002; 121: 2000–8.

24. Antonelli M, Levy M, Andrews PJ, *et al.* Hemodynamic monitoring in shock and implications for management. International Consensus Conference, Paris, France, 27–28 April 2006. *Intensive Care Med* 2007; 33: 575–90.

25. De Backer D, Biston P, Devriendt J, *et al.* Comparison of dopamine and norepinephrine in the treatment of shock. *N Engl J Med* 2010; 362: 779–89.

26. Hinder F, Stubbe HD, Van AH, *et al.* Early multiple organ failure after recurrent endotoxemia in the presence of vasoconstrictor-masked hypovolemia. *Crit Care Med* 2003; 31: 903–9.

27. Myburgh JA, Higgins A, Jovanovska A, *et al.* A comparison of epinephrine and norepinephrine in critically ill patients. *Intensive Care Med* 2008; 34: 2226–34.

Hypovolemic shock

Niels H. Secher and Johannes J. van Lieshout

Summary

Hypovolemic shock is a response to a reduced central blood volume (CBV) whatever its cause – hemorrhage, passive head-up tilt, or other cause – and follows three phases. The first comprises a reduction of CBV initially with reflex increase in heart rate (HR) to approximately 90 bpm and maintained blood pressure (BP) by increased vascular resistance. In the second phase, which corresponds to a reduction of the CBV by about 30%, a Bezold-Jarisch-like reflex ceases sympathetic activity, although plasma adrenaline continues to increase, and together with vagal activation enhances coagulation competence. At this stage of progressive CBV the HR decreases, eventually to extremely low values. In the third phase, BP remains low while HR increases to more than 100 bpm.

To treat hypovolemia, volume substitution can be directed to establish maximal values for stroke volume, cardiac output, or venous oxygen saturation. These variables do not increase when CBV is enhanced in supine healthy humans, and thereby define "normovolemia." The patient's bed can be tilted head-down, and if the mentioned variables then increase significantly, the patient is in need of volume. If not, a volume deficit does not explain the patient's condition. Plasma atrial natriuretic peptide (ANP) also decreases in response to a reduced CBV, and to maintain plasma ANP during major surgery requires a 2.5-liter surplus volume of lactated Ringer's solution. With recording of deviations in central cardiovascular variables, the blood volume can be maintained within 100 ml and provide a comfortable margin to the deficit that affects BP and regional blood flow.

Second only to control of ventilation, intravenous volume administration is the cornerstone physiological treatment modality for anesthesia and intensive care medicine. Providing fluid supports blood volume but, as revealed 70 years ago by Barcroft *et al.* [1] and Gordh [2] in regard to anesthesia, cardiovascular integrity depends on the central blood volume (CBV) rather than on the blood volume as such.

Hypovolemic shock is characterized by a critically reduced CBV, as illustrated when CBV is restrained by actual or simulated gravitational pooling of blood during head-up tilt (HUT) and, for example, lower body negative pressure (LBNP) or limiting venous return by pressure breathing used following thoracic or cardiac surgery to "recruit" the lungs. Experimentally, interventions evaluate the influence of CBV on physiological variables but are also relevant to surgery. For example, shoulder surgery may be carried out with the patient sitting up, and during upper laparoscopic procedures, the patient is tilted at the same time as filling of the inferior caval vein is compressed by abdominal inflation of CO_2 with venous return being further limited by positive-pressure ventilation.

For surgical patients, volume treatment corrects a preoperative volume deficit and attenuates negative influences on CBV by, e.g. hemorrhage, positioning of the patient, anesthesia, and ventilation.[3,4] Volume treatment is most often planned according to a somewhat arbitrary fixed volume regime [5] and to compensate for an eventual blood loss. The treatment is further adjusted by recordings of heart rate (HR) and blood pressure (BP), as introduced to surgery by Cushing in 1903.[6]

Interpretation of the HR and BP responses to a reduced CBV is, however, complex. Cardiovascular variables are regulated and affected by influences other than CBV, including surgical stress and anesthesia.[7] The most accurate recording of fluid balance is probably obtained by physical rather than by physiological variables. For example, thoracic electrical impedance accurately monitors hemorrhage and subsequent administration of the withdrawn amount of blood.[8,9]

To identify that hypovolemia progresses to shock and to specify volume treatment to patients in shock, as well as to patients in general, we address the cardiovascular responses to a reduced CBV followed by a definition of normovolemia as reference for volume treatment. Finally, considerations on the fluid administered to restore the blood volume are mentioned. For an historical account of hypovolemic shock see Beecher [10] and Wiggers,[11] or a more recent summary.[12]

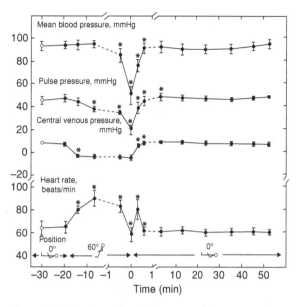

Figure 29.1 Circulatory dynamics in seven subjects at rest and during passive head-up tilt until the onset of (pre)syncopal symptoms, and return to the supine position. Values are mean and SE. * Different from rest. (From Ref. [18], with permission from the American Physiological Society.)

Pre-shock

The cardiovascular response to a reduced CBV is illustrated during tilt table experiments (Figure 29.1). In response to a progressively reduced CBV, cardiovascular variables vary with activation of the autonomic nervous system and are divided into three stages, among which regulation follows the textbook description only in the first stage.[13]

With a moderate reduction of the CBV, mean arterial pressure (MAP) is maintained by peripheral resistance compensating for an approximately 20% reduction in cardiac output (CO).[1] As demonstrated during gravitational stress, MAP is stable at the level of the carotid baroreceptors because reduced distension of the carotid sinus elicits sympathetic excitation. In support, and as an extreme example, the approximately two-fold elevated BP of the giraffe [14] is related to the height of the animal, making its cerebral perfusion pressure similar to that of humans.

In addition, volume and/or pressure receptors within the central circulation that transmit through myelinated nerve fibers respond to a reduced CBV and initiate sympathetic activation. Enhanced sympathetic activity results not only in a relatively stable

MAP but also in an elevated HR,[15] albeit with values typically being lower than 100 bpm (Figure 29.1). Yet values above 100 bpm are recorded occasionally (Figure 29.2), and the HR response to (central) hypovolemia depends on age and does not always reach statistical significance.[16]

Stage II of hypovolemic shock

For volume treatment it is important that the *second stage* of hypovolemic shock represents a reversal of the autonomic response (Figure 29.1). Whereas sympathetic activation dominates the first stage, parasympathetic activity is prevalent during the second stage that is entered when CBV is reduced by 30%.[17] However, sympathetic activity to the adrenal gland is maintained, as identified by a progressive increase in plasma adrenaline.[18] In contrast, plasma noradrenaline reaches a plateau or decreases when central hypovolemia progresses to provoke cerebral hypoperfusion with loss of consciousness. Reduced sympathetic activity is also reflected by muscle sympathetic activity [19] and an increase in muscle oxygenation and explains the fall in peripheral resistance that lowers MAP. The rise in plasma adrenaline is not important with regard to loss of vascular tone.[20]

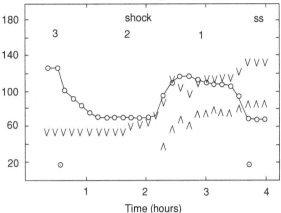

∨ Systolic arterial pressure (mmHg)
○ Heart rate (bpm)
∧ Diastolic arterial pressure (mmHg)

Figure 29.2 Heart rate and systolic and diastolic pressures during surgery for a ruptured abdominal aortic aneurysm. Stages 1–3 of shock indicated. (From Ref. [35], with permission from John Wiley and Sons.) ss, steady state.

Bradycardia

Parasympathetic activity is provoked by a significant reduction in CBV as indicated by plasma pancreatic polypeptide,[18,21] and there is usually a decrease in HR that is blocked by glycopyrron.[15] The bradycardia developed during central hypovolemia may be profound with no ECG activity detected on a monitor and, accordingly, hypovolemia should be suspected whenever "cardiac arrest" manifests in trauma patients, as in patients during and after surgery. Initiation of cardiac resuscitation, including external cardiac compression by applying pressure to the chest, besides positive-pressure ventilation to patients in hypovolemic shock further reduces CBV and could provoke an irreversible stage of shock.

Conversely, immediate restoration of CBV leads to recovery of both circulation and ventilation, within seconds, corresponding to the salutary effects of termination of passive HUT (Figure 29.1), LBNP, or pressure breathing, and indeed by providing ample volume to the patient in shock [21] (Figure 29.2). For surgical patients, therefore, cardiac resuscitation procedures may appear counterproductive unless it is verified that rapid volume infusion is without an effect. If it is not possible to administer such a volume immediately when the patient becomes ill, CBV can, at least partly, be restored by elevating the legs or placing the patient in Trendelenburg's position. Only after such

measures are found futile should a failing circulation be considered of cardiac origin, if not obvious from recording of the ECG.

Unfortunately the bradycardic response to hypovolemia is not regularly included in textbook descriptions (for example Mair [22]). The texts seem to be based on observations derived from acute animal experiments rather than from observations in chronically instrumented conscious animals [7] or in humans.[23] Also it may seem "unreasonable" that vagal activity can be provoked by hemorrhage, but there are also beneficial effects of vagal activity under those circumstances. Vagal activity promotes hemostasis to an extent that it limits blood loss and, conversely, administration of atropine maintains bleeding and can, eventually, be fatal.[24] The second stage of hypovolemic shock may be seen as an attempt by the body to stop bleeding by lowering BP, at the same time as coagulation competence is enhanced by combined increase in vagal activity and plasma adrenaline concentration.

Yet, obviously, not all patients in hypovolemic shock present with a low HR. The bradycardic response to a significantly reduced CBV carries the prerequisite that efferent parasympathetic sinus node activation is intact, and that may not be the case for all patients, as exemplified by those suffering from atrial fibrillation or autonomic dysfunction, e.g. in consequence of diabetes mellitus. Of more general relevance to a surgical environment, vagal tone to the heart is overruled by pain-related sympathetic activity,[25] and many trauma patients are in pain due to crushed tissue. Also, ileus is associated with an elevated HR during hemorrhage.[26]

Pale skin and sympathetic activity

Besides the bradycardic response to stage II hypovolemic shock, it is a characteristic for significant hemorrhage that the skin is pale, as can be observed during a vasovagal syncope, a condition that shares most if not all of the manifestations associated with stage II of hypovolemic shock. Perhaps the pale skin has inspired the notion that peripheral resistance is elevated in response to enhanced baroreceptor activity as the arterial pressure becomes low although peripheral resistance, as mentioned, decreases in reflection of ceased sympathetic activity.

Ceased sympathetic activity reflects that baroreceptor control of BP and HR is eliminated at this stage of shock.[27] Rather than being caused by sympathetic activity during (central) hypovolemia, pale skin reflects a marked (about 25-fold) increase in plasma vasopressin,[28] while a similar reduction in cutaneous blood flow by the increase in plasma angiotensin II is irrelevant to the appearance of the patient.[29] The marked increase in plasma vasopressin, together with lowering of plasma atrial natriuretic peptide (ANP) level, also explains the prolonged low urine production following hypovolemic shock and, conversely, conforms to maintained CO during surgery promoting diuresis. Similarly, cardiac afferent nerves inhibit gastric mobility,[30] which explains why maintained stroke volume of the heart (SV) during surgery reduces postoperative nausea and vomiting (PONV).[31]

The Bezold–Jarisch reflex

Collectively, bradycardia, low vascular resistance, increase in plasma vasopressin, etc., during hemorrhage confirms that a critically reduced CBV is characterized by responses similar to those described in the pharmacological literature as a *Bezold–Jarisch reflex*. However, it remains uncertain which afferent input elicits the reflex. Öberg and White [32] demonstrated the Bezold–Jarisch-like reflex by activation of unmyelinated nerve fibers from the left ventricle and suggested it to be provoked when the heart is emptied of blood. The second stage of hypovolemic shock is associated with only a 10–25% reduction in the diastolic filling of the heart,[33] and yet it remains possible that the most densely innervated apical part of the left ventricle is emptied by a significant reduction in CBV.

A concomitant reduction in HR and BP can, however, also be provoked by hemorrhage following cardiac denervation.[34] Therefore, the specific trigger for the reflex in response to hemorrhage remains in doubt, or it might vary depending on circumstances. The common and clinically relevant finding is that the reflex originates from the central circulation with a contribution from the central nervous system, as when a persons faints when a vein is cannulated.

Stage III of hypovolemic shock

Although stage II of hypovolemic shock may be fatal, there is also a third stage. If the reduction in HR in response to a low CBV is not a terminal event, HR increases again, typically to 120–130 bpm (Figure 29.2),[35] conforming to the tachycardia that

most textbooks hold as a key feature of hypovolemic shock.[22] As demonstrated in animals, sympathetic activity is resumed during severe hemorrhage as indicated by the plasma catecholamine level.[26] It may be that cerebral ischemia, in consequence of prolonged hypotension and a low CO, is important for reactivation of sympathetic activity, and critically reduced cerebral perfusion could indicate that stage III represents a transition to an irreversible stage of shock.[12] However, in contrast to the common descriptions indicating an increase in total peripheral resistance during severe hemorrhage, total peripheral resistance decreases or does not change.[26]

Central vascular pressures during hypovolemic shock

Cardiovascular monitoring of critically ill patients is supplemented by recording of central vascular pressures. In experimental studies, central venous pressure decreases (Figure 29.1) together with mean pulmonary artery and wedge pressures with increasing levels of HUT or LBNP.[17,18]

For clinical evaluation of the circulation during progressive hypovolemia, however, it is a problem that reduction in central vascular pressures relates to the intervention rather than to the well-being of the subject. Although the pressure challenge (HUT or LBNP) may be established, the subject may faint at some later point not preceded by any specific change in central vascular pressure. During sustained HUT or LBNP, the reduction in CBV progresses with accumulation of fluid in the legs [36] and, consequently, CO also decreases, although there is a tendency for the pulmonary artery wedge pressure to increase.[37]

Stable "filling pressures" of the heart do not secure that CO is sufficient to maintain cerebral blood flow and oxygenation, and there are no data to support volume treatment based on central vascular pressure.[38] In fact, for patients, CO is not related to the filling pressures of the heart, although there is a relationship between CO and diastolic filling.[39]

Normovolemia

Patients need volume supplementation during anesthesia and in an intensive care setting, but the strategy remains debated both in regard to the amount that should be provided and to the preferred solutions. What seems established is that for surgery not associated with a significant blood loss, patients should be administered 1 liter of crystalloid.[5] Otherwise, it can be stated only that it is intuitively difficult to defend a volume treatment regime that keeps the patient hypovolemic or one that provides the patient with a volume overload, and yet there is no agreement on the volume load that defines "normovolemia."

With the importance of CBV for circulatory shock, a definition of normovolemia seems desirable, not only to the patient in shock but also to patients throughout the perioperative period, and to patients in general. It appears important that monitoring of the circulation allows for intervention well before cerebral blood flow and oxygenation become affected, and evidence is provided for a volume administration strategy that is accurate within 100 ml.

Cerebral blood flow and oxygenation become affected by a blood loss corresponding to 30% of the (central) blood volume [40] or a blood loss of 1.0–1.5 liters. The proposed volume administration strategy thereby allows volume administration within approximately one-tenth of the volume loss that is significant for brain function.

The impact of a reduced CBV for SV, CO, and thus central or mixed (from the pulmonary artery) venous oxygen saturation (SvO_2) offers monitoring modalities for evaluating the functional consequence of a reduced CBV.

Tilt table experiments

The influence of CBV on flow-related variables is readily illustrated during tilt table experiments. As mentioned, SV, CO, and thus SvO_2 decrease during HUT, while maximal values are obtained during supine rest since, with the increase in central pressures and filling of the heart during the transition from supine to the head-down tilted position, there is no further increase in SV, CO, or SvO_2,[37,41] and SV decreases only during extreme (90°) head-down tilt.[42]

Similarly, healthy non-fasting supine subjects are not volume-responsive with regard to SV.[43] Together, these observations indicate that for supine humans, maximal flow-related variables define normovolemia.

The surgical patient

In contrast to supine healthy subjects, the preoperative patient [3,4] and many patients under intensive care are volume-responsive. To supplement volume is important since any limitation to CO has

consequences for all vascular beds, independent of an eventually large metabolic demand as exemplified by muscle blood flow during exercise.[44] Likewise, cerebral blood flow and oxygenation become affected even with the moderate reduction of CO that is associated with standing up.[40] Even more so, skin, muscle, and notably splanchnic and renal blood flow decrease in response to the elevated sympathetic activity provoked by a limited CBV and thereby CO. Conversely, a volume strategy that secures CO preserves not only splanchnic and renal flows of relevance for surgical healing and diuresis, respectively, but also for cerebral oxygenation, which is widely independent of MAP (Figure 29.3).[45] Thus, it seems evident that the primary focus of volume therapy is to prevent episodes of hypovolemia, and on-line monitoring of flow-related variables makes that possible, with consequences for postoperative complications.[31]

Maintenance of cerebral oxygenation may require a MAP of 90 mmHg, probably because of arteriosclerosis in the vessels that serve the cerebral circulation. Monitoring of cerebral blood flow and/or oxygenation is advocated for older patients and for patients with vascular and/or cardiac disease, also considering that cerebral autoregulation might be compromised by the inhalation agents used for general anesthesia (Figure 29.3).

Evaluation of cerebral oxygenation is relevant especially to cardiac surgery during which the heart–lung machine determines CO. Maintaining cerebral oxygenation, e.g. by increasing the pump speed of the machine, reduces postoperative complications and secures mental well-being.[46] Similarly, maintained cerebral oxygenation is important for reducing complications following other types of surgery, and maintained cerebral oxygenation may be taken as an index for whether handling of the circulation has been adequate.[47]

Titration to establish normovolemia

A problem with directing volume treatment by flow-related variables is their individual variability. For example, the trained athlete has a low resting HR and a compensating large SV that makes it difficult to evaluate whether a given filling of the heart is sufficient to secure a maximal SV.

For CO and SvO_2 the inter-individual variation is smaller, but there remain significant differences among subjects/patients, and only some of

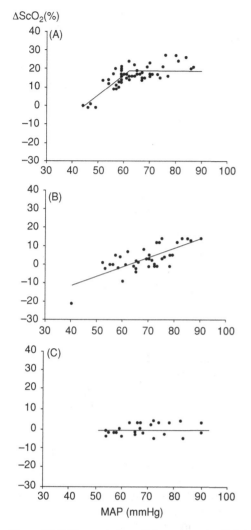

Figure 29.3 Changes in frontal lobe oxygenation (ScO$_2$) and mean arterial pressure (MAP) during anesthesia. Illustrated are three patients, one of whom demonstrated a lower limit of cerebral autoregulation (A); for another no cerebral autoregulation was found (B); and for the third, no lower limit of cerebral autoregulation was detected (C). (Derived from Ref. [45].)

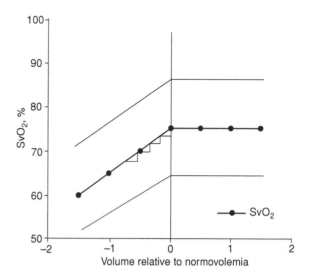

Figure 29.4 Venous oxygen saturation (SvO$_2$) during volume administration. With infusion of 100 ml of volume, SvO$_2$ increases by approximately 1% and administration of volume is continued until SvO$_2$ does not increase further. For individual patients, there are established markedly different relationships between SvO$_2$ and the volume load, but the administration of volume is continued until a maximal value is reached and that may be high, for example in a patient with liver disease or fever.

the variation can be explained. Notably, there are inter-individual differences in CO according to beta-adrenergic polymorphism, with the "Gly–Gly" carrying about a half liter per minute greater CO than the "Arg–Arg" phenotype.[48] In other words, there is a genetic background for why accurate volume administration based on flow-related variables should be individualized.[31] More importantly, however, CO (and thereby SvO$_2$) varies depending on circumstances including type of anesthesia, temperature, and notably disease. Alternatively the volume regime that maintains the plasma (pro)ANP level may be evaluated retrospectively; in that case, it seems to require a surplus of 2.5 liters for major surgery when volume treatment is carried out with lactate Ringer's solution.

Choice of volume treatment

Volume treatment is usually with a crystalloid, eventually supplemented by a (typically synthetic) colloid, considering that administration of blood is an independent risk factor for the surgical patient. Accordingly, initial volume treatment is associated with hemodilution that itself increases CO because of the inverse relationship between CO and hematocrit.[49] To circumvent that limitation to flow-directed volume therapy, a common algorithm requires that SV should be increased by 10% in response to a 200-ml bolus of colloid to justify further administration of volume.[31]

An alternative approach to individualized goal-directed fluid therapy is to take advantage of the observation that SvO$_2$ rather than CO is the regulated variable.[50] Thus, variation in SvO$_2$ is independent of the fluid used for volume administration (a crystalloid, a colloid, or blood products) (Figure 29.4).

Clinical outcome

For patients in hypovolemic shock, the chosen transfusion strategy may be decisive. An attempt may be made to stop bleeding by administration of a pro-hemostatic agent,[51] but the chosen fluid is also important. Synthetic colloid suspensions possess a high intravascular volume expansion effect, but also attenuate coagulation competence and provoke hemorrhage.[52] Alternatively, crystalloids, when administered in a moderate amount, enhance coagulation competence and are recommended for trauma patients. It remains that patients exposed to a massive blood loss require administration of plasma and platelets in addition to red blood cells in order to maintain coagulation competence, and establishing such balanced administration of blood products enhances survival of the trauma patient.[53]

References

1. Barcroft H, Edholm OG, McMichael J, Sharpey-Schafer EF. Posthaemorrhagic fainting; study by cardiac output and forearm flow. *Lancet* 1944; 1: 489–91.

2. Gordh T. Postural circulatory and respiratory changes during ether and intravenous anesthesia. *Acta Chir Scand* 1945; Suppl. 92.

3. Jenstrup M, Ejlersen E, Mogensen T, Secher NH. A maximal central venous oxygen saturation (SvO_{2max}) for the surgical patient. *Acta Anaesthesiol Scand* 1995; 39 (Suppl. 107): 29–32.

4. Bundgaard-Nielsen M, Jørgensen CC, Secher NH, Kehlet H. Functional intravascular volume deficit in patients before surgery. *Acta Anaesthesiol Scand* 2010; 54: 464–9.

5. Bundgaard-Nielsen M, Secher NH, Kehlet H. "Liberal" vs. "restrictive" perioperative fluid therapy – a critical assessment of the evidence. *Acta Anaesthesiol Scand* 2009; 53: 843–51.

6. Cushing HW. On routine determination of arterial tension in operating room and clinic. *Boston Med Surg J* 1903; 148: 250–6.

7. Schadt JC, Ludbrook J. Hemodynamic and neurohumoral responses to acute hypovolaemia in conscious animals. *Am J Physiol* 1991; 260: H305–18.

8. Krantz T, Laurizen T, Cai Y, Warberg J, Secher NH. Accurate monitoring of a blood loss: thoracic electrical impedance during haemorrhage in the pig. *Acta Anaesthesiol Scand* 2000; 44: 598–604.

9. Perko M, Jarnvig IL, Højgaard-Rasmussen N, Eliasen K, Arendrup H. Electric impedance for evaluation of body fluid balance in cardiac surgery patients. *J Cardiothorac Vasc Anesth* 2001; 15: 44–8.

10. Beecher HK. *Resuscitation and Anesthesia for Wounded Men. The Management of Traumatic Shock.* Springfield, IL: CC Thomas, 1949.

11. Wiggers CJ. *Physiology of Shock.* New York: The Commonwealth Fund, 1950.

12. Secher NH, Pawelczyk JA, Ludbrook J (eds.) *Blood Loss and Shock.* London: Edward Arnold, 1994.

13. Secher NH, Jacobsen J, Friedman DB, Matzen S. Bradycardia during reversible hypovolaemic shock: associated neural reflex mechanisms and clinical implications. *Clin Exp Pharm Physiol* 1992; 19: 733–43.

14. Brøndum E, Hasenkam JM, Secher NH, *et al.* Jugular venous pooling during lowering of the head affects blood pressure of the anesthetised giraffe. *Am J Physiol* 2009; 297: R1058–65.

15. Pedersen M, Madsen P, Klokker M, Olesen HL, Secher NH. Sympathetic influence on cardiovascular responses to sustained head-up tilt in humans. *Acta Physiol Scand* 1995; 155: 435–44.

16. Murrell C, Cotter JD, George K, *et al.* Influence of age on syncope following prolonged exercise: differential responses but similar orthostatic intolerance. *J Physiol* 2009; 587: 5959–69.

17. Murray RH, Thomson LJ, Bowers JA, Albreight CD. Hemodynamic effects of graded vasodepressor syncope induced by lower body negative pressure. *Am Heart J* 1968; 76: 799–811.

18. Sander-Jensen K, Secher NH, Astrup A, *et al.* Hypotension induced by passive head-up tilt: endocrine and circulatory mechanisms. *Am J Physiol* 1986; 251: R742–8.

19. Jacobsen TN, Jost CMT, Converse Jr. RL, Victor RG. Cardiovascular sensors: the bradycardic phase in hypovolaemic shock. In: Secher NH, Pawelczyk JA, Ludbrook J. *Blood Loss and Shock*, eds. London: Edward Arnold, 1994: 3–10.

20. Matzen S, Secher NH, Knigge U, Bach FW, Warberg J. Pituitary-adrenal responses to head-up tilt in humans: effect of H_1- and H_2- receptor blockade. *Am J Physiol* 1992; 263: R156–63.

21. Sander-Jensen K, Secher NH, Bie P, Warberg J, Schwartz TW. Vagal slowing of the heart during haemorrhage: observations from 20 consecutive hypotensive patients. *Br Med J* 1986; 292: 364–6.

22. Mair RV. Hypovolemic shock. In: Fauci AS, Braunwald E, Kasper DL, *et al.*, eds. *Harrison's Online.* 17th edn. New York: McGraw-Hill, 2010.

23. Secher NH, Bie P. Bradycardia during reversible haemorrhagic shock – a forgotten observation? *Clin Physiol* 1985; 5: 315–23.

24. Guarini S, Cainazzo MM, Giuliani D, *et al.* Adrenocorticotropin reverses hemorrhagic shock in anesthetized rats through the rapid activation of a vagal anti-inflammatory pathway. *Cardiovasc Res* 2004; 63: 357–65.

25. Sawdon M, Ohnishi M, Little RA, Kirkman E. Naloxone does not inhibit the injury-induced attenuation of the response to severe haemorrhage in the anaesthetized rat. *Exp Physiol* 2009; 94: 641–7.

26. Jacobsen J, Hansen OB, Sztuk F, Warberg J, Secher NH. Enhanced heart rate response to haemorrhage by ileus in the pig. *Acta Physiol Scand* 1993; 149: 293–301.

27. Ogoh S, Volianitis S, Raven PB, Secher NH. Carotid baroreflex function ceases during vasovagal syncope. *Clin Auton Res* 2004; 14: 30–3.

28. Bie P, Secher NH, Astrup A, Warberg J. Cardiovascular and endocrine responses to head-up tilt and vasopressin infusion in man. *Am J Physiol* 1986; 251: R735–41.

29. Sander-Jensen K, Secher NH, Astrup A, *et al.* Angiotensin II attenuates reflex decrease in heart rate and sympathetic activity in man. *Clin Physiol* 1988; 8: 31–40.

30. Abrahamsson H, Thorén P. Vomiting and reflex vagal relaxation of the stomach elicited from heart receptors in the cat. *Acta Physiol Scand* 1973; 88: 8–22.

31. Bundgaard-Nielsen M, Holte K, Secher NH, Kehlet H. Monitoring of perioperative fluid administration by individualized goal-directed therapy. *Acta Anaesthesiol Scand* 2007; 51: 331–40.

32. Öberg B, White S. The role of vagal cardiac nerves and arterial baroreceptors in the circulatory adjustments to hemorrhage in the cat. *Acta Physiol Scand* 1970; 80: 395–403.

33. Jacobsen J, Søfelt S, Fernandes A, *et al.* Reduced left ventricular size at onset of bradycardia during epidural anaesthesia. *Acta Anaesthesiol Scand* 1992; 36: 831–6.

34. Morita H, Vatner SF. Effects of hemorrhage on renal nerve activity in conscious dogs. *Circ Res* 1985; 57: 788–93.

35. Jacobsen J, Secher NH. Heart rate during haemorrhagic shock. *Clin Physiol* 1992; 12: 659–66.

36. Matzen S, Perko GE, Groth S, Friedman DB, Secher NH. Blood volume distribution during head-up tilt induced central hypovolaemia in man. *Clin Physiol* 1991; 11: 411–22.

37. van Lieshout JJ, Harms MPM, Pott F, Jenstrup M, Secher NH. Stroke volume and central vascular pressures during tilt in humans. *Acta Anaesthesiol Scand* 2005; 49: 1287–92.

38. Marik PE, Baram M, Vahid B. Does central venous pressure predict fluid responsiveness? A systemic review of the literature and the tale of seven mares. *Chest* 2008; 134: 172–8.

39. Thys DM, Hillel Z, Goldman ME, Mindich BP, Kapland JA. A comparison of hemodynamic indices derived by invasive monitoring and two-dimensional echocardiography. *Anesthesiology* 1987; 67: 630–4.

40. van Lieshout JJ, Wieling W, Karemaker JM, Secher NH. Syncope, cerebral perfusion and oxygenation. *J Appl Physiol* 2003; 94: 833–48.

41. Jans Ø, Tollund C, Bundgaard-Nielsen M, *et al.* Goal-directed fluid therapy: stroke volume optimization and cardiac dimensions in healthy humans. *Acta Anaesthesiol Scand* 2008; 52: 536–40.

42. Bundgaard-Nielsen M, Sørensen H, Dalsgaard M, Rasmussen P, Secher NH. Relationship between stroke volume, cardiac output and filling of the heart during tilt. *Acta Anaesthesiol Scand* 2009; 53: 1324–8.

43. Bundgaard-Nielsen M, Jørgensen CC, Kehlet H, Secher NH. Normovolaemia defined according to cardiac stroke volume in healthy supine humans. *Clin Physiol Funct Imaging* 2010; 30: 318–22.

44. Secher NH, Volianitis S. Are the arms and legs in competition for cardiac output? *Med Sci Sports Exerc* 2006; 38: 1797–803.

45. Nissen P, Pacino H, Frederiksen HJ, Novovic S, Secher NH. Near-infrared spectroscopy for evaluation of cerebral autoregulation during orthotopic liver transplantation. *Neurocrit Care* 2009; 11: 235–41.

46. Murkin JM, Adams SJ, Novick RJ, *et al.* Monitoring brain oxygen saturation during coronary bypass surgery: a randomized, prospective study. *Anesth Analg* 2007; 104: 51–8.

47. Murkin JM, Arango M. Near-infrared spectroscopy as index of brain and tissue oxygenation. *Br J Anaesth* 2009; 103 (Suppl. 1): 3–13.

48. Snyder EM, Beck HC, Diez NM, *et al.* Arg 16 Gly polymorphism of the β_2-adrenergic receptor is associated with differences in cardiovascular function at rest and during exercise in humans. *J Physiol* 2006; 571: 121–30.

49. Krantz T, Warberg J, Secher NH. Venous oxygen saturation during normovolaemic haemodilution in the pig. *Acta Anaesthesiol Scand* 2005; 49: 1149–56.

50. González-Alonso J, Mortensen S, Dawson EA, *et al.* Erythrocyte and the regulation of human skeletal muscle blood flow and oxygen delivery: role of erythrocyte count and oxygenation state of haemoglobin. *J Physiol* 2006; 572: 295–305.

51. Zaar M, Secher NH, Johansson PI, *et al.* Effects of a recombinant FVIIa analogue, NN1731, on blood loss and survival after liver trauma in the pig. *Br J Anaesth* 2009; 103: 840–7.

52. Rasmussen KC, Johansson PI, Højskov M, *et al.* Hydroxyethyl starch reduces coagulation competence and increases blood loss during major surgery: results from a randomized controlled trial. *Ann Surg* 2014; 259: 249–54.

53. Johansson PI, Ostrowski SR, Secher NH. Management of major blood loss: an update. *Acta Anaesthesiol Scand* 2010; 54: 1039–49.

Chapter

30

Uncontrolled hemorrhage

Robert G. Hahn

Summary

Fluid therapy in hemorrhage strives to restore hemodynamic function and tissue perfusion. However, these goals are not appropriate when there is an injury to a large blood vessel and the hemorrhage has not been stopped surgically (uncontrolled hemorrhage). Clinical situations in which this is the case include penetrating trauma, ruptured aortic aneurysm, and gastric bleeding. Numerous animal experiments in pigs and rats have shown that the low-flow, low-pressure state characterizing serious hemorrhage promotes coagulation, even if a large blood vessel is injured. An immature blood clot is easily washed away if the blood flow rate and the arterial pressure is normalized by infusion fluids. Vigorous fluid therapy then increases both the blood loss and the mortality. The road to optimal survival is to infuse less fluid at lower speed (half volume at half speed is suggested) and aim at a systolic arterial pressure of 90 mmHg. In this situation, the strategy is only to prevent progressive acidosis and irreversible shock. A deviation from normal hemodynamics should be accepted until the source of bleeding has been treated surgically. A sudden drop in arterial pressure during ongoing fluid resuscitation suggests that rebleeding is occurring, and the infusion rate should then be further reduced. There is an unfortunate lack of clinical studies showing that the fluid strategy that has been successful in animal experiments pertains also to humans. However, it is widely accepted in emergency departments and trauma hospitals to resuscitate trauma patients to a lower-than-usual systolic pressure (hypotensive resuscitation).

The anesthetist is taught to compensate hemorrhage with infusion fluids. The aim is to restore the blood volume and thereby also cardiac output, regional blood flow rates, and arterial pressure. However, there are certain situations in which this practice makes the situation worse and can be detrimental to the outcome. These include ongoing major hemorrhage where surgical control cannot be achieved within reasonable time, in particular if a major vessel has been injured. In these situations hemodynamics and outcome do not go hand in hand. Another strategy of fluid treatment should be adopted that favors outcome rather than the hemodynamics.

To correctly identify patients who suffer from uncontrolled hemorrhage is a major clinical challenge. Patients with aortic rupture, gastric bleeding, and traumatic pelvic fracture often fall in this category. The prehospital trauma patient with a penetrating injury is at high risk.

Controlled versus uncontrolled hemorrhage

The normal physiological response to hemorrhage involves vasoconstriction and a reduction of the blood flow rates. After 20% of the blood volume has been lost, the body shifts strategy from a vasoconstriction to vasodilatation, which results in prompt onset of arterial hypotension and hypoperfusion of the tissues. Acidosis develops. Certain vascular beds are closed off from circulation, which causes a reduction of oxygen consumption (shock). The shock becomes irreversible

Clinical Fluid Therapy in the Perioperative Setting, Second Edition, ed. Robert G. Hahn. Published by Cambridge University Press. © Cambridge University Press 2016.

if the bleeding continues and resuscitation therapy with infusion fluids volume is not initiated promptly. In this setting, when the bleeding surface is small or has been stopped by mechanic pressure or surgery, infusion fluids reverse all the components of the shock and are therefore a life-saving therapy.

Clinical experience holds that fluid therapy sometimes can make things worse. The underlying problem is then that fluid therapy interferes with the body's own defense mechanisms. The vasoconstriction of the first phase of hemorrhage (0–20% of the blood volume) aims to reduce the bleeding surface and makes physical action possible by maintaining the arterial pressure. The second phase apparently aims to allow blood clotting by reducing the blood flow rates and the pressure in the circulation. However, an infusion of fluid in this situation raises the blood flow rates and the hydrostatic pressure, and therefore immature blood clots are simply washed away. The hemorrhage escalates and may rapidly become out of control. The infusion fluid becomes a killer instead of a savior.

Studies in pigs

Experimental animal models have been able to provide a better understanding of why infusion fluids sometimes have effects opposite to the intended ones. Many studies have been performed using a swine model in which an uncontrolled hemorrhage is initiated from a tear in the aorta having a width of exactly 5 mm. In this situation there is no vasoconstriction, and the systemic arterial pressure drops within 10 seconds.[1]

Using the aortic tear model, Bickell et al. studied the effects of infusing 3 times as much lactated Ringer's solution as the expected hemorrhage amount over 10 min.[2] Hemodynamic indices dropped markedly when the hemorrhage began, with slight but transient improvement in response to fluid. All pigs that received fluid died ($n = 8$) while all pigs that did not receive any fluid ($n = 8$) survived up to 120 min, when the experiment ended.

Kowalenko et al. studied the effect of the arterial pressure on mortality.[3] Swine were bled from one femoral artery to a mean arterial pressure (MAP) of 30 mmHg before the aortic tear was made. The mortality was 13% and 63% when crystalloid fluid was infused to reach a MAP of 40 mmHg and 80 mmHg, respectively. With no fluid at all, 88% of the animals died. A much larger intraperitoneal hemorrhage was found when fluid was given to reach the highest blood pressure target. Hence, it appeared that the intermediate blood pressure target was most beneficial.

In another study, a slow increase of the MAP to 40, 60, and 80 mmHg by normal saline and blood resulted in a mortality of 11%, 22%, and 78%, respectively. Higher rates were accompanied by larger intraperitoneal hemorrhage volumes.[4] Another research group determined the pressure at which rebleeding starts to be 64 mmHg (systolic 94 and diastolic 45 mmHg). However, the pressure ranges were wide.[5]

Riddez, Johnson, and Hahn developed the aortic tear model by placing a flow probe above and below the aortic tear and monitored the hemorrhage rate as the difference in flow between the two. This technique showed that the rate of the initial hemorrhage decreased in an exponential manner, and stopped within 4 min.[6] The hemorrhage volume during these 4 min averaged 35% of the blood volume. However, rebleeding often occurred and appeared to be a key factor promoting mortality.

When Ringer's acetate was infused slowly, the mortality was 25% in the animals receiving the same amount of fluid as the bled volume, and also in those receiving twice as much, while the mortality was 50% in those animals that received no fluid or 3 times the bled amount. A review of the data on hemorrhage and oxygen consumption suggested that animals that received no fluid died of shock, while massive rebleeding was the cause of death in the group that received the largest fluid volume.[7]

Experiments were also done with a more rapid infusion of the same volume as in the previous study. Here, rebleeding occurred only during the actual infusion.[8]

Hypertonic saline in dextran (HSD) proved to induce rapid massive rebleeding when given in the recommended volume (4 ml/kg over 1 min). The mortality was 60%.[9] However, rebleeding was rarer and the mortality lower (20%) when 1 ml/kg was administered over 5 min.[10]

Studies in small animals

Key findings when transecting the spleen of rats included a high survival when MAP was kept low (50 mmHg) and a progressive increase of the bleeding rate when MAP was raised.[11] A slightly higher MAP (70 mmHg, 100 mmHg is normal) was optimal *after* the hemorrhage had been arrested surgically.[12]

Survival after splenic injury was higher when resuscitation was performed with a mixture of 2/3 of Ringer's lactate and 1/3 of either hydroxyethyl starch (molecular weight 130 kD) or whole blood, as compared with administering Ringer's acetate alone or hydroxyethyl starch alone.[12]

Resuscitation with fresh plasma was more beneficial for survival than with thawed plasma that had been stored for up to 5 days.[13]

Heinius *et al.* studied the effect of hypothermia (30 °C) on uncontrolled hemorrhage in the rat. They exposed the femoral artery in the groin and punctured the vessel with a needle. In hypothermic rats, fluid resuscitation induced more frequent rebleeding events that had longer durations and contained more blood as compared with normothermic animals.[14] However, the mortality was not higher.[15]

In rabbits subjected to splenic injury and mild hypothermia (35 °C), the coagulopathy was more severe with dextran 70 and hetastarch than with 5% human albumin. Mortality rates were 75%, 100%, and 50%, respectively, after resuscitation with these fluids.[16]

Lessons from the animal studies

These animal studies show that rebleeding is rare when fluid therapy is not actively performed. On the other hand, some fluid should apparently be infused to prevent hypovolemic shock. However, ambitious fluid therapy may be detrimental if the bleeding is not yet under control. Infusing fluid at a high rate is more dangerous than providing a large volume. Such infusions increase the blood flow rates and the systemic pressures, which reinitiate bleedings that have successfully been arrested by the coagulation system. Blood clots, which are formed on the outside of the damaged vessels, are immature and can easily be washed away by the resulting sheer stress.

The recommended dose of hypertonic saline dextran (4 ml/kg over 1 min), which might be used for resuscitation in trauma patients, is too large. A smaller amount should be administered over several minutes instead of 1 min if rebleeding events are to be avoided.

The animal studies also teach us that we should not strive for full correction of hemodynamic measures until the bleeding is safely arrested. Until then, a simple rule is to administer *half as much fluid over twice as long a time as usual*. To strive for full correction is futile and dangerous.

The double-probe technique in pigs has shown that rebleeding events are more typically preceded by a rise in aortic blood flow rate than by a rise in arterial pressure. However, the arterial pressure drops soon after the rebleeding has started, and may put an end to the event if the rebleeding is not perpetuated by a continued high infusion rate. During fluid resuscitation the clinician should expect to see a slow rise in arterial pressure, but if a decrease suddenly occurs this is fairly good evidence of a rebleeding event. The used rate of infusion has then been too high. However, instead of turning off the infusion, continue at a lower rate.

Uncontrolled hemorrhage in the clinic

For decades, hypotension has been used in the operating room as a means of reducing blood loss in elective surgery in which transfusion might be needed or bleeding is difficult to remove (such as middle ear surgery).[17] A lower blood pressure clearly reduces the hemorrhage and limits the requirements for erythrocyte transfusions.

A study of 110 trauma victims brought to hospital randomized the patients to a systolic arterial pressure of >100 mmHg while another group was resuscitated to 70 mmHg.[18] There was no difference in mortality (four died in each group). However, those who were resuscitated to 70 mmHg actually had a systolic pressure of 100 mmHg. Still, the rule in emergency departments and trauma hospitals is to resuscitate trauma patients to a lower-than-usual systolic pressure, usually to 90 mmHg.

The occurrence of uncontrolled hemorrhage in prehospital care is not known but has been estimated to be 25% of blunt traumas to the abdomen, chest, and pelvis [19]. In penetrating trauma, the incidence is probably higher. The presence of uncontrolled hemorrhage, which is most common in penetrating injuries, will naturally affect the value of the conventional prehospital fluid therapy.

In 1994, Bickell *et al.* compared the outcomes of almost 600 hypotensive patients, half of whom received crystalloid fluid at the scene of an accident (2.5 liters) while the other half received fluid only after having entered the operating room.[20] The results showed a slight but statistically significant increased survival rate in the delayed resuscitation group (70% versus 62%). Differences were greater in the most severely injured patients (61% versus 48%). The reader, having the animal studies of uncontrolled hemorrhage fresh in the memory, will probably interpret this result to suggest that a rapid infusion of 2.5 liters of crystalloid helped some patients but caused rebleeding in others, whereby the overall effect of the ambitious fluid therapy was nil or even negative. This dual effect of fluid on trauma patients might also explain the lack of positive effect on outcomes of hypertonic saline with and without dextran.[21,22]

Spending time at the scene of an accident to provide infusion fluid is of little real value if the transport time to hospital is 30 min or less. In those situations most patients are better off being rushed to hospital as soon as possible ("scoop-and-run"). Hypovolemic shock should probably be treated with infusion fluids at the scene of the accident ("stay-and-play") only in rural areas where the transport time to hospital exceeds 30 min.

A systolic pressure target of 90 mmHg is suggested in the treatment of the patient with possible uncontrolled hemorrhage. Crystalloid electrolyte fluids are the first-line treatment, while colloid fluids have a limited place.[23]

Fresh whole blood, erythrocytes, and plasma are most likely superior to clear fluids in restoring hemodynamics and facilitate coagulation. Early administration of plasma, in equal proportion to erythrocytes, has been suggested for management of trauma patients,[24,25] and most trauma centers have made uncrossmatched Type-O erythrocytes available for rapid administration to hemorrhaging patients.[26] Hypothermia induces coagulopathy and promotes rebleeding. Therefore, warming the patient with blankets and the use of body-warm infusion fluid is beneficial and might even be life-saving in critical cases. The experiences with early, and even prehospital, transfusion of blood are described in Chapter 32, "Trauma." These can be difficult to practice elsewhere than in a fully equipped trauma hospital. In smaller hospitals, where these practices may not be feasible, crystalloid fluid therapy as outlined in this chapter is the treatment option that the anesthetist has to consider.

References

1. Bickell WH, Bruttig SP, Wade CE. Hemodynamic response to abdominal aortotomy in the anesthetized swine. *Circ Shock* 1989; 28: 321–32.

2. Bickell WH, Bruttig SP, Millnamow GA, O´Benar J, Wade CE. The detrimental effects of intravenous crystalloid after aortotomy in swine. *Surgery* 1991; 110: 529–36.

3. Kowalenko T, Stern S, Dronen S, Wang X. Improved outcome with hypotensive resuscitation of uncontrolled hemorrhagic shock in a swine model. *J Trauma* 1992; 33: 349–53.

4. Stern SA, Dronen SC, Birrer P, Wang X. Effect of blood pressure on hemorrhage volume and survival in a near-fatal hemorrhage model incorporating a vascular injury. *Ann Emerg Med* 1993; 22: 155–63.

5. Sondeen JL, Coppes VG, Holcomb JB. Blood pressure at which rebleeding occurs after resuscitation in swine with aortic injury. *J Trauma* 2003; 54: S110–17.

6. Riddez L, Johnson L, Hahn RG. Early hemodynamic changes during uncontrolled intra-abdominal bleeding. *Eur Surg Res* 1999; 31: 19–25.

7. Riddez L, Johnson L, Hahn RG. Central and regional hemodynamics during fluid therapy after uncontrolled intra-abdominal bleeding. *J Trauma* 1998; 44: 433–9.

8. Riddez L, Hjelmqvist H, Suneson A, Hahn RG. Short-term crystalloid fluid resuscitation in uncontrolled intra-abdominal bleeding in swine. *Prehosp Disaster Med* 1999; 14: 87–92.

9. Riddez L, Hahn RG, Suneson A, Hjelmqvist H. Central and regional hemodynamics during uncontrolled bleeding using hypertonic saline dextran for resuscitation. *Shock* 1998; 10: 176–81.

10. Riddez L, Drobin D, Sjöstrand F, Svensén C, Hahn RG. Lower dose of hypertonic-saline dextran reduces the risk of lethal rebleeding in uncontrolled hemorrhage. *Shock* 2002; 17: 377–82.

11. Li T, Zhu Y, Hu Y, *et al.* Ideal permissive hypotension to resuscitate uncontrolled hemorrhagic shock and the tolerance time in rats. *Anesthesiology* 2011; 114: 111–19.

12. Li T, Zhu Y, Fang Y, Liu L. Determination of the optimal mean arterial pressure for postbleeding resuscitation after hemorrhagic shock in rats. *Anesthesiology* 2012; 116: 103–12.

13. Letourneau PA, McManus M, Sowards K, *et al.* Aged plasma transfusion increases mortality in a rat model of uncontrolled hemorrhage. *J Trauma* 2011; 71: 1115–19.

14. Heinius G, Hahn RG, Sondén A. Hypothermia increases re-bleeding during uncontrolled hemorrhage in the rat. *Shock* 2011; 36: 60–6.

15. Heinius G, Sondén A, Hahn RG. Effects of different fluid regimes and desmopressin on uncontrolled hemorrhage during hypothermia in the rat. *Ther Hypothermia Temp Manag* 2012; 2: 53–69.

16. Kehirabadi BS, Crissey JM, Deguzman R, *et al.* Effects of synthetic versus natural colloid resuscitation on inducing dilutional coagulopathy and increasing hemorrhage in rabbits. *J Trauma* 2008; 64: 1218–28.

17. Sollevi A. Hypotensive anesthesia and blood loss. *Acta Anaesthesiol Scand Suppl* 1988; 89: 39–43.

18. Dutton RP, Mackenzie CF, Scalea TM. Hypotensive resuscitation during active hemorrhage: impact on in hospital mortality. *J Trauma* 2002; 52: 1141–6.

19. Lechleuter A, Lefering R, Bouillon B, *et al*. Prehospital detection of uncontrolled haemorrhage in blunt trauma. *Eur J Emerg Med* 1994; 1: 1–13.

20. Bickell WH, Wall MJ, Pepe PE, *et al*. Immediate versus delayed resuscitation for hypotensive patients with penetrating torso injuries. *N Engl J Med* 1994; 331: 1105–9.

21. Kramer GC, Wade CE, Prough DS. Hypertonic saline dextran: efficacy and regulatory approval. *Acta Anaesthesiol Scand* 1998; 42: 141–4.

22. Bulger EM, May S, Brasel KJ, *et al*. Out-of-hospital hypertonic resuscitation following severe traumatic brain injury: a randomized controlled trial. *JAMA* 2010; 304: 1455–64.

23. James MF. Place of the colloids in fluid resuscitation of the traumatized patient. *Curr Opin Anaesthesiol* 2012; 25: 248–52.

24. Duchesne JC, Hunt JP, Wahl G, *et al*. Review of current blood transfusions strategies in a mature level I trauma center: were we wrong for the last 60 years? *J Trauma* 2008; 65: 272–6.

25. Borgman MA, Spinella PC, Perkins JG, *et al*. The ratio of blood products transfused affects mortality in patients receiving massive transfusions at a combat support hospital. *J Trauma* 2007; 63: 805–13.

26. Dutton RP, Shih D, Edelman BB, Hess JR, Scalea TM. Safety of uncrossmatched Type-O red cells for resuscitation from hemorrhagic shock. *J Trauma* 2005; 59: 1445–9.

Chapter 31

Burns

Folke Sjöberg

Summary

The purpose of fluid treatment for burn-injured patients is to maintain organ perfusion despite major leakage of fluid from the intravascular space. The leakage is due to a sharp reduction of the pressure in the interstitial fluid space (negative imbibition pressure) and an increase of the vascular permeability. Most of the fluid loss due to the first factor takes place within the first 3–4 hours and the bulk of loss from the second factor within 12 hours after the burn.

The formula for plasma volume support most widely used today is the "Parkland" strategy, in which 2–4 ml of buffered Ringer's solution is administered per total body surface area % per kilogram body weight. Half of the calculated volume is given during the first 8 hours after the burn and the other half during the subsequent 16 hours. A colloid rescue strategy should come into play when the fluid volumes provided are very large, and is adequate after 8–12 hours post-burn.

The patient should be in a state of controlled hypovolemia. The combined use of urine output (aim 30–50 ml/h), mean arterial pressure, and the mental state of the patient is gold standard when guiding the fluid therapy. The use of central circulatory parameters increases the risk of fluid overload and does not improve the outcome. The maximal tissue edema reaches a maximum between the first 24 and 48 hours post-burn, and thereafter the added fluid volume is excreted as an ongoing process over 7–10 days.*

* Summary compiled by the Editor.

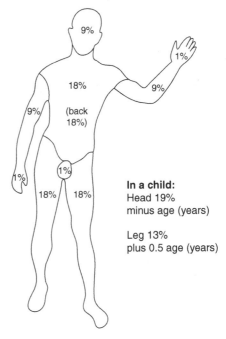

Figure 31.1 Size of the burn in percent of skin surface. According to the "9% rule" the body regions can be divided into areas which are multiples of 9. The calculation is slightly different in a child up to 10 years, because of a relatively larger head and smaller legs.

Seldom within everyday medical practice is there a moment when the need for fluid treatment is so predictable, extensive, and has such large effects on the body fluid balance as it does in the case of the treatment for burns. These fluid needs can most often be predicted from what normally affects burn injury prognosis and outcome, i.e. the extent of the burn on the total body surface (% total body surface area burnt % [TBSA]) and the depth of the burn (Figure 31.1). The total fluid need is also dependent on, and needs to be adjusted by, the size of the individual (kg). If no other complications arise, the fluid treatment is most often directly calculated based on these parameters – in cases when the start of the fluid treatment is delayed after the injury, however, more fluid might be needed.

This chapter first presents the state of the art for burn care, which is then followed by the modern fluid treatment paradigm, i.e. the background for the large fluid needs of these patients. Different fluid treatment strategies will be discussed, and finally some special situations will be presented when there is need for additional knowledge and specialized practice procedures.

Modern burn care

Before addressing the details about burn fluid treatment, there is a need to present the big changes that have occurred recently (in the past 10–20 years) in modern burn care. This will lead to a better comprehension of the advanced medical needs of this patient group and the corresponding fluid treatment strategies.[1]

Incidence

In burn care, in the past 10–20 years there has been a decreasing incidence of burn injuries. This was first described in the United States but has also been shown for most western countries. A very different picture is found in the developing countries and Asia. In general, a decrease of about 30 percent is most often seen in western countries during that time period.[2]

Treatment outcome

At the same time, burn care treatment has significantly been developed and improved. Most obvious is the observation of the significant decrease in hospital mortality for burns, in the range of 70%. However, it is still important to stress that the number of deaths at the scene of the fire is still relatively constant, particularly for Sweden at about 100–120 deaths per year.[2] And these victims most often constitute individuals who are elderly, are physically or mentally disabled, or have drug problems. The reduced hospital mortality rate is claimed to be due to several factors, of which the most important are: modern fluid treatment, aggressive early surgical interventions, improved critical care, and newer and more potent antibiotics and local antimicrobials used in burn wound care.[1]

Another important effect of the early surgical excisional intervention is the length of hospital stay. Length of stay has decreased to approximately 25% of what it was in the 1980s–1990s. At that time, length of stay calculated as the number of days per % body surface area burned was approximately 3–4 days/% TBSA. Today, the corresponding value is less than 1 day/% TBSA for partial thickness burns and approximately 2 days/TBSA% for full thickness burns.[3] When examining mortality rates, they can be depicted as the burned surface area with a 50% predicted mortality risk (lethal dose [LD] 50%). In the mid-1980s the corresponding burn size (LD 50%) was 45% TBSA. Today, and dependent on age, the corresponding burn size for a young person (<60 years old) is 80–90% TBSA burned. The age-adjusted LD 50% are around a Baux index (Age+TBSA%) of 115.[4,5] Another important change in burn care was the introduction of outpatient burn care in the late 1990s; today, patients with burn injuries of up to 10–15% are often routinely treated as outpatients. Outpatient care is also offered for patients with larger burns when most of their open wounds have healed. From this perspective, it is interesting to note that the principles of fluid treatment have not changed since the late 1970s.[1,6,7]

Fluid balance pathophysiology in burns

The purpose of fluid treatment for the burn-injured is to maintain organ perfusion despite major leakage of fluid from the intravascular space. There are mainly two reasons for this fluid loss, which have both been extensively investigated and have a clear temporal pattern:

(a) the negative imbibition pressure in burned tissue;[8,9] and
(b) an increase of the vascular permeability.[10,11]

Negative imbibition pressure

When fluid losses were investigated in experimental models in the 1960s, the fluid loss could not be completely explained by an increase of permeability, and it was postulated that there needed to be another mechanism involved to explain the total fluid loss. In his thesis in 1961, Gösta Arturson predicted that there needed to be another factor involved to explain the total fluid loss in larger burns.[12] He then suggested that the fluid loss from the blood could be explained by a reduction of the interstitial

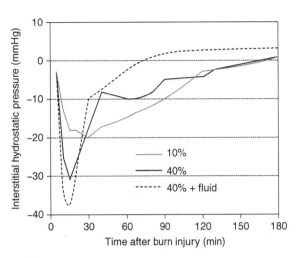

Figure 31.2 Negative imbibition pressure. Schematic drawing of the build-up of negative interstitial fluid pressure depending on the size of a burn injury and whether fluid is administered. Modified from Lund *et al. Am J Physiol* 1988.[8]

tissue pressure. In the 1980s Lund and Reed were able to show in *in vitro* models that there is a build-up of a strong negative interstitial tissue pressure within burn-injured tissue, in the range of −25 to −50 mmHg. This negative gradient, which is called *negative imbibition pressure* and which explains most of the total fluid loss, is most pronounced immediately after the burn and remains for several hours afterwards (Figure 31.2).[8,9] Importantly, most of the total fluid loss seen is lost within these hours, and today we know that this is a reason for early hypovolemia despite the recommended fluid treatment. We will return to this later in the chapter when we discuss the fluid treatment in more detail.

Interestingly, the fluids provided during fluid resuscitation seem to negatively affect the negative imbibition pressure: providing more fluid to the patient leads to a more negative tissue pressure and a larger fluid demand in the tissue, and correspondingly a larger total fluid need for the patient. The mechanism underlying the development of the negative fluid pressure is not fully understood, but it is suggested that it is due to effects on the tissue integrins, which are the components important for regulation of the hydrostatic pressure of the interstitium. The underlying mechanism is that the integrins lose their ability to maintain a positive effect on the pressure: as they are disintegrated by the burn injury to the tissue, their effect is lost and a negative tissue pressure is created. Furthermore, the burn injury effect on the

build-up of a negative tissue imbibition pressure seems to be related to the size of the burn injury, a larger injury leading to a more pronounced negative tissue pressure.[8]

Permeability effects of the burn

It has long been known that burns cause fluid losses from the intravascular space. Another important mechanism is the increase in vascular permeability. Such an effect is seen for a burn injury corresponding to a body surface area of 5% or more. Again, all the details of this effect are yet not elucidated, but there are a number of mediators that have been found to be important. Temporally, in the burn-injured, this effect is also manifested rather early after the injury: most of it is seen within the first 8 hours after the burn. Of the mediators, serotonin [13–15] has been claimed to be the most important from the pathophysiological perspective. Other relevant mediators are: nitric oxide (NO), prostaglandins, and oxygen radicals (see below).[1] Histamine, which historically has been claimed to be important, has recently been questioned.[16]

Another important factor for the fluid loss from the vasculature is the onset of vasodilatation seen in most vascular beds owing to the continuous liberation of pro-inflammatory mediators in injured tissues. This vasodilatation increases the hydrostatic pressure in the microcirculation, leading to fluid loss into the interstitial compartment. It is important, then, to stress that the loss of fluid from the intravascular space affects all the factors that today are claimed as important for the transport of fluid across the capillary/venular wall.

If using the Starling equation to describe the transport of fluid across the capillary, all factors included in the equation are affected negatively (implying a larger fluid loss) in burns. According to the Starling equation, the filtration is dependent on the area of filtration, multiplied by the difference in hydrostatic pressure between capillary and interstitium, minus (the coefficient of filtration) times the difference in colloid osmotic pressure between the capillary and the interstitium. Among these factors, the coefficient of filtration increases greatly, often in the region of 20 times. For the latter parts of the formula, there is an increase in the hydrostatic pressure in the capillary (vasodilatation), together with a decrease in the colloid osmotic pressure in the capillary due to leakage; a decrease in interstitial pressure due to the imbibition pressure; and an increase in the colloid osmotic pressure in the interstitium (due to the leakage of colloid out of the vessels). All of these factors lead to an increase in fluid loss from the vasculature into the tissue. This affects most vascular compartments. The effect on the venular level is claimed to be most important from a quantitative perspective [1] and, although most of the transport across the vascular wall is mediated by smaller molecules, larger proteins are also lost, albeit at a lesser fraction. This is important to note as it underlies the arguments for so-called "colloid rescue" fluid resuscitation in situations of larger burns: this reduces the total colloid loss and corresponding fluid loss, and decreases the risk for compartmental complication.[17]

In clinical practice, the permeability increase is seen in the serum level of albumin, which decreases after the burn as albumin is lost from the intravascular space. It is important also to stress that the intravascular colloid osmotic pressure in the acute phase is dependent not only on albumin but also on the newly synthesized acute phase proteins. Because of uncertainties in the temporal pattern of permeability to proteins locally in the vasculature, no clear advice can be given as to the optimal time when colloids can be administered without the risk of being lost to the interstitium.

There has been an intense debate on when colloids can safely be administered during fluid resuscitation. Today, most burn surgeons would agree that it is adequate to provide colloid after 8–12 hours since the burn if needed to reduce total fluid volume. It is important to understand that providing colloid early may lead to colloid accumulation in the tissue, by early leakage, increasing the risk of higher colloid pressure in the interstitium which in turn increases tissue edema. However, it also needs to be appreciated that only 20% of the crystalloid fluid volume remains intravascularly, and that providing large volumes of crystalloid leads to decreased colloid osmotic pressure intravascularly and thus a further loss of fluid from this compartment. All these effects need to be appreciated when planning the fluid resuscitation for a patient with burns.

Fluid loss in burns – the temporal aspect

When caring for the burn-injured, it is important to examine and discuss the temporal aspects of the fluid loss and the recommended fluid therapy. This is especially the case as recent investigations have shown a clear temporal mismatch between the fluid loss and the fluid volume provided by present guidelines. As previously stated, most of the fluid loss due to the negative imbibition pressure takes place within the first 3–4 hours after the burn. The picture is somewhat different for the fluid loss due to the permeability increase. The most reliable data in humans suggest that this fluid loss occurs from the time of the injury and up to 8 or 10 hours after the burn. Although there is still ongoing debate on this topic, most would agree that the bulk of the loss is during the first 12 hours after the burn.[18,19] One should also take into account the permeability effects of a more or less continuous SIRS (systemic inflammatory response syndrome) reaction that is often seen after the burn, although the magnitude of this is less pronounced if the case is not complicated by sepsis.

Most important is that the present guidelines for fluid resuscitation, especially if based on a pure crystalloid strategy, do not fully account for this early fluid loss, and the patient may be claimed to be in a controlled hypovolemic situation during the first 12–16 hours after the burn. This will be commented on later when discussing the guidelines used for burn fluid resuscitation. In conclusion, it may be stated that the tissue edema reaches a maximum between the first 24 and 48 hours after the burn; this added fluid volume is slowly returned thereafter to the circulation and excreted as urine, often an ongoing process for 7 to 10 days after the burn.

Mediators important for fluid losses

A large number of mediators have been claimed to be important for the underlying mechanisms of fluid losses in burns. Most probable is that there are several that contribute to the fluid loss in different ways. The most important are: nitric oxide (NO), histamine, thromboxanes, prostaglandins (especially PGE2 and F2alpha), serotonin, proteases, oxygen free radicals, eicosanoids, bradykinin, complement factor C3, neuropeptides (especially substance P) and platelet activating factor (PAF), cytokines (interleukin-1,-2,-6,-8, tumor necrosis factor-alpha), and interferons.[1,20] Coagulations and the complement cascade system are thought to be early activated and play a significant role. Interest in the mediators and their possible roles in fluid loss is driven by the hope of finding a blocker that can stop, or reduce, the process. Some attempts have been made in this field, the most successful of which is the use of high-dose vitamin C (as an oxygen radical scavenger), which in a prospective randomized trial showed a reduction in fluid loss in the treatment group.[21–23]

Fluid treatment: practical guidelines

Much of the fluid treatment as we know it today is based on knowledge gained in the 1970s. As long ago as the nineteenth century, there were already theories suggesting that it was the fluid loss, and the corresponding change in the blood, that caused the negative outcomes prevalent at the time. Major breakthroughs in the fluid treatment for burns were made by Underhill who, in the 1920s, started to describe the pathophysiology of the burn injury in more detail. In 1940, following the Cocoanut Grove night-club disaster in Boston, the first attempts to use intravenous fluid treatment in a larger group of injured people were examined. The conclusion was that mortality was significantly lower than expected. In 1953, the first fluid formula to be based on burn size and patient weight was introduced by Evans.[1,20]

The formula most widely used today is the one that was published in 1973 by Charles Baxter, then working at the Parkland Memorial Hospital in Dallas. The formula states, based on experimental findings in dogs and humans, that 2–4 ml of Ringer's solution per total burnt percent of body surface area (TBSA%) and kilogram body weight should be provided. Half of the calculated volume is given during the first 8 hours after the burn and the other half during the subsequent 16 hours. The main advantages are easily attainable fluid (Ringer's lactate), low cost, and a treatment strategy that is easy to start and follow. A number of other formulae have been presented over the years, but none has the global impact of the "Parkland" strategy. Some of the alternatives are listed in Table 31.1.[1,20] Today, few centers in Europe or the United States use strategies other than the Parkland option.[24]

Endpoints for the fluid treatment

As for many medical treatments, there are endpoints for the fluid treatment to be aimed at. This has been increasingly important for burn care, as over-resuscitation can have significant negative effects on the burned tissue (extensive tissue edema) and even lead to complications such as compartment syndrome

Table 31.1 Fluid treatment formulae

Formula	Contains
Main programs	
Parkland	Lactated Ringer's solution 2–4 ml/kg per TBSA% Half of the fluid volume is given in the first 8 h and the remaining volume during the next 16 h
Modified Brooke	Lactated Ringer's solution 2 ml/kg per TBSA% Half of the fluid volume is given in the first 8 h and the remaining volume during the next 16 h
Colloid-based alternatives	
Evans	Sodium chloride solution 1.0 ml/kg per TBSA% + colloid 1.0 ml/kg per TBSA% + 2,000 ml 5% glucose solution
Brooke	Lactated Ringer's solution 1.5 ml/kg per TBSA% + colloid 0.5 ml/kg + 2,000 ml 5% glucose solution
Slater	Lactated Ringer's solution 2,000 ml per 24 h + fresh frozen plasma 75 ml/kg per 24 h
Dextran-based	
Demling	Dextran 40 in isotonic saline solution (2 ml/kg per hour in 8 h) + Ringer's lactate in a volume sufficient to produce 30 ml of urine per hour + fresh frozen plasma (0.5 ml/kg per hour from 8 h to 26 h after the burn injury) Conventional crystalloid therapy during the first 8 h
Hypertonic formulae	
Monafo	Ringer's lactate containing 250 mmol Na per liter. Volume sufficient to produce urine 30 ml/h
Warden	Ringer's lactate + 50 mmol sodium bicarbonate (total 180 mEq sodium per liter) with an aim to produce 30–50 ml/h urine volume for the first 8 h. Thereafter, Ringer's lactate to maintain diuresis

and, at one of its extremes, the abdominal compartment syndrome.

There has even been a term coined for the issue of over-resuscitation in burns – "fluid creep." Although it has been repeatedly discussed, the underlying reason for this increase in fluid provided is not quite clear. A number of explanations have been provided that state that the risk of over-resuscitation, especially with crystalloid solution, can be minimized.[25,26]

Firstly, with increasing survival rates, even patients with very large burns can survive today. In 1960, the Baux index (age plus TBSA%) was used to provide a mortality risk estimate; for example, a 30-year-old with a burn size of 50% faced a 80% mortality risk. Today the lethal dose that leads to a 50% mortality risk (LD 50) has a Baux index of 115. Given these changes, it can be appreciated that the fluid volumes provided according to the resuscitation formulae have increased and, correspondingly, negative effects of large fluid volumes such as extensive tissue edema can be anticipated. Therefore, a colloid rescue strategy should come into play when the fluid volumes provided are large.[17]

Secondly, in modern times more patients are initially intubated and sedated prior to arrival to the hospital. Both sedation and positive-pressure ventilation lead to larger fluid needs to maintain the arterial pressure.[27]

Thirdly, and most importantly, invasive monitoring has become a treatment standard, and this leads to a significant risk of over-resuscitating the patient. This is because, when utilizing the Parkland crystalloid fluid regimen, the patient is hypovolemic during the first 12–18 hours after burn. This has been well documented, and it is important to stress that the strategy is to maintain a controlled hypovolemic situation, by the use of this formula and aiming at 30–50 ml/h urine output. The central circulatory parameters (e.g. intrathoracic blood volume index when using a PiCCO system, wedge pressure in the case of a pulmonary artery catheter, or stroke volume/cardiac output by echocardiography) should herald hypovolemia during this specific time period. When assessing the circulation at 18 hours after injury by these measures, the central parameters have normalized. In clinical practice today, urine output is the gold standard, and added to that is mean arterial pressure and the mental state of the patient. The use of central circulatory parameters for burn resuscitation does not improve outcome but increases the risk of fluid overload.[18,28,29]

Fact square

In the Parkland strategy, burn fluid resuscitation is performed with Ringer's lactate 2–4 ml/kg per TBSA%. Treatment endpoint is urine production 0.5–1.0 ml/kg per hour, together with a mean arterial pressure >70 mmHg, and the patient should be mentally alert.

Situations in which Parkland strategy should be modified and specific interventions needed

Very large burns or burns that need very large fluid volumes

When the needs rapidly exceed that calculated by the formulae (2–4 ml/kg per TBSA%), it is mandatory to use either albumin or plasma (i.e. colloid rescue treatment) alone or in conjunction with the crystalloid to reduce the risk of an abdominal compartment syndrome. The clinician should be observant for the early need for escharotomy (i.e. skin incisions to reduce tissue pressure in circumferential burns on the thorax or extremities). Adding colloid should preferably be performed no earlier than 8 hours after the burn if possible, to reduce the risk of colloid deposition in the tissues due to the "capillary leak." One publication states [26] that the risk of abdominal compartment syndrome increases significantly when fluid volumes of about 300 ml/kg per 24 hours are exceeded. When in doubt, start assessing abdominal compartment pressure according to standard ICU procedures. Albumin and plasma are both effective in reducing tissue edema, but research indicates a larger pressure-reducing effect on using plasma.

Inhalation injuries

Previously in the burns literature it was stated that the presence of smoke inhalation injury leads to an increased fluid need, and many textbooks suggested administering increased fluid, in the range of an extra 1–2 ml/kg per TBSA%. However, recent publications do not support an extra need for fluid volume, and there is also at least a theoretical issue of keeping the lung "dry" to optimize gas exchange.[25]

Electrical injuries: chromogens in urine

Another occasion on which the fluid need may be difficult to predict, and for which there are often very large needs, is in cases of high-voltage (>1,000 volts) electrical injuries. These injuries constitute approximately 5–10% of the burn injuries at a burn center. The explanation for the large fluid need is two-fold: firstly, the total tissue volume that is injured is often significantly larger in electrical injuries than in isolated skin injuries. Other tissues such as muscle and bone may be involved, and the burn that is seen at the skin level is only a minor part of the total tissue injury. Secondly, both free hemoglobin and myoglobin are circulated in the blood, and these have a toxic effect on the kidneys. In order to reduce this toxicity, increased urine output is recommended, together with alkalizing the urine by adding sodium bicarbonate to the resuscitation fluid. Urine pH should be maintained at approximately 7 and the urine volumes at 100–200 ml/h.[1,20]

Table 31.2 Daily maintenance fluid need for children

100 ml/kg up to a body weight of 10 kg

Above 10 kg weight, add 50 ml/kg in the weight range of 11–20 kg

Above 20 kg weight, add 20 ml for each extra kg

Example: Maintenance fluid for a child of 28 kg: 1,000 ml + 500 ml + 160 ml, i.e. total 1,660 ml per 24 h

Burns in children

There are several issues when treating burn injuries in children that need to be given special attention. Firstly, owing to the thinner skin of the child, there is a larger risk that the burn becomes deeper. Secondly, the larger ratio of skin area to body mass means that the child is more prone to hypothermia. Thirdly, there is a larger risk for hypoglycemia owing to smaller glycogen deposits. Fourthly, the relative size of the airway is smaller, increasing the risk for an upper airway obstruction due to tissue edema. The larger skin area to body mass ratio leads to more fluid being needed in the resuscitation. This is accomplished by providing 3–4 ml/kg per TBSA% and also adding the normal 24 h fluid maintenance need of the child (see Table 31.2).

Very extensive burns: maintaining organ perfusion and temperature, and dealing with the sodium load

In cases of very large burns (>50 TBSA%, and mainly full thickness), specific conditions apply beyond the regular fluid treatment and the early "colloid rescue":

There is often a need for pressure support treatment by use of inotropes (for example noradrenaline/vasopressin or dobutamine infusion). In addition to the circulatory problem, there might be toxic effects from the burn-injured tissue on the heart, as evidenced by leakage of troponin to the circulatory system.[30]

The temperature issue also needs to be mentioned. In very large burns, the usual temperature regulation is almost completely absent because of the skin injury, and these patients need active warming with convective (fluid-based) heating systems. Just using hot air or air-based heaters will not suffice.[31]

As a consequence of the large fluid volume provided, there might also be a sodium problem depending on the limited fluid elimination capacity of the kidneys. For example, in the case of a 70% burn in an adult of 70 kg, and using the Parkland strategy without colloids, about 20 liters of lactated Ringer's solution will be provided. This adds a significant sodium load to the individual (20 liters × 130 mosmol Na/l, which equals 2,600 mosmol of Na). Given that the kidneys have a ceiling effect for sodium excretion (usually in the range of 500 mosmol/24 hours) it is not uncommon that there are increased serum sodium levels (>160 mosmol/l) observed on days 5–10 after the injury. The consequence of this has not been extensively studied, but many burn centers add glucose-containing fluids when the total fluid volume exceeds 10 liters to reduce this risk.

Fluid treatment and early tangential excision of the burn wound

As surgical techniques have evolved, many burn centers now practice very early tangential excision. During such a procedure, all full thickness and deep second-degree burns are surgically excised. A few years ago, many centers performed the excision irrespective of the burn injury size. Today this is less common, and the procedure is instead staged in several surgeries with 20% TBSA excision per surgery (thus a 40% burn would be excised in two surgeries of 20% each). This leads to a significant blood loss during the fluid resuscitation period. In general, for most centers, the blood loss is estimated to be in the range of 0.3 unit of packed red cells per TBSA% excised: that is, a blood loss of approximately 7 units for an excision of 20% TBSA. On these occasions it is important that the anesthesia and surgical teams co-operate well and that there is adequate monitoring of the patient.[1,20] Plasma and platelet infusions are often added to optimize coagulation.

Future prospects

It is surprising that current fluid treatment for burns still rests on a 40-year-old strategy, even though more knowledge and better techniques exist to support its use today. There is a significant need for improvement, possibly through blocking the process of fluid loss from the circulation, or by developing new resuscitation fluids. Although it was hoped that starch-based solutions, by containing molecules of larger sizes, would reduce the fluid losses, they have been found to be detrimental to kidney function and have therefore been abandoned in this respect.[32]

References

1. Herndon D. *Total Burn Care*. 4th edn. Saunders, Elsevier; 2012.

2. Akerlund E, Huss FR, Sjoberg F. Burns in Sweden: an analysis of 24,538 cases during the period 1987–2004. *Burns* 2007; 33(1): 31–6.

3. Engrav LH, Heimbach DM, Rivara FP, *et al.* Harborview burns–1974 to 2009. *PLoS One* 2012; 7(7): e40086.

4. Galeiras R. Critical care of the burn patient. *Crit Care Med* 2010; 38(4): 1225; author reply 1225–6.

5. Galeiras R, Lorente JA, Pertega S, *et al.* A model for predicting mortality among critically ill burn victims. *Burns* 2009; 35(2): 201–9.

6. Baxter CR. Sixth National Burn Seminar. Fluid therapy of burns. *J Trauma* 1967; 7(1): 69–73.

7. Baxter CR. Fluid volume and electrolyte changes of the early postburn period. *Clin Plast Surg* 1974; 1(4): 693–703.

8. Lund T, Wiig H, Reed RK. Acute postburn edema: role of strongly negative interstitial fluid pressure. *Am J Physiol* 1988; 255(5 Pt 2): H1069–74.

9. Lund T, Wiig H, Reed RK, Aukland K. A 'new' mechanism for oedema generation: strongly negative interstitial fluid pressure causes rapid fluid flow into thermally injured skin. *Acta Physiol Scand* 1987; 129(3): 433–5.

10. Vlachou E, Gosling P, Moiemen NS. Microalbuminuria: a marker of endothelial dysfunction in thermal injury. *Burns* 2006; 32(8): 1009–16.

11. Vlachou E, Gosling P, Moiemen NS. Microalbuminuria: a marker of systemic endothelial dysfunction during burn excision. *Burns* 2008; 34(2): 241–6.

12. Arturson G. Pathophysiological aspects of the burn syndrome with special reference to liver injury and alterations of capillary permeability. *Acta Chir Scand Suppl* 1961; Suppl 274: 1–135.

13. Ferrara JJ, Franklin EW, Choe EU, *et al.* Serotonin receptors regulate canine regional vasodilator responses to burn. *Crit Care Med* 1995; 23(6): 1112–16.

14. Holliman CJ, Meuleman TR, Larsen KR, *et al.* The effect of ketanserin, a specific serotonin antagonist, on burn shock hemodynamic parameters in a porcine burn model. *J Trauma* 1983; 23(10): 867–71.

15. Samuelsson A, Abdiu A, Wackenfors A, Sjoberg F. Serotonin kinetics in patients with burn injuries: a comparison between the local and systemic responses measured by microdialysis – a pilot study. *Burns* 2008; 34(5): 617–22.

16. Johansson J, Backryd E, Granerus G, Sjoberg F. Urinary excretion of histamine and methylhistamine after burns. *Burns* 2012; 38(7): 1005–9.

17. O'Mara MS, Slater H, Goldfarb IW, Caushaj PF. A prospective, randomized evaluation of intra-abdominal pressures with crystalloid and colloid resuscitation in burn patients. *J Trauma* 2005; 58(5): 1011–18.

18. Bak Z, Sjoberg F, Eriksson O, Steinvall I, Janerot-Sjoberg B. Hemodynamic changes during resuscitation after burns using the Parkland formula. *J Trauma* 2009; 66(2): 329–36.

19. Sjoberg F. The 'Parkland protocol' for early fluid resuscitation of burns: too little, too much, or … even … too late …? *Acta Anaesthesiol Scand* 2008; 52(6): 725–6.

20. Jeschke MG, Kamolz LP, Sjöberg F, Wolf SE (eds.) *Handbook of Burns*. 1st edn. Wien: Springer; 2012.

21. Matsuda T, Tanaka H, Hanumadass M, *et al.* Effects of high-dose vitamin C administration on postburn microvascular fluid and protein flux. *J Burn Care Rehabil* 1992; 13(5): 560–6.

22. Matsuda T, Tanaka H, Yuasa H, *et al.* The effects of high-dose vitamin C therapy on postburn lipid peroxidation. *J Burn Care Rehabil* 1993; 14(6): 624–9.

23. Tanaka H, Lund T, Wiig H, *et al.* High dose vitamin C counteracts the negative interstitial fluid hydrostatic pressure and early edema generation in thermally injured rats. *Burns* 1999; 25(7): 569–74.

24. Greenhalgh DG. Burn resuscitation: the results of the ISBI/ABA survey. *Burns* 2010; 36(2): 176–82.

25. Saffle JI. The phenomenon of "fluid creep" in acute burn resuscitation. *J Burn Care Res* 2007; 28(3): 382–95.

26. Oda J, Yamashita K, Inoue T, *et al.* Resuscitation fluid volume and abdominal compartment syndrome in patients with major burns. *Burns* 2006; 32(2): 151–4.

27. Mackie DP, Spoelder EJ, Paauw RJ, Knape P, Boer C. Mechanical ventilation and fluid retention in burn patients. *J Trauma* 2009; 67(6): 1233–8; discussion 1238.

28. Holm C, Mayr M, Tegeler J, *et al.* A clinical randomized study on the effects of invasive monitoring on burn shock resuscitation. *Burns* 2004; 30(8): 798–807.

29. Holm C, Melcer B, Horbrand F, *et al.* Arterial thermodilution: an alternative to pulmonary artery catheter for cardiac output assessment in burn patients. *Burns* 2001; 27(2): 161–6.

30. Bak Z, Sjoberg F, Eriksson O, Steinvall I, Janerot-Sjoberg B. Cardiac dysfunction after burns. *Burns* 2008; 34(5): 603–9.

31. Kjellman BM, Fredrikson M, Glad-Mattsson G, Sjoberg F, Huss FR. Comparing ambient, air-convection, and fluid-convection heating techniques in treating hypothermic burn patients, a clinical RCT. *Ann Surg Innov Res* 2011; 5(1): 4.

32. Bechir M, Puhan MA, Fasshauer M, *et al.* Early fluid resuscitation with hydroxyethyl starch 130/0.4 (6%) in severe burn injury: a randomized, controlled, double-blind clinical trial. *Crit Care* 2013; 17(6): R299.

Chapter

32

Trauma

Joshua D. Person and John B. Holcomb

Summary

In the United States, injury is the leading cause of death among individuals between the ages of 1 and 44 years, and the third leading cause of death overall. Approximately 20% to 40% of trauma deaths occurring after hospital admission are related to massive hemorrhage and are therefore potentially preventable with rapid hemorrhage control and improved resuscitation techniques. Over the past decade, the treatment of this population has transitioned into a damage control strategy with the development of resuscitation strategies that emphasize permissive hypotension, limited crystalloid administration, early balanced blood product transfusion, and rapid hemorrhage control. This resuscitation approach initially attempts to replicate whole blood transfusion, utilizing an empiric 1:1:1 ratio of plasma:platelets:red blood cells, and then transitions, when bleeding slows, to a goal-directed approach to reverse coagulopathy based on viscoelastic assays. Traditional resuscitation strategies with crystalloid fluids are appropriate for the minimally injured patient who presents without shock or ongoing bleeding. This chapter will focus on the assessment and resuscitation of seriously injured trauma patients who present with ongoing blood loss and hemorrhagic shock.

The resuscitation of massively bleeding patients has changed markedly over the past century. The use of blood banking and the transfusion of injured patients originated during World War I when it was found to decrease mortality in bleeding and severely injured soldiers.[1] Whole blood was the sole transfusion product until the 1960s and 1970s when component therapy was adopted in the western world.

The next 40 years saw patients resuscitated initially with large volumes of crystalloid and colloid followed by packed red blood cells (RBCs), with limited transfusion of plasma, platelets, and cryoprecipitate based on laboratory values. In hindsight, this approach led to substantial iatrogenic resuscitation injury, and a growing body of literature developed indicating that aggressive resuscitation with large volumes of crystalloid led to cardiac and pulmonary complications, abdominal compartment syndrome, gastrointestinal dysmotility, coagulopathy, and disturbances of immunological and inflammatory mediators.[2]

After major trauma and shock, capillary permeability increases with a resultant decrease in the plasma colloid osmotic pressure and loss of intravascular fluid into the interstitial space. In response to decreased pressure and intravascular hypovolemia, volume returns from the extravascular space in an attempt to re-expand the vascular space and maintain blood pressure.[3,4] The rationale of large-volume crystalloid resuscitation was related to the theory that tissue injury resulted in sequestration of fluid into the traumatized area, with a resultant decrease in extracellular volume that should be replaced with fluids, the so-called "third space concept." This theory has been refuted by several studies which demonstrated that postoperatively, there is a net "no change" or increase in the extracellular volume.[4–7] Trauma also leads to endothelial cell dysfunction and an increase in proinflammatory cytokines, which is exacerbated by proinflammatory crystalloid administration, and leads to the initiation of an exaggerated inflammatory response with resultant fluid overload and tissue edema.[8]

In the past decade, there has been a philosophical change in the way severely injured trauma patients are resuscitated which focuses on the early balanced transfusion of blood products and limited crystalloid use. This approach focuses on repairing the endothelium, maintaining intravascular volume, and decreasing edema.

Triage and initial assessment

The triage and initial assessment of injury severity in trauma patients is primarily driven by abnormalities of physiological variables such as blood pressure and heart rate. Basic vital signs are easily obtainable in the field and may provide insight as to whether or not a patient is "clinically stable." This data is used in the prehospital setting to determine the patient's mode of transport, destination of treatment, treatment priority, and need for potentially life-saving interventions. When grossly abnormal, vital signs serve as reliable indicators for early diagnostic and therapeutic decision making after injury. However, they can be problematic in many cases as normal physiological compensatory mechanisms may mask the true degree of injury and tissue hypoperfusion. These compensatory mechanisms, especially in young healthy patients, allow for a significant reduction in central circulating blood volume, stroke volume, and cardiac output to occur well before changes in blood pressure develop.[9] Patients may appear "clinically stable" when in fact they are approaching cardiovascular collapse. Hypotension in trauma patients was classically defined as a systolic blood pressure (SBP) of less than 90 mmHg. More recent literature suggests that a SBP of 90 mmHg does not represent the onset of circulatory failure, but rather the clinical manifestation of physiological decompensation associated with advanced hemorrhagic shock and impending cardiovascular collapse. A SBP of <110 mmHg may be a more clinically relevant definition of hypotension in trauma patients as it is at this threshold that tissue hypoperfusion begins to develop, as evidenced by increasing base deficit, with resultant increase in mortality, ICU length of stay, complications, and ventilator days.[10] To overcome the well-described limitations of blood pressure and heart rate, accurate non-invasive methods of delineating the compensated shock state need to be developed and validated.

Intravascular volume depletion, with or without associated hypotension, leads to the physiological state of shock which is characterized by tissue malperfusion and the inability to maintain aerobic metabolism. There are several different mechanisms by which the shock state can be produced after trauma. Hypovolemia due to massive blood loss is the most likely etiology and the leading cause of death after injury. Other causes must also be considered and rapidly treated, including blunt myocardial damage leading to cardiogenic shock, spinal cord injury with resultant vasodilation and distributive shock, or obstructive shock secondary to tension pneumothorax or pericardial tamponade. Acute blood loss, if not expeditiously treated with hemorrhage control and restoration of intravascular volume, will lead to hemodynamic instability, tissue malperfusion, cellular hypoxia, multisystem organ failure, and death.

The two most commonly used laboratory markers in assessing tissue hypoperfusion and the development of anaerobic metabolism in trauma are serum lactate and base deficit. Both tests are easily obtainable and provide quick results which can help guide resuscitative efforts. Base deficit represents the number of mEq/l of additional base that must be added to a liter of blood to normalize the pH and is calculated directly from the blood gas analyzer from the pCO_2, pH, and HCO_3^- values as applied to a standard nomogram.

Changes in base deficit occur early in hemorrhage and will often precede alterations in hemodynamic parameters such as blood pressure, urine output, and pH.[11] Normal values for base deficit vary among institutions but tend to be greater than -2 mmol/l. A significant base deficit has been shown to be a marker of mortality in several studies.[12–14] Mortality starts increasing when base deficit is >4, and when ≥ 8 mmol/l has predicted a 25% mortality rate in trauma patients less than 55 years old without head injury.[15] Lactate is a by-product of anaerobic metabolism and is often considered a marker for tissue hypoxia. It is produced by the conversion of pyruvate to lactate after glycolysis by the enzyme lactate dehydrogenase. Although lactate can be elevated in several other conditions, its use to guide resuscitation by lactate clearance has been validated in several studies. Both the initial lactate value and the time to normalization of lactate levels are predictive of mortality, with 100% mortality in ICU patients who fail to achieve normal levels.[16–20]

While blood volume varies with age and physiological state, the average adult blood volume represents approximately 7% of body weight (70 ml/kg of body weight). For a 70 kg individual, estimated blood volume is approximately 5 liters. There are many potential sites of major hemorrhage following injury. Injury to the base of the skull or neck can lead to rapid exsanguination from major vascular structures which are frequently difficult to control and can also lead to difficulty in securing a reliable airway owing to swelling and distortion of normal anatomy. Injuries to the chest can cause parenchymal lung or great vessel injury resulting in hemothorax, which is easily identified with standard chest X-ray. Penetrating cardiac injury can rapidly cause cardiovascular collapse secondary to pericardial tamponade or massive exsanguination. In the peritoneal cavity, hepatic, splenic, and mesenteric injuries can lead to massive hemoperitoneum if not rapidly controlled either in the operating room or interventional radiology suite. Bleeding in the retroperitoneal space from injuries to the great abdominal vessels, renal lacerations, or pelvic fractures with associated damage to pelvic vessels can be difficult to diagnose as ultrasound examination and peritoneal lavage are not reliable diagnostic tools. Extremity injury, such as a penetrating wound or open fracture of the proximal leg or upper arm, may cause massive bleeding from damage to arterial and venous structures. More commonly, and frequently overlooked, a closed fracture of the femur can easily hide 2–3 units of blood without obvious physical exam findings of ongoing bleeding.

In modern trauma centers, facilities and personnel are available to address each of these injuries. When patients present with multiple serious injuries, diagnostic and therapeutic dilemmas arise in properly sequencing the plan of care between advanced imaging studies and operative or angiographic intervention. For this reason, advanced trauma care centers with focused hybrid operating suites are becoming more common, allowing patients to be moved directly from the emergency department to the hybrid resuscitation area where all imaging and interventions can occur simultaneously and in one location. It is very likely that as this capability becomes more common, time to hemostasis after multisystem injury will decrease and survival will improve.

Massive transfusion

Traditionally, massive transfusion has been defined as the administration of 10 or more units of RBCs over a 24-hour period. Several alternative definitions

have been proposed, including transfusion of an entire blood volume over 24 hours, 10 units over 6 hours, 5 units over 4 hours, 8 or more units over 12 hours, or 3 or more units over a 1-hour period.[21] Older definitions suffered from significant bias, and have been replaced with rate-based definitions that quantify transfusion requirement over shorter time periods. Regardless of definition, this patient population represents the most critically injured and those most likely to die secondary to massive hemorrhage. In a civilian hospital setting, the incidence of trauma patients receiving massive transfusion ranges between 1% and 3% of all admissions. The mortality of trauma patients who receive massive transfusion is between 20% and 50%.[22–26] Also of critical importance is that these patients die quickly after admission, with the median time to death from hemorrhage of 2 hours.[26] These high mortality rates, especially in those patients who die very soon after admission, are frequently associated with the "lethal triad" that follows severe trauma, characterized by hypothermia, metabolic acidosis, and coagulopathy.[27] Historically, both hypothermia and acidosis were aggressively treated, without a specific focus on coagulopathy. In recent years it has become understood that trauma-induced coagulopathy (TIC) is a multifactorial event which is strongly associated with increased mortality. It is important to promptly recognize those patients who develop TIC, and focus all resuscitative efforts on reversing and preventing any exacerbation of this coagulopathy. The exact etiology of TIC is unclear but the systemic shedding of the glycocalyx and resultant increased permeability of the endothelium is at least partially responsible. Hemorrhagic shock leads to systemic endothelial injury and dysfunction that causes disturbances in coagulation, vascular leak, edema, inflammation, and tissue injury, termed "endotheliopathy of trauma." Plasma has been shown to repair endothelial tight junctions, decrease paracellular permeability, and restore the glycocalyx, while crystalloids have no effect. The exact mechanism is unknown, but resuscitating with plasma appears to help repair the vascular endothelium, minimizing edema and avoiding the iatrogenic resuscitation injury associated with large volumes of crystalloid administration.[28,29]

Historically, blood product components were infused in a serial fashion. Many liters of crystalloid were infused first, then moving to RBCs and then adding plasma when the entire blood volume was substituted, followed by the addition of platelets when two blood volumes were substituted. This strategy was problematic as the dilution of coagulation factors and platelets by large volumes of crystalloid and RBCs led to further coagulopathy and ongoing bleeding. This transfusion strategy was challenged early in the new millennium, primarily by US military experiences with combat injuries in Iraq, where thawed AB fresh frozen plasma was administered together with RBCs and platelets from the start of resuscitation.[30]

In 2007, Borgman *et al.* found a survival advantage in massively transfused patients utilizing a balanced transfusion strategy.[31] The transfusion of a 1:1:1 balanced ratio of blood product components (plasma:platelets:RBCs) became the foundation for the strategy described as "damage control resuscitation" (DCR). At the same time that combat surgeons were developing this concept, Johansson and colleagues in Copenhagen were implementing a similar approach, based on their transfusion experience with ruptured aortic aneurysms.[32] The DCR approach has been examined and validated by multiple authors, and has undergone evaluation in single- and multicenter retrospective studies, multicenter observational studies, and recently a prospective and randomized multicenter study.[31,33–35] The pragmatic randomized optimal plasma and platelet ratio (PROPPR) study evaluated 680 patients randomized to either a 1:1:1 or a 1:1:2 ratio. The authors found that there was no mortality difference at 24 hours and 30 days, but more patients in the 1:1:1 group achieved hemostasis and fewer experienced death due to exsanguination by 24 hours. There was a significant difference ($p = 0.02$) in mortality at 3 hours and this difference persisted over the ensuing 30 days. No other safety differences were identified between the two groups despite the increased use of plasma and platelets transfused in the 1:1:1 group. These results have been viewed favorably and many guidelines now recommend starting transfusion with a 1:1:1 approach in massively bleeding patients.[36]

At our center, the Texas Trauma Institute, we have 4 units of universal donor liquid plasma and RBCs available in the emergency department at all times. If the door is opened to the refrigerator housing these units, the massive bleeding protocol is activated and 6 units of RBCs, 6 units of plasma, and a 6 pack of platelets are delivered automatically to the emergency department. The goal of this protocol is to keep these products readily available for transfusion at the patient's bedside until hemostasis is achieved.

We utilize an active performance improvement process to review each bleeding protocol activation, ensuring optimal efficiency of this critical pathway.

Measuring coagulation

The recent paradigm shift in the resuscitation of massively bleeding patients has also been associated with a change in the way that coagulation parameters in trauma patients are measured. Historically, conventional tests such as international normalized ratio (INR), prothrombin time (PT), partial thromboplastin time (PTT), platelet count, and fibrinogen levels were used to identify those patients with traumatic coagulopathy who were in need of blood product transfusion. These tests are problematic as they were not designed to guide resuscitation efforts or comprehensively describe coagulation function, and are poorly associated with bleeding and transfusion requirements. Furthermore, they are often clinically irrelevant in massively bleeding patients as the results take a prolonged time period to return. The optimal coagulation test used to guide resuscitation in critically injured patients would be a rapid assay based on whole blood that more accurately reflects the integrated function of all aspects of the coagulation system.

The cell-based model of hemostasis, which emphasizes both the importance of tissue factor as the initiator of coagulation as well as cellular elements such as platelets, replaced the classical cascade model of coagulation in the mid-1990s. According to the cell-based model, hemostasis occurs in three phases: *initiation*, *amplification*, and *propagation*, with the magnitude of thrombin generation determining the hemostatic capacity of the formed clot.[37] This integrated model of coagulation is now widely accepted, and the viscoelastic hemostatic assays (VHAs) are felt to reflect this approach more accurately than the conventional tests described above.

VHAs such as thromboelastography (TEG) and rotational thromboelastometry (ROTEM) have historically been used to guide resuscitation in cardiac and transplant centers, and are now frequently being used in the trauma population. These assays produce a tracing based on viscoelastic properties of a whole blood sample and represent components of the coagulation system including plasma proteins and fibrinogen function, thrombin burst, platelet function, and the fibrinolytic system. Compared with conventional coagulation tests, results are available faster, cheaper, and provide a more global assessment of the functional aspects of intravascular coagulation.[38] They have also been shown to predict increased risk of pulmonary embolism following major trauma.[39] Rapid thromboelastography (r-TEG) can be implemented with computer software packages that allow the tracing to be monitored in real-time in the trauma bay, operating room, or intensive care unit as the test is being performed in the laboratory. This capability provides the clinician with clinically useful data that can be acted upon before the entire test is finalized and reported. When compared with conventional coagulation tests this technology provides more rapid results and has proven to be clinically superior, identifying patients with an increased risk of needing early RBC, plasma, and platelet transfusions, and those with excessive fibrinolysis. With a similar cost profile, it is feasible to replace conventional coagulation tests with VHAs in trauma patients.[31] However, in the rapidly bleeding patient the VHAs still do not return data fast enough for clinical utility. Rates of transfusion easily approach several units every 5 min, and the rate of death from hemorrhagic shock is highest in the first hour after admission. In these patients minutes really do make a difference, and it is in this scenario that the empiric 1:1:1 transfusion approach is utilized. Unfortunately, VHAs do not reveal any direct data about endotheliopathy of trauma and reveal limited information about platelet function. Newer coagulation tests should integrate these important data points, providing a more comprehensive picture of TIC.

Hemorrhage control

In the prehospital setting, the use of tourniquets, hemostatic dressings, pelvic binders, and hypotensive resuscitation efforts to minimize and prevent ongoing blood loss is central to the model of damage control resuscitation. Trauma patients that have bleeding controlled are much easier to resuscitate. Historically, the prehospital approach to hypotensive trauma patients included the prompt administration of large volumes of isotonic intravenous fluids. More recently, most centers have adopted the practice of "permissive hypotension" prior to operative control of bleeding, which is used to prevent the disruption of clot formation and exacerbation of ongoing hemorrhage. The use of excessive crystalloid not only further dilutes coagulation factors, exacerbates endothelial damage, and increases edema, but the associated increase in

blood pressure can also "pop the clot," leading to further hemorrhage. Consistent with this approach, a randomized trial of prehospital hypotensive resuscitation for penetrating torso injuries found that when compared with the standard prehospital crystalloid resuscitation group, those patients who were randomized to receive no fluids prior to arrival in the operating room had less intraoperative blood loss, increased survival, and shorter hospital length of stay.[40]

Because so many patients exsanguinate before reaching the hospital, newer methods of prehospital abdominal hemorrhage control are needed. An interesting experimental option is the use of a novel intraabdominal self-expanding polyurethane foam which can be instilled into the peritoneal cavity in order to provide temporary control of non-compressible hemorrhage in the prehospital setting.[41] Clinical trials are being reviewed by regulatory bodies, and if successful could significantly alter this landscape. The use of catheter-based interventions for control of noncompressible torso hemorrhage is also an area of active clinical research. Resuscitative endovascular balloon occlusion of the aorta (REBOA), initially described in the 1950s, has been more frequently utilized over the past several years as non-vascular surgeons become more comfortable with endovascular techniques. This procedure can be performed in the emergency department and provides rapid temporary control of abdominal and pelvic hemorrhage until definitive hemostasis is achieved, without the need for a resuscitative thoracotomy with cross-clamping of the aorta.[42]

Prehospital transfusion

Optimal prehospital care is based on the logistically feasible extension of hospital care that can be effectively delivered. As the resuscitation of bleeding trauma patients in the hospital has shifted away from a crystalloid-based resuscitation to a balanced blood product approach, the use of prehospital transfusion has developed. Why would we infuse crystalloids in the prehospital setting when they are avoided in the hospital? Following the lead of the recent military experience, several civilian trauma centers have placed RBCs and plasma on their helicopters. Several retrospective studies have demonstrated a benefit with prehospital transfusion of RBCs and plasma including lower overall transfusion requirements, decreased coagulopathy, improved early survival, and negligible wastage of blood products.[43–45].

We start transfusion with a plasma first approach, and 85% of prehospital transfused patients have continued transfusion in the hospital. These small retrospective studies have generated significant interest, and there are now several ongoing prospective and observational studies. While current studies are evaluating liquid products, future randomized studies will include the use of dried blood products. This exciting area of investigation is rapidly expanding and is extremely important. Bringing blood products to the point of injury will likely improve survival.

Bringing it all together

Starting at the point of injury and continuing into the emergency department, evaluation with an emphasis on rapid identification and treatment of active hemorrhage should ensue. All devices that are effective in controlling external compressible hemorrhage are utilized. If the patient has had transfusion started prehospital, the massive bleeding protocol is automatically activated and products are waiting in the emergency department when the patient arrives. Diagnosis is made via a thorough physical examination, assessment of vital signs and response to initial resuscitation, brief radiographic studies to include plain films of the chest and pelvis, and ultrasound of the mediastinum and peritoneal cavity to evaluate for signs of occult hemorrhage (Focused Assessment with Sonography in Trauma, FAST). VHA assessment of coagulation parameters (TEG, ROTEM), hemoglobin level, and blood gas analysis is obtained on all seriously injured patients.

Our group utilizes the Assessment of Blood Consumption (ABC) score both on the helicopter and in the emergency department to help guide the initiation of transfusion. The ABC score is a rapid nonlaboratory-dependent tool that can accurately predict those patients who will require massive transfusion. Patients are given one point each for: penetrating mechanism, initial SBP of ≤90 mmHg, initial heart rate of ≥120 bpm, and positive FAST exam. An ABC score of ≥2 is 75% sensitive and 86% specific for predicting massive transfusion.[46]. The ABC scoring system is utilized to help predict which patients will require massive transfusion as physician gestalt has proved to be less accurate.[47] After complete evaluation, hemodynamically stable patients can have resuscitation guided by the returning VHAs. Patients who present hypotensive or in shock, or have an ABC score ≥2, should have large-bore i.v. access obtained and have the massive bleeding protocol initiated, initially receiving a 1:1:1 ratio-driven resuscitation with rapid control of hemorrhage sought in the operating room or interventional radiology suite. It is critical to have resuscitation and hemorrhage control interventions occur simultaneously, with minimal time spent in the emergency department in these most critically ill patients. Ideally, less than 15 min should be spent in the evaluation phase, and the patient should move to definitive hemorrhage control very quickly. We feel that this provides optimal resuscitation of the endothelium. Response to resuscitation should be closely monitored (heart rate, blood pressure, urine output, base deficit, lactate levels, etc.) and when bleeding slows so that laboratory values return in a clinically useful time period, resuscitation should transition from a ratio-driven approach to a goal-driven approach guided by VHAs. The TEG Ly30 can assess for hyperfibrinolysis in a whole blood sample by measuring the percentage of maximal clot strength that has been dissolved 30 min after maximum amplitude (MA) has been reached. Mortality from trauma rises as fibrinolysis increases to ≥3% as evidenced by TEG Ly30.[48] In our center, those patients who are hyperfibrinolytic (>3%) with ongoing hemorrhage, and are within a 3-hour window from injury, receive tranexamic acid according to the CRASH2 trial dose.[49–51] When bleeding stops and resuscitation is complete, TEG values are usually near normal. Utilizing the concepts described above has resulted in a 30% decrease in death from hemorrhage over the past 7 years.

References

1. Stansbury LG, Hess JR. Putting the pieces together: Roger I. Lee and modern transfusion medicine. *Transfus Med Rev* 2005; 19: 81–4.

2. Cotton BA, Guy JS, Morris JA Jr, *et al.* The cellular, metabolic, and systemic consequences of aggressive fluid resuscitation strategies. *Shock* 2006; 26: 115–21.

3. Holte K, Sharrock NE, Kehlet H. Pathophysiology and clinical implications of preoperative fluid excess. *Br J Anaesth* 2002; 89: 622–32.

4. Gutelius JR, Shizgal HM, Lopez G. The effect of trauma on extracellular water volume. *Arch Surg* 1968; 97: 206–14.

5. Nielsen OM, Engell HC. Extracellular fluid volume and distribution in relation to changes in plasma colloid osmotic pressure after major surgery. A randomized study. *Acta Chir Scand* 1985; 151: 221–5.

6. Virtue RW, LeVine DS, Aikawa JK. Fluid shifts during the surgical period: RISA and S35 determinations following glucose, saline or lactate infusion. *Ann Surg* 1966; 63: 523–8.

7. Nielsen OM, Engell HC. The importance of plasma colloid osmotic pressure for interstitial fluid volume and fluid balance after elective abdominal vascular surgery. *Ann Surg* 1986; 203: 25–9.

8. Powers KA, Zurawska J, Szaszi K, *et al.* Hypertonic resuscitation of hemorrhagic shock prevents alveolar macrophage activation by preventing systemic oxidative stress due to gut ischemia reperfusion. *Surgery* 2005; 137: 66–74.

9. Gutierrez G, Reines HD, Wulf-Gutierrez ME. Clinical review: hemorrhagic shock. *Crit Care* 2004; 8: 373–81.

10. Eastridge BJ, Salinas J, McManus JG, *et al.* Hypotension begins at 110 mm Hg: redefining "hypotension" with data. *J Trauma* 2007; 63: 291–7.

11. Davis JW, Kaups KL, Parks SN. Base deficit is superior to pH in evaluating clearance of acidosis after traumatic shock. *J Trauma* 1998; 44: 114–18.

12. Davis JW. The relationship of base deficit to lactate in porcine hemorrhagic shock and resuscitation. *J Trauma* 1994; 36: 168–72.

13. Bannon MP, O'Neill CM, Martin M, *et al.* Central venous oxygen saturation, arterial base deficit, and lactate concentration in trauma patients. *Am Surg* 1995; 61: 738–45.

14. Sauaia A, Moore FA, Moore EE, *et al.* Early predictors of postinjury multiple organ failure. *Arch Surg* 1994; 129: 39–45.

15. Rutherford EJ, Morris JA, Reed GW, *et al.* Base deficit stratifies mortality and determines therapy. *J Trauma* 1992; 33: 417–23.

16. McNelis J, Marini CP, Jurkiewicz A, *et al.* Prolonged lactate clearance is associated with increased mortality in the surgical intensive care unit. *Am J Surg* 2001; 182: 481–5.

17. Weil MH, Afifi AA. Experimental and clinical studies on lactate and pyruvate as indicators of the severity of acute circulatory failure (shock). *Circulation* 1970; 41: 989–1001.

18. Abramson D, Scalea TM, Hitchcock R, *et al.* Lactate clearance and survival following injury. *J Trauma* 1993; 35: 584–8.

19. Manikis P, Jankowski S, Zhang H, *et al.* Correlation of serial blood lactate levels to organ failure and mortality after trauma. *Am J Emerg Med* 1995; 13: 619–22.

20. Jeng JC, Jablonski K, Bridgeman A, Jordan MH. Serum lactate, not base deficit, rapidly predicts survival after major burns. *Burns* 2002; 28: 161–6.

21. Savage SA, Zarzaur BL, Croce MA, Fabian TC. Redefining massive transfusion when every second counts. *J Trauma Acute Care Surg* 2013; 74: 396–400.

22. Wudel JH, Morris JA, Yates K, *et al.* Massive transfusion: outcome in blunt trauma patients. *J Trauma* 1991; 31: 1–7.

23. Como JJ, Dutton RP, Scalea TM, *et al.* Blood transfusion rates in the care of acute trauma. *Transfusion* 2004; 44: 809–13.

24. Malone DL, Dunne J, Tracy JK, *et al.* Blood transfusion, independent of shock severity, is associated with worse outcomes in trauma. *J Trauma* 2003; 54: 898–905.

25. Huber-Wagner S, Qvick M, Mussack T, *et al.* Massive blood transfusion and outcome in 1062 polytrauma patients: a prospective study based on the trauma registry of the German trauma society. *Vox Sang* 2007; 92: 69–78.

26. Sauaia A, Moore FA, Moore EE, *et al.* Epidemiology of trauma deaths: a reassessment. *J Trauma* 1995; 38: 185–93.

27. Cosgriff N, Moore EE, Sauaia A, *et al.* Predicting life-threatening coagulopathy in the massively transfused trauma patient: hypothermia and acidosis revisited. *J Trauma* 1997; 42: 857–61.

28. Holcomb JB, Pati S. Optimal trauma resuscitation with plasma as the primary resuscitative fluid: the surgeon's perspective. *Hematology Am Soc Hematol Educ Program* 2013; 2013: 656–9.

29. Pati S, Matijevic N, Doursout MF, *et al.* Protective effects of fresh frozen plasma on vascular endothelial permeability, coagulation, and resuscitation after hemorrhagic shock are time dependent and diminish between days 0 and 5 after thaw. *J Trauma* 2010; 69: S55–63.

30. Holcomb JB, Jenkins D, Rhee P, *et al.* Damage control resuscitation: directly addressing the early coagulopathy of trauma. *J Trauma* 2007; 62: 307–10.

31. Borgman MA, Spinella PC, Perkins JG, *et al.* The ratio of blood products transfused affects mortality in patients receiving massive transfusions at a combat support hospital. *J Trauma* 2007; 63: 805–13.

32. Johansson PI, Stensballe J, Rosenberg I, *et al.* Proactive administration of platelets and plasma for patients with a ruptured abdominal aortic aneurysm: evaluating a change in transfusion practice. *Transfusion* 2007; 47: 593–8.

33. Holcomb JB, Wade CE, Michalek JE, *et al.* Increased plasma and platelet to red blood cell ratios improves outcome in 466 massively transfused civilian trauma patients. *Ann Surg* 2008; 248: 447–58.

34. Holcomb JB, del Junco DJ, Fox EE, *et al.* The prospective, observational, multicenter, major trauma transfusion (PROMMTT) study; comparative effectiveness of a time-varying treatment with competing risks. *JAMA Surg* 2013; 148: 127–36.

35. Cotton BA, Reddy N, Hatch QM, *et al.* Damage control resuscitation is associated with a reduction in resuscitation volumes and improvement in survival in 390 damage control laparotomy patients. *Ann Surg* 2011; 254: 598–605.

36. Holcomb JB, Tilley BC, Baraniuk S, *et al.* Transfusion of plasma, platelets, and red blood cells in a 1:1:1 vs. a 1:1:2 ratio and mortality in patients with severe trauma. The PROPPR randomized clinical trial. *JAMA* 2015; 313: 471–82.

37. Hoffman M, Cichon LJ. Practical coagulation for the blood banker. *Transfusion* 2013; 53: 1594–602.

38. Holcomb JB, Minei KM, Scerbo ML, *et al.* Admission rapid thromboelastography can replace conventional coagulation tests in the emergency department. Experience with 1974 consecutive trauma patients. *Ann Surg* 2012; 256: 476–86.

39. Cotton BA, Minei KM, Radwan ZA, *et al.* Admission rapid thrombelastography predicts development of pulmonary embolism in trauma patients. *J Trauma Acute Care Surg* 2012; 72: 1470–5.

40. Bickell WH, Wall MJ Jr, Pepe PE, *et al.* Immediate versus delayed fluid resuscitation for hypotensive patients with penetrating torso injuries. *N Engl J Med* 1994; 331: 1105–9.

41. Rago AP, Larentzakis A, Marini J, *et al.* Efficacy of a prehospital self-expanding polyurethane foam for noncompressible hemorrhage under extreme operational conditions. *J Trauma Acute Care Surg* 2015; 78: 324–9.

42. Holcomb JB, Fox EE, Scalea TM, *et al.* Current opinion on catheter-based hemorrhage control in trauma patients. *J Trauma Acute Care Surg* 2014; 76: 888–93.

43. Holcomb J, Donathan D, Cotton B, *et al.* Prehospital transfusion of plasma and red blood cells in trauma patients. *Prehosp Emerg Care* 2015; 19: 1–9.

44. Brown J, Sperry J, Fombona A, *et al.* Pre-trauma center red blood cell transfusion is associated with improved early outcomes in air medical trauma patients. *J Am Coll Surg* 2015; 5: 797–808.

45. Brown J, Cohen M, Minei J, *et al.* Pretrauma center red blood cell transfusion is associated with reduced mortality and coagulopathy in severely injured patients with blunt trauma. *Ann Surg* 2015; 5: 997–1005.

46. Nunez TC, Voskresensky IV, Dossett LA, *et al.* Early prediction of massive transfusion in trauma: simple as ABC (assessment of blood consumption)? *J Trauma* 2009; 66: 346–52.

47. Pommerening MJ, Goodman MD, Holcomb JB, *et al.* Clinical gestalt and the prediction of massive transfusion after trauma. *Injury* 2015; 46: 807–13.

48. Cotton BA, Harvin JA, Kostousouv V, *et al.* Hyperfibrinolysis at admission is an uncommon but highly lethal event associated with shock and prehospital fluid administration. *J Trauma Acute Care Surg* 2012; 73: 365–70.

49. Johansson PI, Stensballe J, Oliveri R, *et al.* How I treat patients with massive hemorrhage. *Blood* 2014; 124: 3052–8.

50. CRASH-2 Trial collaborators. Shakur H, Roberts I, *et al.* Effects of tranexamic acid on death, vascular occlusive events, and blood transfusion in trauma patients with significant haemorrhage (CRASH-2): a randomised, placebo-controlled trial. *Lancet* 2010; 376: 23–32.

51. Harvin JA, Peirce CA, Mims MM, *et al.* The impact of tranexamic acid on mortality in injured patients with hyperfibrinolysis. *J Trauma Acute Care Surg* 2015; 78: 905–9.

Chapter

33

Absorption of irrigating fluid

Robert G. Hahn

Summary

Absorption of irrigating fluid can occur in endo-scopic surgeries. The complication is best known from transurethral prostatic resection and tran-scervical endometrial resection. When monopolar electrocautery is used, the irrigation is performed with electrolyte-free fluid containing glycine, or mannitol or sorbitol. With bipolar electrocautery the irrigating fluid is usually isotonic saline. Inci-dence data on fluid absorption and associated adverse effects show great variation, but absorp-tion in excess of 1 liter usually occurs in 5% to 10% of the operations and causes symptoms in 2–3 patients per 100 operations.

The pathophysiology of the complications aris-ing from absorption of electrolyte-free irrigating fluids is complex. Symptoms can be related to metabolic toxicity, cerebral edema, and circula-tory effects caused by rapid massive fluid overload. Available data on absorption of isotonic saline suggest that symptoms are likely when the volume exceeds 2 liters.

Ethanol monitoring is the most viable of the methods suggested for monitoring of fluid absorp-tion in clinical practice. By using an irrigating fluid that contains 1% of ethanol, updated information about fluid absorption can be obtained at any time perioperatively by letting the patient breathe into a hand-held alcolmeter.

Treatment of massive fluid absorption is sup-portive with regard to ventilation, hemodynam-ics, and well-being. Hypertonic saline is indicated when electrolyte-free fluids are used, while diuret-ics should be withheld until the hemodynamic situation has been stabilized. In contrast, absorp-tion of isotonic saline should (logically) be treated with diuretics as saline does not cause osmotic diuresis and is not distributed to the intracellular space.

A number of different sterile water solutions are employed for irrigation in connection with various operative procedures. Medical aspects of these are pri-marily of interest when used during endoscopy. Here, these solutions dilate the operating field and wash away debris and blood. A potential complication of such irrigation is absorption of the fluid by the patient, even to the extent that symptoms ensue. The rate and vol-ume of fluid absorbed, as well as the type of fluid used, are of importance to the appearance of this iatrogenic complication.

Patients developing overt symptoms due to absorp-tion of irrigating fluid were first described in con-nection with transurethral resection of the prostate (TURP). The complication was named "transurethral resection (TUR) syndrome" and was proved during the 1940s to be due to uptake of more than 3 liters of ster-ile water used for irrigation. An intense effort started to add various non-electrolyte solutes to the sterile water for the purpose of preventing fluid absorption from causing hemolysis-induced renal failure. In the mid-1950s the hemolysis problem had disappeared, but other types of adverse effects continued to appear. Since then, several hundred life-threatening and even fatal TUR syndromes have been reported.[1]

The TUR syndrome might also develop in other operations, including transcervical resection of the endometrium (TCRE), transurethral resection of bladder tumors, cystoscopy, arthroscopy, rectal tumor surgery, vesical ultrasonic lithotripsy, and percutaneous nephrolithotripsy.

The most common irrigating fluids used today contain one or two solutes, such as glycine, sorbitol, or mannitol, to prevent hemolysis in case of absorption. These fluids are intended for *monopolar* electrocautery, i.e. when current travels between the tip of the resectoscope to an electrode placed on the patient's hip or back.

With *bipolar* electrocautery the current travels only across the tip of the resectoscope, and electrolyte-containing solutions (most often isotonic saline) can then be used. This technique was introduced early in the new millennium and is slowly taking over the market for electrocautery. The use of saline has paramount influence over the type of adverse effects that can be expected if absorption occurs.

Sterile water is still often used during cystoscopy as it provides superior vision for the urologist. Although perforations do occur, absorption of irrigating fluid during cystoscopy is very rare.

Mechanisms

Irrigating fluid is most often absorbed directly into the vascular system during TURP and TCRE, and implies that a vein has been severed by the electrosurgery. The event usually starts in the middle or at the end of the surgery, and continues until it is completed.[2]

Extravasation occurs after perforations of anatomic structures with the resectoscope. The perforated tissue is the prostatic capsule in TURP, the uterine wall in TCRE, and the bladder wall during cystoscopy and transurethral resection of bladder tumors. Extravasation is the predominant route of absorption during renal stone surgery.[3]

Smoking is the only constitutional patient factor associated with large-scale fluid absorption during TURP,[4] which is probably due to anoxia-induced enlargement of the prostate vessels. Transurethral resection in prostate cancer is associated with the same incidence of fluid absorption as those with benign tissue.[2] Fluid absorption increases with the extent of the resection, since the exposure to the fluid then becomes prolonged.[2]

During TCRE, fluid absorption occurs more often when fibroids are resected.[5] Some extravasation via the Fallopian tubes can be expected to occur because the fluid pressure used is much higher than during TURP (about 150 mmHg versus 15–40 mmHg).[6]

Incidence and clinical presentation

Electrolyte-free fluid

Symptoms of fluid absorption occur in between 1% and 8% of TURPs performed when glycine is used as the irrigating solution.[1] Absorption in excess of 1 liter is associated with a statistically increased risk of symptoms.[7] This has been reported in between 5% and 20% of TURPs performed.[2,8] Extravasation is the cause in about 20% of these patients.[7] Fluid absorption seems to be slightly more common during TCRE and percutaneous stone surgery than during TURP.[9,10]

The incidence and severity of symptoms for increasing amounts of absorbed fluid have been best established for glycine solution during TURP. Olsson *et al.* [7] recorded an average of 1.3 symptoms from the circulatory and nervous systems in each TURP during which very little or no fluid was absorbed (0–300 ml). This figure increased to 2.3 symptoms per operation when between 1 and 2 liters of glycine 1.5% was taken up, while 5.8 symptoms developed when the absorption exceeded 3 liters. The dose-dependent increase in the number of symptoms has been confirmed in later prospective studies.[8,11]

During surgery, the patient may experience transient prickling and burning sensations in the face and neck, suffer chest pain, become restless, and complain of headache. Bradycardia and arterial hypotension are very common signs of volume overload, which occasionally progress to pulmonary edema.

Nausea and arterial hypotension followed by vomiting and low urinary output are typical symptoms in the postoperative period.[7,8,11] Absorption of a few hundred milliliters is associated with transient cognitive dysfunction,[12] while apparent confusion might occur after absorption of 1–2 liters,[13] which, with larger absorption volumes, eventually results in coma.[14]

Abdominal pain is a common first sign of extravasation, which is further associated with a higher incidence of arterial hypotension and poor urinary output.[15]

Mild TUR syndromes are incomplete and easily overlooked. A drop in arterial pressure at the end of surgery combined with nausea is the most common presentation. The severe TUR syndrome is rare and occurs perhaps in 0.1–0.5% of operations. A French review of 24 severe TUR syndromes showed neurological (92%) and cardiovascular symptoms (54%), visual disturbances (42%), digestive symptoms (25%), and renal failure (21%). The mortality rate was 25%.[16]

Electrolyte-containing fluid

There is only scarce information about the incidence and symptomatology of fluid absorption when endoscopic resection is performed with the bipolar technique. There is a widespread belief among urologists that all adverse effects including the TUR syndrome have disappeared because hyponatremia does not occur when isotonic saline is used for irrigation. It is true that the parts of the TUR syndrome that are due to hyponatremia, such as brain edema and epileptic seizures, no longer can occur. However, a few publications using ethanol as the tracer show that fluid absorption still occurs, and suggest that the problem is underestimated by the medical community.

One study reported saline absorption that exceeded 500 ml in 2% of 185 TURP patients [17] and another 16% of 55 patients undergoing high-power laser prostate vaporization, of which one patient with the largest absorption (>2 liters) showed agitation and dyspnea.[18] Likewise, in a further study, saline absorption occurred in 44% and the volume exceeded 1 liter in 20% of the patients (maximum 3.5 liters). Three patients had symptoms, consisting of depressed consciousness, mild dyspnea, and low oxygen saturation.[19] Absorption averaged as much as 900 ml in a study in which TURP was compared with transurethral enucleation.[20]

In addition to observations made during and after prostate surgery, there is much information about dose-dependent adverse effects of isotonic saline to be found from the literature where saline has been given by intravenous infusion. However, fluid absorption might occur much faster than infusion fluids are normally administered, which raises special concerns. Up to 2.4 liters over 10 min has been reported.[21]

The irrigating solutions

Glycine is an amino acid with a dose-dependent half-life of between 40 min and several hours, which is probably due to intracellular accumulation.[22] Glycine is an inhibitory neurotransmittor in the retina, and absorption sometimes causes visual disturbances

or transient blindness, which always resolve within 24 hours.

Elimination occurs by direct cleavage in the liver, which is a process that yields ammonia. Those who absorb glycine may develop hyperammonemic encephalopathy, which is associated with blood ammonia concentrations >100 µmol/l (normal range 10–35).[23] A genetic disposition seems to be involved, since only 15–20% of a group of volunteers had a rise in blood ammonia when challenged by glycine overload.[24]

Absorption of glycine solution induces osmotic diuresis, whereby 5–10% of an excess dose becomes excreted along with electrolytes, including sodium. This creates an absolute loss of sodium from the body, which undoubtedly prolongs the hyponatremia that always results from dilution of the extracellular fluid (ECF) with electrolyte-free irrigating fluid. Glycine is usually marketed in a 1.5% solution, which is slightly hypo-osmotic.

A review of the mortality, symptoms, and biochemical disturbances after experimental infusions and absorption of glycine in animals, volunteers, and patients shows that glycine solution is associated with the worst outcome of the electrolyte-free irrigating fluids.[25] However, sterile water was not included in the comparison because of too scarce data.

Mannitol is an isomer of glucose that is marketed as a 3% or 5% solution, of which the latter is iso-osmotic. The elimination half-life is 100–130 min but is markedly longer in patients with a raised serum creatinine concentration. Mannitol cannot be metabolized and is excreted unchanged in the urine. The lack of reabsorption causes osmotic diuresis. Circulatory symptoms following absorption of mannitol 3% are as common as for glycine 1.5%, but neurological symptoms are rare.[8]

Sorbitol is metabolized to fructose and glucose in the liver with a half-life of 30 min. Overload with sorbitol may be complicated by lactic acidosis,[26] and intolerance to a metabolite, fructose, can be life-threatening. In commercial solutions sorbitol is often combined with mannitol in a 5:1 or 2:1 ratio.

Sterile water causes hemolysis and renal damage if absorbed into the blood. Therefore this irrigating solution should only be used without electrocautery, i.e. for visual inspections.

These hypo-osmotic irrigating fluids hydrate the ECF space but also add water to the intracellular fluid (ICF). Volume expansion of the ICF becomes more apparent with time when glycine and sorbitol are used as solutes as they undergo intracellular metabolism.

Isotonic saline is used for irrigation with the bipolar resection technique. Infusion of 2–3 liters of normal saline in volunteers was followed by mental changes and discomfort from swelling.[27,28] Normal saline also gives rise to hyperchloremic metabolic acidosis and inhibits kidney function due to its high amount of chloride.[29]. Other adverse effects are not fluid-specific but probably follow the same course as the balanced Ringer's solutions when given in progressively larger volumes. However, many symptoms of "TUR syndrome" known from the absorption of electrolyte-free fluid seem to be absent.[30].

Pathophysiology

The TUR syndrome induced by an electrolyte-free irrigating fluid has a complex pathophysiology.[1] Key elements comprise a two-stage cardiovascular disturbance, hyponatremia, and cerebral edema.

The cardiovascular response to fluid absorption consists of transient hypervolemia with increased central hemodynamic pressures, which level off within 15 min. This phase might involve chest pain, dyspnea, and acute pulmonary edema on the operating table.

Hypervolemia is followed by a hypokinetic phase with low cardiac output, hypovolemia, and low arterial pressure.[31] Disturbances of heart function include bradycardia and depression of the ST segment and the T wave. Cardiac function is also impaired by fluid-induced damage to the myocardium.[32–34] Glycine causes more damage to the myocardium than other fluids.[32]

The existence of hypovolemia is the part of the pathophysiology that has been most difficult to explain. Causes include that rapidly absorbed fluid that has distributed to the interstitial fluid space does not return to the plasma,[31] which is probably due to loss of stiffness of the interstitial gel when overwhelmed by massive amounts of fluid. The absorbed fluid then accumulates in lacunae in the tissues. There is also an osmotic-driven uptake of fluid to the cells because irrigating fluids are usually hypo-osmotic, and both glycine and sorbitol are distributed intracellularly. The intracellular uptake is aggravated by the osmotic diuresis that is induced by all electrolyte-free irrigating fluids because this diuresis causes a net loss of sodium from the body. These factors, together with transiently increased bleeding, make the TUR

syndrome a hypovolemic condition that promotes low-flow circulation, arterial hypotension and possibly cardiovascular shock 10–15 min after the absorption has stopped.

Hyponatremia (<120 mmol/l) is a feared but invariable consequence of absorption of electrolyte-free irrigating fluid.[14] Hyponatremia is aggravated by osmotic diuresis, which attracts sodium ions despite the presence of hyponatremia.

Hyponatremia is typically accompanied by hypo-osmolality (reduction by 10–25 mosmol/kg) since most irrigating fluids are hypo-osmolar. These changes promote brain edema, which lowers consciousness a few hours after the surgery.

Serum potassium often increases transiently by 15–25% and a moderately severe metabolic acidosis develops. The risk of urosepsis is increased.[8]

The kidneys ultimately swell in response to large amounts of irrigating fluid, which is followed by poor urinary output and ultimately by renal damage and anuria. Absorption of sterile water exerts a more direct toxic effect on the kidneys which is due to the accompanying hemolysis.

Death from the TUR syndrome is caused by cardiovascular collapse and shock during the hypokinetic hemodynamic phase, or else by cerebral herniation resulting from brain edema.[16]

Comparisons between the different irrigating fluids show that mannitol solution is better than glycine with respect to tissue damage [32] and mortality [35] (animals) and symptoms (volunteers [36] and patients [8]).

Isotonic saline does not cause brain edema, but the experience of this fluid with regard to other symptoms during endoscopic surgery is limited. Besides abdominal discomfort and nausea,[27] large amounts of saline promote the development of pulmonary edema.

Animal experiments show that replacing electrolyte-free irrigating fluids with normal saline reduces, but does not eliminate, tissue damage [34] and mortality.[37] In any event, symptoms of the TUR syndrome are a smaller issue when using normal saline as the irrigant instead of glycine 1.5%,[30] which rates worst in comparison with other fluids.[25,32,35,36]

Measuring fluid absorption

Absorption of electrolyte-free irrigating fluid can be estimated by measuring *serum sodium* at the very end of surgery. The correlation between the decrease in serum sodium from the preoperative value and volume of irrigant absorbed is somewhat dependent on the period of time during which absorption has occurred. However, a good estimate can be obtained by taking a decrease of 5–6 mmol/l to represent absorption of 1 liter of fluid during TURP, and that 10–12 mmol/l corresponds to absorption of twice as much volume.[36,38]

The hyponatremic response to fluid absorption in females undergoing TCRE is stronger, and 1 liter of fluid corresponds to a reduction of approximately 10 mmol/l in serum sodium. In both groups of patients, the drop in serum sodium is only 1/3 as large at the end of surgery in response to fluid that has been absorbed by extravasation.[38]

The possibility of assessing fluid absorption by serum sodium does not exist when using isotonic saline, although the addition of glucose up to a concentration of 0.5% in the saline solution can serve as replacement.[39]

The *volumetric fluid balance* is based on a calculation of the difference between the amount of irrigating fluid used and the volume recovered. Positive values are regarded as absorption. The accuracy is moderately good, and errors up to 1 liter can be made due to variations in bag-to-bag content, spillage on the floor, and the addition of blood and urine to the irrigating fluid returns. The volumetric fluid balance is less prone to error during TCRE.

Ethanol has been added to the irrigating fluid to a concentration of 1% and the measured body concentration used an index of fluid absorption. Measurements of the ethanol level in exhaled breath can be made during surgery with relatively little effort. The sensitivity is superior to the other two methods (approximately 100 ml is detected) and has the benefit of being non-invasive. Ethanol monitoring has been well evaluated worldwide and is an excellent educational tool for urologists-in-training.[38] The method might also be used during TCRE.[9] An example of how a pattern of ethanol changes look during an operation with fluid absorption is shown in Figure 33.1.

One important issue is that the anesthetist must be aware of how the alcolmeter is calibrated (for blood or breath) to consult the correct nomogram when obtaining an estimate of how much fluid that has been absorbed. A challenge is that intravascular and extravascular absorption give rise to different patterns and levels of breath ethanol concentrations. The extravascular type gives a slowly rising

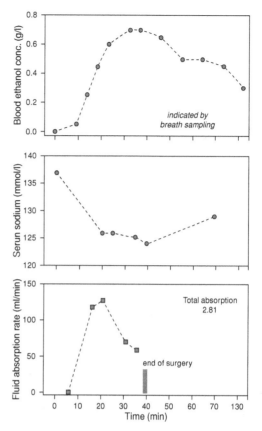

Figure 33.1 Blood ethanol concentration as indicated in the breath (top); serum sodium (middle); and the fluid absorption rate as obtained by careful measurements of the volumetric fluid balance corrected from blood loss over 5- or 10-min periods (bottom) in one patient undergoing transurethral resection of the prostate. The route of fluid uptake is intravascular. From Ref. [48], reproduced courtesy of *Acta Anaesthesiologica Scandinavica*.

ethanol concentration that remains high when irrigation has stopped (Figure 33.2). With the more common intravascular type of fluid absorption, elevations of the breath ethanol concentration can occur much faster and a drop is seen within a few minutes after the irrigation has stopped.

Measuring serum sodium has the purpose of confirming that fluid absorption is the cause of the symptoms. On the other hand, non-invasive methods that can be repeated perioperatively, such as volumetric balance and the ethanol method, open up the possibility of preventing large-scale fluid absorption from occurring. Once data indicate that 1 liter of fluid has been absorbed it is suggested that the operation should be concluded earlier than planned, and after 2 liters it becomes even more important to stop surgery. An

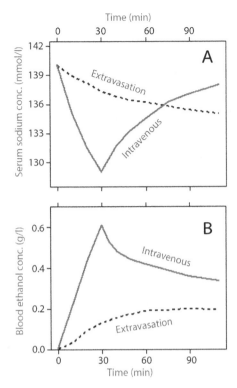

Figure 33.2 Expected course of serum sodium (**A**) and blood ethanol concentration (**B**) (the latter measured in the expired breath) during and after TURP during which absorption of 2 liters of irrigating fluid containing glycine 1.5% and ethanol 1% has occurred over 30 min, depending on the route of absorption.

early indication that irrigating fluid has been absorbed allows the optimal level of postoperative care to be chosen and also the initiation of the earliest possible treatment.

Nomograms for how to estimate fluid absorption are shown in Figures 33.3 and 33.4. Regression equations have also been developed for calculation of fluid absorption in the scientific setting (see Box 33.1).

Prevention

Fluid absorption and blood loss is reduced, but not eliminated, by vaporizing rather than resecting tissue.

The irrigating fluid used during TURP might be evacuated through a suprapubic trocar. This allows the use of continuous irrigation at a low fluid pressure, which speeds up the operation but increases the use of irrigating fluid. Low-pressure irrigation limits or prevents fluid absorption as long as the outflow is not obstructed by debris and blood clots.

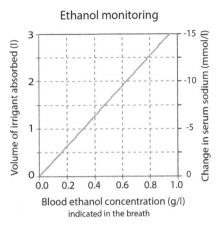

Figure 33.3 Nomogram for quick reference between the volume of irrigant absorbed and the breath ethanol concentration (calibrated to blood ethanol) and, if the fluid is electrolyte-free, the corresponding decrease in serum sodium. The volume of irrigant absorbed is given from the average absorption time during TURP, which is 20 min. The median absolute residual error is 146 ml and R^2 for the regression is 0.80. From Ref. [48], reproduced courtesy of *Acta Anaesthesiologica Scandinavica*.

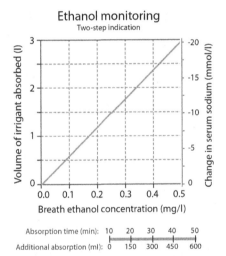

Figure 33.4 Nomogram for estimating the volume of irrigant absorbed from the breath ethanol concentration (not calibrated to blood ethanol) at any time during TURP. If the fluid is electrolyte-free, the corresponding decrease in serum sodium is also predicted. To estimate intravascular fluid absorption, first use the upper nomogram and add the effect of distribution and elimination by using the scale below. The median absolute residual error is 118 ml and R^2 for the regression 0.90. The accompanying decrease in serum sodium inflicted by the use of electrolyte-free irrigating fluid is obtained directly from the upper nomogram. From Ref. [48], reproduced courtesy of *Acta Anaesthesiologica Scandinavica*.

Fluid absorption varies between surgeons and depends on their skill in avoiding prostatic capsule perforations or the opening up of venous sinuses.

Box 33.1 How to calculate fluid absorption from a regression equation

An equation recommended for scientific reports is one that is based on 10-min measurements throughout 90 TURPs [49]. Here, the equation gives the absorbed volume in 10-min increments that must be summed to give the total absorption:

$$\text{Absorption (ml)} = \sum (2{,}140 + 3{,}430 \text{ ethanol}_i)$$
$$\times \Delta \text{ethanol} + (44 + 806 \text{ ethanol}_i)$$

where ethanol$_i$ is the blood ethanol concentration as indicated in the breath at the beginning of the 10-min period, and Δethanol is the change in concentration during that 10-min period.

Assume that we have a TURP operation in which one ethanol measurement is made at the end of three successive 10-min periods. The readings are 0.15, 0.25, and 0.30 g/l. When the reading is zero, the equation should not be applied. Inserting the data series given above, this equation provides the following output for the three 10-min periods mentioned above:

Absorption = $(2{,}140 + 3{,}430 \times 0) \times 0.15 +$
$(44 + 806 \times 0) = 321 + 44 = 365$ ml
Absorption = $(2{,}140 + 3{,}430 \times 0.15) \times 0.10 +$
$(44 + 806 \times 0.15) = 265 + 165 = 430$ ml
Absorption = $(2{,}140 + 3{,}430 \times 0.25) \times 0.05 +$
$(44 + 806 \times 0.25) = 150 + 246 = 396$ ml

The total absorption during the 30-min surgical procedure is the sum of these three 10-min calculations, i.e. 365, (365 + 430) = 795, and finally (365 + 430 + 396) = 1,191 ml. The median absolute residual error is approximately 100 ml, and the equation can also be applied for decreasing concentrations, as some ongoing absorption is needed to maintain an already elevated ethanol level. Decreasing ethanol concentrations can be handled by letting Δethanol attain negative values. Continued absorption is needed to maintain a raised ethanol level, and more is required to maintain a high concentration than a low because most of the decrease is due to distribution. Arrested absorption typically results in a rapid fall in the ethanol level provided that absorption has occurred by the intravascular route.

From [48], reproduced courtesy of *Acta Anaesthesiologica Scandinavica*.

There is a belief among urologists that dangerous fluid absorption during TURP can be prevented by limiting the operating time to 1 hour. However, the odds for absorption involve a similar likelihood over time, which accumulates to a gradually increased total risk.[2]. Hence, massive fluid absorption might already be at hand after 20 min of surgery.

Placing the irrigating fluid bag at low height above the operating table is of little help because urologists tend to operate at a much lower fluid pressure than made possible by the bag height.[40,41]

The bipolar resection technique allows the use of normal saline for irrigation, and is often claimed to prevent the TUR syndrome. Experience with fluid overload during bipolar resection is still limited. There is no reason to believe that fluid absorption will be less frequent, but the TUR syndrome is likely to have a different appearance.

Treatment

The TUR syndrome requires general supportive measures if breathing and/or consciousness are affected. Severe hypotension should be treated promptly with colloid volume loading, intravenous calcium, and adrenergic drugs.

Hypertonic saline should be infused when the hemodynamics is under control. The indication requires either that symptoms have developed or that the serum sodium concentration has fallen to below 120 mmol/l, which corresponds to absorption of approximately 3.5 liters of fluid. Hypertonic saline combats cerebral edema and expands the plasma volume, reduces cellular swelling, and increases urinary excretion.

Both experimental [42] and clinical [43,44] studies support the usefulness of treating the TUR syndrome with hypertonic saline. Above all, raising the serum sodium level is most essential in menstruating women because they are more prone to develop brain damage from hyponatremia than other patients.

Rapid correction of chronic hyponatremia might induce pontine myelinolysis but this is not the experience with acute hyponatremia. An infusion of 250 ml of 7.5% NaCl can be started slowly and another bag added later if necessary. Raising the serum sodium level by 1 mmol/l per hour has been suggested as a safe rate,[44] but hypertonic saline has not been reported to induce pontine myelinolysis when given faster. Treatment should stop when serum sodium has reached 130 mmol/l as there is a risk of over-correction.

Diuretic treatment is imperative in case pulmonary edema or renal failure develops. However, such drugs aggravate hypotension and hyponatremia and should therefore be withheld until the hemodynamic situation is under control and a drip of hypertonic saline is ongoing. The value of diuretics has not been evaluated in randomized clinical studies, but without diuretics absorbed electrolyte-free irrigating fluid in excess of 1 liter is strongly associated with a positive fluid balance 24 hours after TURP.[45] Hypertonic mannitol might be superior to furosemide if used early on after the surgery.[46]

Massive extravasation to the periprostatic or intraperitoneal spaces can be treated with surgical drainage. Here, electrolytes from the ECF enter the pool of irrigating fluid more quickly than the pool is absorbed by the circulation.[47] Hence, surgical drainage removes electrolytes from the body and they need to be replaced. Special attention should be given to the high risk of arterial hypotension and associated oliguria.[15]

Large-scale fluid absorption with normal saline is a possibility during bipolar resection. Treatment should probably be limited to general supportive measures and diuretics. Hypertonic saline is not indicated.

References

1. Hahn RG. Fluid absorption in endoscopic surgery (review). *Br J Anaesth* 2006; 96: 8–20.

2. Hahn RG, Ekengren J. Patterns of irrigating fluid absorption during transurethral resection of the prostate as indicated by ethanol. *J Urol* 1993; 149: 502–6.

3. Gehring H, Nahm W, Zimmermann K, *et al.* Irrigating fluid absorption during percutaneous nephrolithotripsy. *Acta Anaesthesiol Scand* 1999; 43: 316–21.

4. Hahn RG. Smoking increases the risk of large-scale fluid absorption during transurethral prostatic resection. *J Urol* 2001; 166: 162–5.

5. Istre O. Transcervical resection of the endometrium and fibroids: the outcome of 412 operations performed over 5 years. *Acta Obstet Gynecol Scand* 1996; 75: 567–74.

6. Olsson J, Berglund L, Hahn RG. Irrigating fluid absorption from the intact uterus. *Br J Obstet Gynaecol* 1996; 103: 558–61.

7. Olsson J, Nilsson A, Hahn RG. Symptoms of the transurethral resection syndrome using glycine as the irrigant. *J Urol* 1995; 154: 123–8.

8. Hahn RG, Sandfeldt L, Nyman CR. Double-blind randomized study of symptoms associated with absorption of glycine 1.5% or mannitol 3% during transurethral resection of the prostate. *J Urol* 1998; 160: 397–401.

9. Olsson J, Hahn RG. Ethanol monitoring of irrigating fluid absorption in transcervical resection of the endometrium. *Acta Anaesthesiol Scand* 1995; 39: 252–8.

10. Istre O. Transcervical resection of the endometrium and fibroids: the outcome of 412 operations performed over 5 years. *Acta Obstet Gynecol Scand* 1996; 75: 567–74.

11. Hahn RG, Shemais H, Essén P. Glycine 1.0% versus glycine 1.5% as irrigating fluid during transurethral resection of the prostate. *Br J Urol* 1997; 79: 394–400.

12. Nilsson A, Hahn RG. Mental status after transurethral resection of the prostate. *Eur Urol* 1994; 26: 1–5.

13. Tuzin-Fin P, Guenard Y, Maurette P. Atypical signs of glycine absorption following transurethral resection of the prostate: two case reports. *Eur J Anaesth* 1997; 14: 471–4.

14. Henderson DJ, Middleton RG. Coma from hyponatraemia following transurethral resection of the prostate. *Urology* 1980; 15: 267–71.

15. Hahn RG. Transurethral resection syndrome from extravascular absorption of irrigating fluid. *Scand J Urol Nephrol* 1993; 27: 387–94.

16. Radal M, Jonville Bera AP, Leisner C, Haillot O, Autret-Leca E. Effets indésirables des solutions d'irrigation glycollées. *Thérapie* 1999; 54: 233–6.

17. Fagerström T, Nyman CR, Hahn RG. Complications and clinical outcome 18 months after bipolar and monopolar transurethral resection of the prostate. *J Endourol* 2011; 25: 1043–9.

18. Hermanns T, Fankhauser CD, Hefermehl LJ, *et al.* Prospective evaluation of irrigating fluid absorption during pure transurethral bipolar plasma vaporisation of the prostate using expired-breath ethanol measurements. *BJU Int* 2013; 112: 647–54.

19. Hermanns T, Grossman NC, Wettstein MS, *et al.* Absorption of irrigating fluid occurs frequently during high power 532 nm laser vaporization of the prostate. *J Urol* 2015; 193: 211–16.

20. Ran L, He W, Zhu Z, Zhou Q, Gou X. Comparison of fluid absorption between transurethral enucleation and transurethral resection for benign prostate hyperplasia. *Urol Int* 2013; 91: 26–30.

21. Hahn RG. Early detection of the TUR syndrome by marking the irrigating fluid with 1% ethanol. *Acta Anaesthesiol Scand* 1989; 33: 146–51.

22. Hahn RG. Dose-dependent half-life of glycine. *Urol Res* 1993; 21: 289–91.

23. Hoekstra PT, Kahnoski R, McCamish MA, Bergen W, Heetderks DR. Transurethral prostatic resection syndrome – a new perspective: encephalopathy with associated hyperammonaemia. *J Urol* 1983; 130: 704–7.

24. Hahn RG, Sandfeldt L. Blood ammonia levels after intravenous infusion of glycine with and without ethanol. *Scand J Urol Nephrol* 1999; 33: 222–7.

25. Hahn RG. Glycine 1.5% for irrigation should be abandoned. *Urol Int* 2013; 91: 249–55.

26. Treparier CA, Lessard MR, Brochu J, Turcotte G. Another feature of TURP syndrome: hyperglycaemia and lactic acidosis caused by massive absorption of sorbitol. *Br J Anaesth* 2001; 87: 316–19.

27. Hahn RG, Drobin D, Ståhle L. Volume kinetics of Ringer's solution in female volunteers. *Br J Anaesth* 1997; 78: 144–8.

28. Williams EL, Hildebrand KL, McCormick SA, Bedel MJ. The effect of intravenous lactated Ringer's solution versus 0.9% sodium chloride solution on serum osmolality in human volunteers. *Anesth Analg* 1999; 88: 999–1003.

29. Scheingraber S, Rehm M, Sehmisch C, Finsterer U. Rapid saline infusion produces hyperchloremic acidosis in patients undergoing gynecologic surgery. *Anesthesiology* 1999; 90: 1265–70.

30. Yousef AA, Suliman GA. Elashry OM, *et al*. A randomized comparison between three types of irrigating fluids during transurethral resection in benign prostatic hyperplasia. *BMC Anesthesiol* 2010; 10: 7.

31. Hahn RG, Gebäck T. Fluid volume kinetics of dilutional hyponatremia; a shock syndrome revisited. *Clinics* 2014; 69: 120–7.

32. Hahn RG, Nennesmo I, Rajs J, *et al*. Morphological and X-ray microanalytical changes in mammalian tissue after overhydration with irrigating fluids. *Eur Urol* 1996; 29: 355–61.

33. Hahn RG, Zhang W, Rajs J. Pathology of the heart after overhydration with glycine solution in the mouse. *APMIS* 1996; 104: 915–20.

34. Hahn RG, Olsson J, Sótonyi P, Rajs J. Rupture of the myocardial histoskeleton and its relation to sudden death after infusion of glycine 1.5% in the mouse. *APMIS* 2000; 108: 487–95.

35. Olsson J, Hahn RG. Survival after high-dose intravenous infusion of irrigating fluids in the mouse. *Urology* 1996; 47: 689–92.

36. Hahn RG, Stalberg HP, Gustafsson SA. Intravenous infusion of irrigating fluids containing glycine or mannitol with and without ethanol. *J Urol* 1989; 142: 1102–5.

37. Olsson J, Hahn RG. Glycine toxicity after high-dose i.v. infusion of glycine 1.5% in the mouse. *Br J Anaesth* 1999; 82: 250–4.

38. Hahn RG. Ethanol monitoring of irrigating fluid absorption (review). *Eur J Anaesth* 1996; 13: 102–15.

39. Piros D, Fagerström T, Collins JW, Hahn RG. Glucose as a marker of fluid absorption in bipolar transurethral surgery. *Anesth Analg* 2009; 109: 1850–5.

40. Hahn RG, Ekengren J. Absorption of irrigating fluid and height of the fluid bag during transurethral resection of the prostate. *Br J Urol* 1993; 72: 80–3.

41. Ekengren J, Zhang W, Hahn RG. Effects of bladder capacity and height of fluid bag on the intravesical pressure during transurethral resection of the prostate. *Eur Urol* 1995; 27: 26–30.

42. Bernstein GT, Loughlin KR, Gittes RF. The physiologic basis of the TUR syndrome. *J Surg Res* 1989; 46: 135–41.

43. Ayus JC, Krothapalli RK, Arieff AI. Treatment of symptomatic hyponatremia and its relation to brain damage. *N Engl J Med* 1987; 317: 1190–5.

44. Ayus JC, Arieff AI. Glycine-induced hypo-osmolar hyponatremia. *Arch Intern Med* 1997; 157: 223–6.

45. Hahn RG. Total fluid balance during transurethral resection of the prostate. *Int Urol Nephrol* 1996; 28: 665–71.

46. Crowley K, Clarkson K, Hannon V, McShane A, Kelly DG. Diuretics after transurethral prostatectomy: a double-blind controlled trial comparing frusemide and mannitol. *Br J Anaesth* 1990; 65: 337–41.

47. Olsson J, Hahn RG. Simulated intraperitoneal absorption of irrigating fluid. *Acta Obstet Gynecol Scand* 1995; 74: 707–13.

48. Hahn RG. Fluid absorption and the ethanol monitoring method. *Acta Anaesthesiol Scand* 2015; 59: 1081–93.

49. Hahn RG. Calculation of irrigant absorption by measurement of breath alcohol level during transurethral resection of the prostate. *Br J Urol* 1991; 68: 390–3.

34 Adverse effects of infusion fluids

Robert G. Hahn

Summary

Adverse effects may arise if an infusion fluid diverges from the body fluids with respect to osmolality or temperature. Coagulation becomes impaired when the fluid-induced hemodilution is approximately 40%. Infusion of 2–3 liters of crystalloid fluid prolongs the gastrointestinal recovery time, while 6–7 liters promotes poor wound healing, pulmonary edema, and pneumonia. In abdominal surgery, suture insufficiency and sepsis become more common. However, a liberal fluid program in the postoperative period probably does not increase the number of complications.

Isotonic saline probably shares these adverse effects with the balanced crystalloid fluids, but adds on a tendency to metabolic acidosis and slight impairment of the kidney function (−10%). Glucose solutions may induce hyperglycemia and post-infusion rebound hypoglycemia. Glucose 5% without electrolytes increases the risk of postoperative subacute hyponatremia.

Adverse effects associated with colloid fluids include anaphylactic reactions, which occur in approximately 1 out of 500 infusions. To reduce this problem when dextran is used, pretreatment with a hapten inhibitor (dextran 1 kDa) should be employed. Hyperoncotic colloid solutions may cause pre-renal anuria in dehydrated patients. The indications for hydroxyethyl starch have been limited, owing to impairment of kidney function in severely ill patients.

Edema from a colloid is most clearly associated with inflammation-induced acceleration of the capillary escape rate. A factor promoting peripheral edema from crystalloid fluids is that volume expansion negatively affects the viscoelastic properties of the interstitial fluid gel. The slow excretion of crystalloid fluid during anesthesia and surgery also contributes to the development of edema.

Fluids administered by intravenous infusion are associated with adverse effects of different types. These include problems arising from hypothermia, electrolyte composition, infused volume or rate of infusion, or anaphylactoid/toxic effects.

Many of these problems have already been described in this book because they are important guides when tailoring fluid therapies. This chapter sums up the issues that the anesthetist should consider.

Osmolality and temperature

Isotonic and nearly isotonic crystalloid solutions are non-toxic and do not cause immunological reactions. Hypertonic fluids often cause pain at the site of infusion and may induce local inflammation resulting in thrombophlebitis. Injection of a small amount (1 ml) of local anesthetic is usually sufficient to curtail this pain. Infusion in a large vein is recommended if a lengthy infusion is planned and the osmolality of the fluid is >600 mosmol/kg.

Infusion of fluid at room temperature may cause shivering, which increases the oxygen consumption. In volunteers, crystalloid fluid at 18 °C as compared with 36 °C stimulated release of atrial natriuretic peptides and increased the urinary excretion.[1]

A reduction of the body temperature is very common during surgery, but the cause is then multifactorial. Normal thermoregulation is impaired by general anesthesia and the almost naked patient is exposed to cold air (radiant heat loss), air currents (convective heat loss), and cold instruments (conductive heat loss).[2] The greatest heat loss occurs during the first hour of surgery during surgery and is due to evaporation from skin preparatory solutions and exposure of viscera. A plateau in body temperature is commonly seen after 2–4 hours of surgery.[3]

Infusion fluids contribute to the development of hypothermia by increasing the conductive heat loss. One liter of intravenous fluid at room temperature increases the loss by 16 kcal, and one liter of blood at 4 °C is 30 kcal.[1] Irrigation of body cavities, such as the bladder, may give rise to exceptional fluid-induced heat losses due to the large fluid volumes used; in transurethral prostate surgery it is not uncommon to irrigate the bladder with 15–20 liters of fluid.

The use of blankets to cover the body and warming of the infusion fluids prevent serious reductions of the body temperature during surgery. Continuous warming of the fluid is recommended since the temperature drops fast after being taken out from a heater; in one study of 3-liter bags the temperature decreased by 0.1 °C per minute.[4]

The problem arising in a patient who has become hypothermic (35 °C and below) is a larger blood loss due to coagulopathy. Plasma behaves "as if it lacked clotting factors."[3] In the postoperative care unit, the patient will experience postoperative thermal discomfort and feel cold. As normal thermoregulatory responses return, vasoconstriction and shivering may ensue, which is uncomfortable and delays discharge.

Hemostatic effects

All infusion fluids impair coagulation by dilution of the plasma proteins, of which some are important to the coagulation cascade. However, crystalloids (and possibly gelatin) actually strengthen the coagulation until the blood has been diluted by 40%, whereafter coagulopathy gradually develops. The reason is that the effects of coagulation inhibitors (antithrombin, protein C, and alpha-2-macroglobulin) decrease with progressive dilution while the hemodilution must be quite severe for the activity of the promotors of coagulation, such as thrombin, to be reduced.

The first critical point is when the plasma concentration of the precursor of thrombin, fibrinogen, drops below 1 g/l from the normal range of 1.5–3.0 g/l (when estimating this decrease, the anesthetist must consider that the relative decrease in plasma protein concentration from an infusion fluid is almost twice as large as the concomitant decrease in blood hemoglobin concentration). With further hemodilution, the concentrations of the other coagulation factors become critical, and finally the thrombocytes. Hemostatic problems get worse if excessive hemodilution is combined with hypothermia.

To prevent coagulopathy, all colloid fluids have a maximum recommended dose that can be infused per 24 hours. This dose is 3.5 liters for hydroxyethyl starch (HES) 130/0.4 and 1.5 liters for dextran 70. Starch preparations with larger molecules have about the same maximum dose as dextran. The maximum doses are not only explained by the long-lasting dilution of the coagulation proteins, but also by changes in plasma viscosity and microcirculatory flow. Toxic effects on certain coagulation factors have also been proposed. However, the evidence for a clinical effect is scarce, except possibly for dextran, which reduces platelet adhesiveness and increases the lysability of blood clots.[5] On the other hand, these effects contribute to the usefulness of dextran in preventing venous thromboembolism during surgery.

A more detailed account of the effects of infusion fluids on the coagulation system can be found in Chapter 9, "Fluids and coagulation."

Crystalloid fluids

Small amounts of *balanced crystalloid fluids* are not associated with adverse effects, but high infusion rates and large volumes are.

In patients with heart failure, high infusion rates may precipitate pulmonary edema owing to acute expansion of the plasma volume. Distribution of fluid to perivascular tissue might also explain the impairment of pulmonary function (forced vital capacity) occurring in healthy volunteers with a mean age of 63 years after infusion of 40 ml/kg of crystalloid fluid.[6]

Adverse effects that develop also in the young and healthy are related to the distribution of the fluid. Crystalloid fluid distributes preferentially to interstitial tissues with high compliance for volume expansion, such as the subcutis, the lungs, and the gastrointestinal tract. Infusion of Ringer's acetate at a rate of 1.6 ml/kg per minute (2 liters over 15 min in an adult) caused swelling sensations in the face and arms, as well as slight dyspnea, in young women.[7]

Infusing 2 liters of Ringer's acetate in laparoscopic cancer patients delayed the gastrointestinal recovery time by 2 days.[8] A meta-analysis of restrictive/liberal fluid studies of open abdominal surgery showed that providing between 1.75 and 2.75 liters of crystalloid fluid during the surgery reduced the number of surgical complications.[9]

A study of cystectomy patients reported that the gastrointestinal and cardiac complications were more common, and the hospital time longer, when 8.8 ml/kg per hour instead of 3.5 ml/kg per hour of crystalloid fluid was infused. Here, the treatment program in the low-volume group included a low-dose noradrenaline infusion to maintain the arterial pressure.[10] A study of major abdominal surgery showed that administering 4 ml/kg per hour resulted in fewer postoperative complications than 12 ml/kg per hour.[11]

Increasing the crystalloid fluid load to 6–7 liters opens a more severe scenario of adverse effects. Pulmonary edema may develop that is occasionally fatal, and can arise several days after any surgery.[12] In colon surgery, wound infection, suture insufficiency, bleeding, pulmonary edema, and pulmonary infections become more common for this load than for the use of 3 liters of fluid.[13] Larger fluid volumes are associated with a weight increase of several kilos, which might persist for 4–5 days postoperatively.

In contrast to the intraoperative period, a restrictive crystalloid fluid program during the postoperative period did not reduce the number of complications. One study found just the opposite.[14] This might be explained by the fact that fluid given after surgery is readily excreted at this stage.[15] In contrast, the crystalloid fluid infused during anesthesia and surgery is eliminated very slowly, the half-life being at least 10 times longer than after surgery (300–400 min versus 20–40 min).

Isotonic saline is associated with specific adverse effects due to the non-physiological electrolyte composition. These include metabolic acidosis, impairment of kidney function, possibly abdominal pain, and a higher incidence of postoperative complications.[16,17] These negative effects are hardly noticeable after infusion of 1 liter of saline but clearly noticeable after 2 liters, when blood pH can be expected to

have arrived at the lower end of the normal interval and the renal blood flow and the glomerular filtration rates have been reduced by 10–15%. The cause of the acidosis is that the surplus of chloride ions in isotonic saline decreases the plasma strong ion difference ($SID = [Na^+] + [K^+] + [Ca^{2+}] + [Mg^{2+}] - [Cl^-] -$ [other strong anions]) by diluting the body fluids with a solution having a SID of zero. Moreover, there is all reason to believe that isotonic saline shares the more general adverse effects of crystalloid fluids that are associated with the rate of infusion and volume overload and have been described above.

Glucose solutions always carry a risk of inducing hyperglycemia. The capacity to handle exogenous glucose shows a four-fold reduction in the course of surgery (see Chapter 4, "Glucose solutions"). Plasma glucose >9–10 mmol/l promotes infection, while >12 mmol/l results in osmotic diuresis and poorer neurological outcome in the case of cardiac arrest. Glucose solutions should normally be half-isotonic with regard to electrolytes, as glucose-free fluids may induce subacute hyponatremia, which presents with neurological disturbances (confusion, dizziness, balance problems) 2–3 days after the surgery. The pathophysiology is multifactorial and typically includes at least two of the following factors: electrolyte-free fluids by intravenous infusion and by mouth (soft drinks etc.), vasopressin release after a marked intraoperative drop in arterial pressure, medication with diuretics, and some impairment of kidney function. The serum sodium concentration is <130 mmo/l when symptoms appear.

Treatment of subacute hyponatremia consists of slow restoration of the serum sodium level (1–2 mmol/l per hour) with isotonic saline, occasionally with hypertonic saline. Titration of the serum sodium level during treatment is mandatory to prevent the increase being too fast. All neurological symptoms resolve if the diagnosis is made promptly and followed by judicious restoration of the serum sodium level.

Glucose solutions that are given reasonably fast should not be turned off abruptly, as the body has difficulty in adapting to the new situation and hypoglycemia easily develops 30–45 min later (Figure 34.1A). If parturients are given glucose, the rate of infusion should not exceed 1 liter per 6 hours, as hypoglycemia may otherwise develop in the baby soon after delivery. This complication might occur during minor surgery (Figure 34.1B) but becomes progressively more unlikely with more extensive surgery (Figure 34.1C, D).

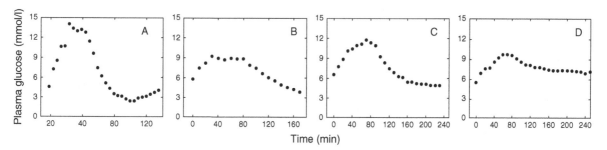

Figure 34.1 A: Rebound hypoglycemia in a young male volunteer who received 14 ml/kg of glucose 5% over 45 min. **B**: Rebound hypoglycemia in a 19-year-old who received 3.3 ml/kg of glucose 2.5% over 20 min and then half that rate over 60 min during inguinal hernia surgery. **C**: Plasma glucose in a 31-year-old male who received 3.3 ml/kg of glucose 2.5% over 80 min during laparoscopic cholecystectomy. **D**: Slow elimination of glucose in a 73-year-old male who received 3.3 ml/kg of glucose 2.5% over 20 min and then half that rate over 60 min during open colon surgery.

Bicarbonate is usually marketed in a hypertonic solution (600–800 mosmol/kg). Bicarbonate may be use to combat life-threatening acidosis. The use of bicarbonate solutions is quite limited because the rational treatment of acidosis is to seek and treat the underlying cause. The end product in the metabolism is carbon dioxide and water, which means that administration of bicarbonate increases breathing, which is an issue for patients with pulmonary disease.

Colloid fluids, general

All colloid fluids are associated with a risk of anaphylaxis. The risks, as quantified in a French multicenter study of almost 20,000 patients, were 0.35% for gelatin, 0.27% for dextran, 0.10% for albumin, and 0.06% for HES. The reactions were considered to be severe in 20% of the patients.[18] Reactions were more common in males and tripled in patients with known drug allergy. These reactions make it necessary to have drugs for acute treatment of anaphylaxis at hand when providing a colloid fluid. In many countries, a hapten inhibitor in the form of a very small dextran molecule (1 kDa) is available, which greatly reduces the number of allergic reactions to dextran and further makes those that develop very mild.

Mild allergic reactions show as a feeling of warmth in the skin, possibly together with erythema and itching. Nausea may develop. More severe reactions consist of various degrees of arterial hypotension and bronchospasm.

All colloid fluids, but particularly the hyperoncotic preparations such as 10% HES and dextran 40, may induce pre-renal anuria in dehydrated patients.[19,20] This problem might in part be due to tissue deposition of the colloid molecules. A more simplistic explanation is that the filtration pressure in the glomeruli becomes insufficient when the colloid osmotic pressure in the plasma is artificially increased at the same time as the hydrostatic pressure is low.

Colloid fluids, specific

Large amounts of *albumin* place a metabolic burden on the patient, as the protein is split into amino acids that are incorporated into new proteins or used as energy. The nitrogen content can be difficult to excrete for patients with impaired kidney function. The long half-life of exogenous albumin (2 weeks) can make peripheral edema particularly long-lasting. This is a concern in diseases, such as sepsis, in which the increased capillary leakage rate might be greater than the capacity of the lymphatic system to remove the colloid. Albumin should be avoided in head injury, where normal saline is a better choice for intravenous volume support.[21]

Hydroxyethyl starch undergoes a sequential metabolism but a smaller fraction of the molecules accumulates in the reticuloendothelial system, where it can be found even after several years. Repeated infusions of starch over several days can cause long-standing (1–2 years) and troublesome itching that is probably due to tissue deposition of starch.[22] Several weeks may elapse between HES exposure and the onset of pruritus. There is some evidence that HES (Voluven) has a higher tendency than crystalloid fluid to cause nausea and vomiting after laparoscopic surgery.[23]

HES is associated with a dose-dependent increased likelihood of renal impairment and need for renal-replacement therapy. This has been shown in septic patients [24–26] and in patients subjected to general intensive care.[27] The same findings have not been made when HES is used in the operating room.

During aortic repair HES is even better than gelatin in preserving the kidney function,[28] which is opposite to the findings made in septic patients.[24]

Dextran does not leave any metabolic residues in the body. The risk of severe anaphylactic reactions is a concern, and infusing this colloid without first injecting a hapten inhibitor must be questioned practice. Dextran colloid improves microcirculatory flow which gives rise to "oozing," i.e. that cut surfaces bleed from a larger number of capillaries. Already by 1988 there were 10 randomized controlled trials available of dextran as a drug for the prevention of thromboembolism; pooling of the data showed an incidence of 15.6% among dextran-treated patients and 24.2% in the controls.[29]

Gelatin has been claimed to reduce the function of fibronectin, a plasma factor of importance to wound healing and phagocytosis.[30] The clinical importance of this finding is unclear. Well-known problems associated with gelatin mainly consist of anaphylactic reactions, which often are histamine-dependent. Most reactions present as urticaria or transient fever, but severe allergic edema may also occur. There is cross-reactivity between different preparations of gelatin.[31]

Peripheral edema

All infusion fluids may cause postoperative weight gain and peripheral edema. The mechanisms are partially known but include the following:

Colloid fluids induce peripheral edema when inflammation-induced shedding of the endothelial glycocalyx increases the capillary leak of proteins. The leakage, which also includes the macromolecules of the colloid solution, must be transported back to the plasma by the lymphatic system, which may be overwhelmed by the increased burden. In septic shock, one can reckon with a four-fold increase of the capillary leakage rate. Hence, colloid-induced peripheral edema develops because of a discrepancy between capillary leakage rate and the capacity of the lymphatic system, whereby a surplus of fluid is held in the interstitium by oncotic forces ("queue theory") instead of being excreted.

There is experimental evidence to support that peripheral edema can also develop without an increase of the capillary escape rate. The cause is probably the vastly different half-lives for the infused colloid macromolecules than for their associated plasma volume

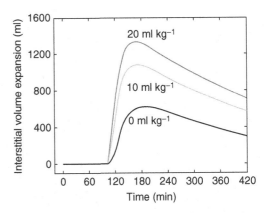

Figure 34.2 Volume expansion of the interstitial fluid space when 20 ml/kg of Ringer's acetate is infused over 30 min in 10 male volunteers (mean body weight 79 kg) beginning at 105 min, preceded by an infusion of either no starch, or 10 or 20 ml/kg of hydroxyethyl starch 130/0.4, between 0 and 30 min. The crystalloid fluid has a preferential peripheral distribution when preceded by starch. From Ref. [32].

expansion. The former half-life is much longer than the latter, showing that the macromolecules reside outside the bloodstream for a considerable time after an infusion. Although the infusion may cause an appropriate diuretic response during which the entire infused volume is excreted, even slowly leaking macromolecules increase the colloid osmotic pressure of the interstitial fluid space, which is normally only half of that measured in the plasma.[1] In the interstitium, their oncotic strength binds fluid volume from subsequently infused crystalloids. This phenomenon can be regarded as an interaction effect between a colloid and a crystalloid; as an example, infusing Ringer's acetate almost 2 hours after Voluven was followed by a much more peripheral accumulation of fluid and a smaller urinary excretion than when Ringer's acetate was infused alone (Figure 34.2).[32]

Crystalloid fluid is often said to cause peripheral edema because such fluid is distributed over the entire extracellular fluid space. This view is simplistic since large parts of the interstitial fluid space have very low compliance to volume expansion, some low enough to be virtually impossible to expand with isotonic crystalloid fluids. These parts include bone tissue, the brain, and organs surrounded by a tight capsule. Crystalloid fluid accumulates preferentially in interstitial areas with the highest compliance to volume expansion, such as the skin and gastrointestinal tract. Volume kinetic studies suggest that crystalloid fluid usually fills 2/3 of the expected size of the interstitial fluid space.

Studies showing a 20%/80% distribution of crystalloid fluid between the plasma and the interstitium never take the urinary excretion into account. A more correct figure after a 30-min equilibration period would be 20%/50%/30% (plasma/interstitium/urine) in a volunteer and 30%/60%/10% during surgery. However, the amount that resides in the interstitium is smaller with slow infusions and higher with rapid infusions.

Edema is rarely an issue in volunteer experiments because the urinary excretion is very prompt. However, anesthesia and surgery are associated with marked fluid retention. Here, the half-life of balanced crystalloids increases from 20–50 min to several 100 min. This adds to the volume expansion of both the plasma and the interstitial fluid space, and therefore promotes edema.

A second mechanism that promotes edema from crystalloid fluid is that the fibers of the interstitial fluid matrix lose elasticity when volume-expanded, whereby fluid deposited in the interstitial fluid gel has difficulty in returning to the plasma. The interstitium behaves like a filled balloon that does not return to its original size when deflated. If the fluid that remains in the plasma is excreted, the altered elasticity of the interstitial fibers gives rise to the paradoxical situation in which peripheral edema is present alongside hypovolemia. The lost elasticity is dependent on the rate of infusion and is quite apparent after infusion of crystalloid fluid at the rate of 50 ml/min for 30 min (about 2 liters). The anesthetist who wants to limit this problem should provide a continuous infusion at a rate no faster than 10 ml/min, where actually very little of the infused fluid even enters the interstitial fluid space because of the compliance issue.[33,34] Very large volumes of crystalloid fluid even break up the interstitial fluid matrix, and the fluid forms lacunae in the interstitium, which makes it very difficult to recruit and make available for excretion.[35,36] This break-up of the interstitium is best studied in isolated lung preparations.[37,38] The situation might be expected to be worsened by the fact that albumin, which is normally excluded from parts of the interstitium, can penetrate into opened parts of the interstital gel and bind fluid by its oncotic strength.[39]

How much the complex neuroendocrine response to trauma contributes to the development of peripheral edema is difficult to quantify. The response includes a rise in plasma glucose, which recruits fluid from the intra- to the extracellular fluid space, and elevations of water-retaining hormones such as

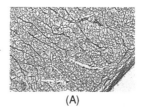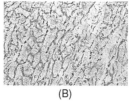

(A)   (B)

Figure 34.3 A: Normal cytoarchitecture of a pig's heart after receiving 150 ml/kg of mannitol 3% over 90 min. Lumina of the vessels are preserved (×200; field of view 300 μm). **B**: Destroyed cytoarchitecture in the subendocardium in a mouse that died after receiving 300 ml/kg of isotonic saline over 60 min. The reticular fibers are fragmented and degenerated (×600; field of view 100 μm). Light microscopy with Gordon and Sweet's silver impregnation for reticulum fibers. Photographs were taken in the course of the studies reported in Refs. [43] and [42].

aldosterone, vasopressin, and cortisol. Beta-1-adrenergic stimulation acts to retain fluid in the extracellular fluid space. Alpha-1-adrenergic stimulation increases the rate of elimination of infused crystalloid fluid,[40,41] as does the rise in atrial natriuretic peptide concentration occurring from vigorous plasma volume expansion. None of these hormones specifically changes the distribution of fluid to the interstitium except for atrial natriuretic peptide, which, together with activation of the inflammatory cascade, increases the capillary leakage of macromolecules (e.g. proteins) from the plasma. At the same time, the atrial natriuretic peptide and probably also inflammation increase the urinary excretion, and thus the total effect on the body may consist mainly of a reduction of the plasma volume.

A special mechanism that promotes peripheral edema is found in burns. Here, there is a marked drop in the interstitial hydrostatic pressure, which more or less suctions fluid from the intravascular space to peripheral tissues.

Death from overhydration has been studied in animals. The hearts of mice receiving large amonts of isotonic saline show changes similar to those occurring from irrigating fluid, namely severe interstitial dilatation with fluid lacunae that compress the capillary lumina, making blood flow difficult.[42] Rupture and fragmentation are common features of this process (Figure 34.3).

References

1. Tølløfsrud S, Bjerkelund CE, Kongsgaard U, *et al.* Cold and warm infusion of Ringer's acetate in healthy volunteers: the effects on haemodynamic parameters,

transcapillary fluid balance, diuresis and atrial peptides. *Acta Anaesthesiol Scand* 1993; 37: 768–73.

2. Morrison RC. Hypothermia in the elderly. *Int Anesthesiol Clinics* 1988; 26: 124–33.

3. Doufas AG. Unintentional perioperative hypothermia. In: Lobato EB, Gravenstein N, Kirby RR, eds. *Complications in Anesthesiology*. Philadelphia: Lippincott Williams & Wilkins 2008, 636–46.

4. Hahn RG. Cooling effect from absorption of pre-warmed irrigating fluid in transurethral prostatic resection. *Int Urol Nephrol* 1993; 25: 265–70.

5. Bergqvist D. Dextran and haemostasis. *Acta Chir Scand* 1982; 148: 633–40.

6. Holte K, Jensen P, Kehlet H. Physiologic effects of intravenous fluid administration in healthy volunteers. *Anesth Analg* 2003; 96: 1504–9.

7. Hahn RG, Drobin D, Ståhle L. Volume kinetics of Ringer's solution in female volunteers. *Br J Anaesth* 1997; 78: 144–8.

8. Li Y, He R, Ying X, Hahn RG. Ringer's lactate, but not hydroxyethyl starch, prolongs the food intolerance time after major abdominal surgery; an open-labelled clinical trial. *BMC Anesthesiol* 2015; 15: 72.

9. Varadhan KK, Lobo DN. Symposium 3: A meta-analysis of randomised controlled trials of intravenous fluid therapy in major elective open abdominal surgery: getting the balance right. *Proc Nutr Soc* 2010; 69: 488–98.

10. Wuethrich PY, Burkhard FC, Thalmann GN, Stueber F, Studer UE. Restrictive deferred hydration combined with preemptive norepinephrine infusion during radical cystectomy reduces postoperative complications and hospitalization time. *Anesthesiology* 2014; 120: 365–77.

11. Nisanevich V, Felsenstein I, Almogy G, *et al.* Effect of intraoperative fluid management on outcome after intraabdominal surgery. *Anesthesiology* 2005; 103: 25–32.

12. Arieff AI. Fatal postoperative pulmonary edema. Pathogenesis and literature review. *Chest* 1999; 115: 1371–7.

13. Brandstrup B, Tonnesen H, Beier-Holgersen R, *et al.* Effects of intravenous fluid restriction on postoperative complications: comparison of two perioperative fluid regimens. A randomized assessor-blinded multicenter trial. *Ann Surg* 2003; 238: 641–8.

14. Vermeulen H, Hofland J, Legemate DA, Ubbink DT. Intravenous fluid restriction after major abdominal surgery: a randomized blinded clinical trial. *Trials* 2009; 10: 50.

15. Holte K, Hahn RG, Ravn L, *et al.* Influence of liberal vs. restrictive fluid management on the elimination of a postoperative intravenous fluid load. *Anesthesiology* 2007; 106: 75–9.

16. Stenvinkel P, Saggar-Malik AK, Alvestrand A. Renal haemodynamics and tubular sodium handling following volume expansion with sodium chloride (NaCl) and glucose in healthy humans. *Scand J Clin Lab Invest* 1992; 52: 837–46.

17. Wilkes NJ, Woolf R, Mutch M, *et al.* The effects of balanced versus saline-based hetastarch and crystalloid solutions on acid–base and electrolyte status and gastric mucosal perfusion in elderly surgical patients. *Anesth Analg* 2001; 93: 811–16.

18. Laxenaire MC, Charpentier C, Feldman L. Anaphylactoid reactions to colloid plasma substitutes: incidence risk factor mechanisms. A French multicenter prospective study. *Ann Fr Anesth Reanimat* 1994; 13: 301–10.

19. Moran M, Kapsner C. Acute renal failure associated with elevated plasma oncotic pressure. *N Engl J Med* 1987; 317: 150–3.

20. Haskell LP, Tannenberg AM. Elevated urinary specific gravity in acute oliguric renal failure due to hetastarch administration. *NY State J Med* 1988; 88: 387–8.

21. The SAFE Study Investigators. Saline or albumin for fluid resuscitation in patients with traumatic brain injury. *N Engl J Med* 2007; 357: 874–84.

22. Bork K. Pruritus precipitated by hydroxyethyl starch: a review. *Br J Dermatol* 2005; 152: 3–12.

23. Hayes I, Rathore R, Enohumah K, *et al.* The effect of crystalloid versus medium molecular weight colloid solution on post-operative nausea and vomiting after ambulatory gynecological surgery – a prospective randomized trail. *BMC Anesthesiol* 2012; 12: 15.

24. Schortgen F, Lacherade LC, Bruneel F, *et al.* Effects of hydroxyethyl starch and gelatine on renal function in severe sepsis: a multicentre randomised study. *Lancet* 2001; 357: 911–16.

25. Brunkhorst FM, Engel C, Bloos F, *et al.* Intensive insulin therapy and pentastarch resuscitation in severe sepsis. *N Engl J Med* 2008; 358: 125–38.

26. Perner A, Haase N, Guttormsen AB, *et al.* Hydroxyethyl starch 130/0.42 versus Ringer's acetate in severe sepsis. *N Engl J Med* 2012; 367: 124–34.

27. Myburgh JA, Finfer S, Bellomo R, *et al.* Hydroxyethyl starch or saline for fluid on intraoperative oliguria resuscitation in intensive care. *N Engl J Med* 2012; 367: 1901–11.

28. Mahmood A, Gosling P, Vohra RK. Randomized clinical trial comparing the effects on renal function of hydroxyethyl starch or gelatine during aortic aneurysm surgery. *Br J Surg* 2007; 94: 427–33.

29. Clagett GP, Reisch JS. Prevention of venous thromboembolism in general surgical patients. *Ann Surg* 1988; 208: 227–40.

30. Brodin B, Hesselvik F, von Schenck H. Decrease of plasma fibronectin concentration following infusion of gelatin-based plasma substitute in man. *Scand J Clin Lab Invest* 1984; 44: 529–33.

31. Russell WJ, Fenwick DB. Anaphylaxis to Haemaccel and cross reactivity to Gelofusin. *Anaesth Intensive Care* 2002; 30: 481–3.

32. Hahn RG, Bergek C, Gebäck T, Zdolsek J. Interactions between the volume effects of hydroxyethyl starch 130/0.4 and Ringer's acetate. *Crit Care* 2013; 17: R104.

33. Zdolsek J, Li Y, Hahn RG. Detection of dehydration by using volume kinetics. *Anesth Analg* 2012; 115: 814–22.

34. Hahn RG, Drobin D, Zdolsek J. Distribution of crystalloid fluid changes with the rate of infusion: a population-based study. *Acta Anaesthesiol Scand* 2016; Jan 13: doi: 10.1111/aas.12686.

35. Guyton AC. Interstitial fluid pressure. II. Pressure-volume curves of interstitial space. *Circ Res* 1965; 16: 452–60.

36. Guyton AC, Granger HJ, Taylor AE. Interstitial fluid pressure. *Physiol Rev* 1971; 51: 527–63.

37. Lai-Fook SJ, Toporoff B. Pressure–volume behavior of perivascular interstitium measured in isolated dog lung. *J Appl Physiol* 1980; 48: 939–46.

38. Goldberg HS. Pulmonary interstitial compliance and microvascular filtration coefficient. *Am J Physiol* 1980; 235: H189–98.

39. Parker JC, Falgout HJ, Oarker RE, Granger N, Taylor AE. The effect of fluid volume loading on exclusion of interstitial albumin and lymph flow in the dog lung. *Circ Res* 1979; 45: 440–50.

40. Ewaldsson CA, Vane LA, Kramer GC, Hahn RG. Adrenergic drugs alter both the fluid kinetics and the hemodynamic responses to volume expansion in sheep. *J Surg Res* 2006; 131: 7–14.

41. Li Y, Zhu HB, Zheng X, *et al*. Low doses of esmolol and phenylephrine act as diuretics during intravenous anesthesia. *Crit Care* 2012; 16: R18.

42. Hahn RG, Olsson J, Sótonyi P, Rajs J. Rupture of the myocardial histoskeleton and its relation to sudden death after infusion of glycine 1.5% in the mouse. *APMIS* 2000; 108: 487–95.

43. Sandfeldt L, Riddez L, Rajs J, *et al*. High-dose intravenous infusion of irrigating fluids containing glycine and mannitol in the pig. *J Surg Res* 2001; 95: 114–25.

Index

Printed in the United States
by Baker & Taylor Publisher Services